Forensic DNA Typing Protocols

METHODS IN MOLECULAR BIOLOGY™

John M. Walker, SERIES EDITOR

METHODS IN MOLECULAR BIOLOGY™

Forensic DNA Typing Protocols

Edited by

Angel Carracedo

Institute of Legal Medicine
University of Santiago de Compostela
Galicia, Spain

HUMANA PRESS ✳ TOTOWA, NEW JERSEY

© 2005 Humana Press Inc.
999 Riverview Drive, Suite 208
Totowa, New Jersey 07512

www.humanapress.com

This publication is printed on acid-free paper. ∞
ANSI Z39.48-1984 (American Standards Institute)

Permanence of Paper for Printed Library Materials.

Production Editor: Robin B. Weisberg
Cover illustration from Fig. 5 in Chapter 10, "Universal Tag Arrays in Forensic SNP Analysis," by Marie Allen and Anna-Maria Divne.
Cover design by Patricia F. Cleary

For additional copies, pricing for bulk purchases, and/or information about other Humana titles, contact Humana at the above address or at any of the following numbers: Tel.: 973-256-1699; Fax: 973-256-8341; E-mail: humana@humanapr.com; or visit our Website: www.humanapress.com

Printed in the United States of America. 10 9 8 7 6 5 4 3 2 1

eISBN 1-59259-867-6

Library of Congress Cataloging-in-Publication Data

Forensic DNA typing protocols / edited by Angel Carracedo.
    p. ; cm. -- (Methods in molecular biology, ISSN 1064-3745 ; v. 297)
  Includes bibliographical references and index.
  ISBN 1-58829-264-9 (alk. paper)
  1. DNA fingerprinting. 2. Forensic genetics.
  [DNLM: 1. DNA Fingerprinting--methods. 2. Polymorphism, Single Nucleotide--genetics.
QZ 52 F715 2005] I. Carracedo, Angel. II. Series: Methods in molecular biology (Clifton, N.J.) ; v. 297.
  RA1057.55.F67 2005
  614'.1--dc22

                                  2004010563

Preface

The discovery of polymorphisms in repetitive DNA by Dr. Alec Jeffreys and coworkers in 1985 has had a tremendous impact on forensic genetics. Since then we have witnessed a revolution in the field of forensic identification, and different markers and technologies for DNA typing have moved at a breathtaking pace.

Rapid advances in technology, from serological or electrophoretic analysis of protein polymorphisms to direct investigation of the underlying DNA polymorphisms, occurred in a very short space of time in the mid-1980s. Consequently, the incorporation of modern molecular biological techniques in the forensic genetic laboratory has resulted in major benefits for justice.

DNA analysis has become the standard method applied by most forensic genetic labs, especially in criminal forensic casework (e.g., analysis of stains and hairs, identification of human remains, and paternity testing). Polymerase chain reaction (PCR)-based DNA typing systems have made it possible to analyze DNA obtained from only a few cells as well as from highly degraded human samples (recently demonstrated by the identification of relatively old human remains). The potential of DNA typing has made possible the resolution of immigration problems and complicated paternity testing cases when the father is not available. Rapid identification of individuals in mass disaster using DNA typing has also been possible. Computerized DNA databases for the identification of criminal offenders have been created in some countries.

Owing to these many impressive applications, the media have taken great interest in DNA profiling, mainly because of the value of the evidence presented through DNA profiling in certain well-known legal cases.

Initially, the use of DNA profiling was very controversial in some countries, perhaps because of a hasty introduction of this new methodology. Ironically, however, this has contributed to a much more reliable use of DNA profiling.

Two parallel upheavals concerning the introduction of DNA typing technology have been accountable for the aforementioned: the introduction of quality control and accreditation schemes and, in particular, the spreading use of the statistics in the evaluation of DNA evidence. Also, progress in standardizing the tests has proven even more important than the technical advances.

In addition to the DNA revolution, the evolution and development of DNA markers and technologies themselves have been rapid and spectacular. In only a few years we have progressed from the original multilocus DNA fingerprint analysis of DNA minisatellites, through single locus probe analysis of specific minisatellites, to a host of systems based on the PCR technique.

Microsatellites or short-tandem repeats (STRs) have been almost completely substituted for minisatellites in forensic labs. STRs were first analyzed in manual electrophoretic systems. The introduction of fluorescent-based technology and the use of DNA sequencers have revolutionized the field, allowing the typing of large multiplexes, as well as the automation of the typing procedure. Commercially available and robust multiplexes with up to 15 STRs are routinely used by most of the forensic labs.

But new markers and methods of detection have been proposed, and the most important new advances are the introduction of the use of mtDNA and Y chromosome polymorphisms and especially the new use of single nucleotide polymorphisms (SNPs). It is now clear that SNP typing will be of prime importance in the field, owing to the potential advantages of this type of marker, especially for the analysis of degraded samples.

Because STR typing is familiar in all the forensic labs and the typing protocols are well established, we have decided to focus *Forensic DNA Typing Protocols* on the newer methods and technologies forensic scientists use to solve certain types of cases and to implement these new DNA typing methods in their laboratories. In addition, we have included a chapter on how to create large STR multiplexes, since some labs are interested in the design of STR multiplexes for specific purposes (e.g., STRs with short amplicons for degraded samples; pentanucleotide STRs for the analysis of mixtures).

Forensic DNA Typing Protocols provides protocols for the major methods of DNA analysis that have been recently introduced for identity testing, including Y chromosome, mtDNA, and SNP typing. Chapters with protocols for new applications in the forensic genetics labs—such as species identification or typing of CYP polymorphisms for the analysis of adverse reactions to drugs—have also been included. Ancient DNA is another field of forensic and anthropological interest where there is a need for well-tested protocols from laboratories with extensive experience in the field; two chapters are devoted to this topic. Finally, proper DNA quantification is a crucial requirement for the analysis of critical forensic samples, including mixtures, and new methods based on real-time PCR are now available. For this reason two chapters including protocols for DNA quantification of forensic samples and for the determination of the number of amelogenin gene copies have been added.

I am indebted to Professor John Walker, the series editor, for his helpful encouragement and patience, but I especially owe my thanks to all the contributing authors who have made this book possible.

Angel Carracedo

Contents

Contributors

ANTONIO ALONSO • *Instituto Nacional de Toxicología, Servicio de Biología, Madrid, Spain*

VANESA ÁLVAREZ-IGLESIAS • *Institute of Legal Medicine, Faculty of Medicine, University of Santiago de Compostela, Santiago de Compostela, Galicia, Spain*

CÍNTIA ALVES • *Instituto de Patologia e Imunologia Molecular da Universidade do Porto, Porto, Portugal*

MARIE ALLEN • *Department of Genetics and Pathology, Uppsala University, Uppsala, Sweden*

HANNA ANDRÉASSON • *Department of Genetics and Pathology, Uppsala University, Uppsala, Sweden*

KLAUS BENDER • *Institut für Rechtsmedizin, Mainz, Germany*

CLAUS BØRSTING • *Department of Forensic Genetics, Institute of Forensic Medicine, University of Copenhagen, Copenhagen, Denmark*

MARÍA BRIÓN • *Institute of Legal Medicine, Faculty of Medicine, University of Santiago de Compostela, Santiago de Compostela, Galicia, Spain*

JOHN M. BUTLER • *Biotechnology Division, National Institute of Standards and Technology, Gaithersburg, MD*

CRISTIAN CAPELLI • *Institute of Legal Medicine, Catholic University of Rome, Rome, Italy*

ANGEL CARRACEDO • *Institute of Legal Medicine, Faculty of Medicine, University of Santiago de Compostela, Santiago de Compostela, Galicia, Spain*

ANNA-MARIA DIVNE • *Department of Genetics and Pathology, Uppsala University, Uppsala, Sweden*

KRISTINA FAHR • *Bruker Daltonik GmbH, Leipzig, Germany*

LEONOR GUSMÃO • *Instituto de Patologia e Imunologia Molecular da Universidade do Porto, Porto, Portugal*

CHRISTINE KEYSER-TRACQUI • *Laboratoire d'Anthropologie Moléculaire, Institut de Médecine Légale, Strasbourg, France*

SILVANO KÖCHL • *Institute of Legal Medicine, University of Innsbruck, Innsbruck, Austria*

MARKUS KOSTRZEWA • *Bruker Daltonik GmbH, Leipzig, Germany*

MARÍA VICTORIA LAREU • *Institute of Legal Medicine, Faculty of Medicine, University of Santiago de Compostela, Santiago de Compostela, Galicia, Spain*

JAMES LEE • *Department of Forensic Science, Central Police University, Kuei-San, Taoyuan, Taiwan, Republic of China*

ADRIAN LINACRE • *Forensic Science Unit, University of Strathclyde, Glasgow, UK*

BERTRAND LUDES • *Laboratoire d'Anthropologie Moléculaire, Institut de Médecine Légale, Strasbourg, France*

PABLO MARTÍN • *Instituto Nacional de Toxicología. Servicio de Biología, Madrid, Spain*

NIELS MORLING • *Department of Forensic Genetics, Institute of Forensic Medicine, University of Copenhagen, Copenhagen, Denmark*

HARALD NIEDERSTÄTTER • *Institute of Legal Medicine, University of Innsbruck, Innsbruck, Austria*

WALTHER PARSON • *Institute of Legal Medicine, University of Innsbruck, Innsbruck, Austria*

CHRISTOPHER PHILLIPS • *Institute of Legal Medicine, Faculty of Medicine, University of Santiago de Compostela, Santiago de Compostela, Galicia, Spain*

CLARA RUIZ PONTE • *Institute of Legal Medicine, Faculty of Medicine, University of Santiago de Compostela, Santiago de Compostela, Galicia, Spain*

BEATRIZ QUINTÁNS • *Institute of Legal Medicine, Faculty of Medicine, University of Santiago de Compostela, Santiago de Compostela, Galicia, Spain*

ANTONIO SALAS • *Institute of Legal Medicine, Faculty of Medicine, University of Santiago de Compostela, Santiago de Compostela, Galicia, Spain*

JUAN J. SANCHEZ • *Department of Forensic Genetics, Institute of Forensic Medicine, University of Copenhagen, Copenhagen, Denmark*

PAULA SÁNCHEZ-DIZ • *Institute of Legal Medicine, Faculty of Medicine, University of Santiago de Compostela, Santiago de Compostela, Galicia, Spain*

BEATRIZ SOBRINO • *Institute of Legal Medicine, Faculty of Medicine, University of Santiago de Compostela, Santiago de Compostela, Galicia, Spain*

FRANK TSCHENTSCHER • *Institut für Rechtsmedizin, Universitaetsklinikum Essen, Essen, Germany*

PETER M. VALLONE • *Biotechnology Division, National Institute of Standards and Technology, Gaithersburg, MD*

1

Forensic DNA-Typing Technologies

A Review

Angel Carracedo and Paula Sánchez-Diz

Summary

Since the discovery of deoxyribonucleic acid (DNA) profiling in 1985, forensic genetics has experienced a continuous technical revolution, both in the type of DNA markers used and in the methodologies or its detection. Highly informative and robust DNA-typing systems have been developed that have proven to be very effective in the individualization of biological material of human origin. DNA analysis has become the standard method in forensic genetics used by laboratories for the majority of forensic genetic expertise and especially in criminal forensic casework (stain analysis and hairs) and identification.

Key Words: DNA analysis; DNA profiling; DNA typing; forensic genetics.

1. Introduction

Deoxyribonucleic acid (DNA) profiling, or typing, as it is now known, was first described in 1985 by Alec Jeffreys and co-workers *(1)* ,and it has had a tremendous impact in forensic genetics. Prior to that time, all forensic genetic casework (e.g., paternity testing, criminal casework, individual identification) was performed using classical serological genetic markers. Blood groups, human leukocyte antigen (HLA), and polymorphic protein and enzymes were used for solving forensic genetic casework using immunological and electrophoretic methodologies. These genetic markers were nevertheless limited when it was necessary to analyze minimal or degraded material, which is commonly involved in forensic cases. It was, in addition, difficult to analyze biological material other than blood, and therefore the information obtained from hair, saliva, and even semen in rape cases was rather limited.

From: *Methods in Molecular Biology, vol. 297: Forensic DNA Typing Protocols*
Edited by: A. Carracedo © Humana Press Inc., Totowa, NJ

Because the polymorphic proteins and enzymes were infrequent, it was necessary to obtain as much information as possible. For this reason, sophisticated electrophoretic methods, such as isoelectric focusing, immobilines, or hybrid isoelectric focusing, were developed and applied. Despite these methods, the information that the forensic geneticists were able to report in many cases was clearly insufficient.

Since the discovery of polymorphisms in repetitive DNA by Jeffreys et al. *(1)*, highly informative and robust DNA-typing systems have been developed that are quite powerful for the individualization of biological material of human origin.

DNA typing has advantages over traditional protein, the first of which being it is more informative and can be analyzed in minute or degraded material because DNA is physically much more resistant to degradation than proteins. In addition, the same DNA genotype can be obtained from any tissue (i.e., blood, saliva, semen, hair, skin, bones), whereas the analysis of protein markers is restricted to cells where these proteins are expressed.

DNA analysis has become the standard method in forensic genetics used by laboratories for the majority of forensic genetic expertise and especially in criminal forensic casework (stain analysis and hairs) and identification.

2. DNA Polymorphisms

Hidden in the approx 3 billion base pairs of DNA of the haploid human genome are an estimated 35,000 genes *(2)*. All human genes are encoded in approx 10% of the human genome. Thus, the great majority (more than 90%) of the human genome represents "noncoding" parts of the genome because they do not contain genetic information directly relevant for protein synthesis. Genetic variation is rather limited in coding DNA with the exception of the HLA region. This is the result of the fact that expressed genes are subjected to selection pressure during evolution to maintain their specific function. In contrast, the noncoding part of the genome is not mainly controlled by selection pressure, and thus mutations in these regions are usually kept and transmitted to the offspring, leading to a tremendous increase in genetic variability. Therefore, these regions are very appropriate for forensic genetics because they are very informative and at the same time not useful for drawing conclusions about the individual other than for identification purposes.

An important percentage of the noncoding DNA (30%) consists of repetitive sequences that can be divided into two classes: tandemly repetitive sequences and interspersed elements. The majority of forensic typing systems in current use are based on genetic loci with tandem repetitive DNA sequences.

Tandemly repeated sequences can be found in satellite DNA, but from the forensic point of view, regions of repetitive DNA much shorter than satellite

DNA are much more interesting. These regions can be classified into minisatellites *(1)* and microsatellites or short tandem repeat (STRs) *(3,4)*. Minisatellites, otherwise known as variable number of tandem repeats (VNTR) loci *(5)*, are composed of sequence motifs ranging from around 15 to 50 bp in length, reiterated tandemly for a total length of 500 bp to 20 Kb. STRs are much shorter. The repeat unit ranges from 2 to 6 bp for a total length between 50 and 500 bp.

In addition, minisatellites and STRs have differences in their distribution in the human genome and probably in their biological function. Thus, minisatellites are more common in subtelomeric regions, whereas STRs are widely distributed throughout the human genome, occurring with a frequency of one locus every 6–10 kb *(6)*. The origin of the variability seems to be different as well. Although unequal crossing over and even gene conversion *(7)* are involved in the variability of minisatellites, replication slippage is mainly involved in the origin of the variability in microsatellites *(8)*.

The genetic variation between individuals in these minisatellites and STR systems is mainly based on the number of tandemly arranged core repeat elements, but it is based also on differences in the DNA sequence itself because the repeats can have slight differences in the sequence.

3. DNA-Typing Methods

Technologies used for DNA typing for forensic purposes differ in their ability to differentiate two individuals and in the speed and sensitivity with which results can be obtained. The speed of analysis has dramatically improved for forensic DNA analysis. DNA testing that previously took more than 1 wk can now be performed in a few hours.

Southern blotting with multi-locus and single-locus (SLP) DNA probes have been used for paternity testing and forensic stain typing, and they are still used (especially SLPs) by a few laboratories working in paternity testing

Briefly, the technique is as follows: First, the DNA is extracted and then cut by a specific enzyme (usually *Hinf*I in Europe and *Hae*III in the United States) into many small fragments. A tiny fraction of those fragments include the particular minisatellite to be analyzed. The fragments are then separated by electrophoresis in submarine agarose gels using TAE or TBE as buffers. After an appropriate length of time, the fragments migrate different distances in the electric field, depending mainly on their sizes, with the smaller ones migrating more rapidly. DNA fragments are then chemically treated to separate the double strands into single ones.

Because the gels are difficult to work with, the single-stranded fragments are then transferred directly to a nylon membrane, to which they adhere. This process is called Southern blotting, named after its inventor *(9)*. The next step is to flood the membrane with a single-stranded probe, which will hybridize with the DNA fragments that contain the target minisatellite sequence and adhere to it. The membrane is then washed several times to remove any probe that does not bind to this specific DNA sequence.

Probes can be labeled using isotopic or nonisotopic methods. Nonisotopic chemiluminescent methods are more popular than isotopic ones.

Whatever the labeling method is, the nylon membrane usually is placed on an x-ray film, with the final result of an autoradiograph with the bands of the minisatellite clearly impressed in the film. The process requires several days for sufficient radioactive decay to produce a visible band on the film.

Originally, multilocus probes were proposed for forensic genetic analysis. However, this type of probe was not very successful in the forensic field because despite its informativeness, statistical problems of evaluation of the evidence in cases of match and standardization problems arose. For these reasons, this probe was substituted in the forensic field by the analysis of VNTRs using SLPs under high-stringency conditions.

Until the introduction of STR analysis by polymerase chain reaction (PCR), minisatellite analysis with single-locus probes was very popular in forensic laboratories. Nowadays, it is still used in some laboratories, particularly for paternity testing analysis.

The main advantage of SLP analysis is the enormous variability of some of the minisatellites and the adequate knowledge of the mutation rate in some of them. The main disadvantages are the time needed for the analysis and especially the need for the relatively large amount of nondegraded DNA required for SLP typing. Because DNA extracted from forensic specimens is often degraded because of environmental conditions, these techniques have often failed to produce reliable results. PCR has overcome these difficulties, and it has strongly enhanced the usefulness of DNA profiling techniques in forensic science.

PCR is a technique for the in vitro amplification of specific DNA sequences by the simultaneous primer extension of complementary strands of DNA. The PCR method was devised and named by Mullis and colleagues at the Cetus Corporation *(10)*, although the principle had been described in detail by Khorana et al. *(11)* more than a decade earlier. The use of PCR was limited until heat-stable DNA polymerases became available. DNA polymerases conduct the synthesis off a complementary strand of DNA in the 5' to 3' direction using a single-stranded template, but starting from a double-stranded region. The PCR uses the same principle but uses two primers, each complementary to opposite strands of the region of DNA that have been denatured by heating. The primers are arranged so that each primer extension reaction directs the synthesis of DNA toward the other. This results in the novo synthesis of the region flanked by the two primers.

Automated temperature cyclers (usually called thermocyclers) allow the exact control of successive steps of denaturation, annealing of the primers, and extension (when the DNA polymerase extends the primer by using a complementary strand as a template). All these three steps constitute a cycle, and a normal PCR reaction consists of 20–25 cycles, allowing the formation of 2^{20-25} molecules from a single molecule of template DNA.

Most PCR-based typing systems allow alleles to be identified as discrete entities, thus avoiding most of the statistical issues that arise in matching and binding SLPs bands and making standardization easier. Also, apart from the increased sensitivity inherent in any PCR technique, it is more likely to be successful in analyzing old or badly degraded material mainly because of the small size of some of the DNA polymorphisms (SNPs and STRs) susceptible to analysis by PCR *(12,13)*.

Once PCR has been used to generate a large number of copies of a DNA segment of interest, different approaches may be taken to detect genetic variation within the segment amplified. Because 10^6 or more copies of the target sequence can be produced, it is possible to use nonisotopic methods of detection. A number of imaginative methods for PCR product detection have been described.

The first one was the use of sequence-specific oligonucleotide (SSO) probes *(14)* to detect variation in HLA–class II genes, especially in the HLA DQA1 system *(15)*. An SSO probe is usually a short oligonucleotide (15–30 nucleotides in length) with a sequence exactly matching the sequence of the target allele. The SSO probe is mixed with dissociated strands of PCR product under very stringent hybridization conditions such that the SSO and the PCR product strand will be hybridized if there is a perfect sequence complimentary but will not be if there are different sequences. The classical format for the use of SSO probes is to spot dissociated PCR product strands onto a nitrocellulose or nylon membrane and to probe the membranes with labeled SSO; because of the fact that the samples are spotted as a "dot" on the membrane, this format is known as dot blotting. A reverse dot-blot format is much more commonly used *(16)*. With this format (which has its antecedents in affinity chromatography), the SSO is immobilized on the membrane and is used to capture PCR products containing biotin label in the primers. Several genetic loci can be analyzed by this technology using commercially available kits. The AmpliType PM PCR amplification kit (Perkin-Elmer, Foster City, CA) was very popular in forensic laboratories some years ago. With this kit, the loci HLA DQA1, LDLR, GYPA, HBGG, D7S8, and GC are amplified in a multiplex fashion. The last five loci listed are typed simultaneously in a single reverse dot-blot strip containing ASO probes; HLA DQA1 must be typed in a separate strip. The system was validated for forensic analysis *(17)*, and it is still used by some laboratories although most of them currently prefer to use more informative STR systems.

The efforts of forensic scientists have mainly addressed the amplification of fragment-length polymorphisms. The minisatellite D1S80 (pMCT118) was the first to be applied to the forensic routine *(18)*, but these systems have been substituted by STRs. The analysis of STRs by PCR is now the method of choice for forensic identification. Dinucleotide STRs are the most common STRs in the human genome and are the genetic markers most commonly used for linkage analysis, although they are not being used in forensic science. The reason is that analysis of these STRs has been affected by strand slippage during amplification, producing artifactual stutter bands *(19)*. Nevertheless, tetra and pentanucleotide repeats appear to be less prone to slippage and are more suitable for forensic purposes. The percent of stutters is very interesting to identify and select ideal STRs for forensic purposes because having a low percentage of stutters is critical for the analysis of mix stains. Some tetranucleotide STRs (such as TH01) are known to have a good behavior regarding these characteristics, but pentanucleotides are ideal systems for analyzing mixtures.

According to its structure, STRs range from the extremely complex STRs to the most simple *(20)*. Complex STRs have the advantages of hypervariability. Simple STRs have the advantages of easy standardization and low mutation rates. Mutation events are more frequent in the male germ line, and the rates of different loci can differ by several orders of magnitude, the structure and length being the most influential factors in the rate *(21)*. In addition to the characteristics already mentioned, the selection of ideal STRs for forensic purposes include the analysis of other artifactual bands, the robustness, and the size. In general, short sizes are desirable because the size of the amplified product is critical in degraded samples, and small fragments can be amplified when larger fragments failed *(13)*.

Another important fact is the possibility of amplifying multiple STR loci in a single multiplex reaction. This coupled with the direct detection of amplified products to polyacrylamide gels, makes STR DNA profiling amenable to automation. For this reason, the ability to be included in multiplexes is another characteristic that should be analyzed for the selection of good STRs for forensic purposes.

STRs were firstly analyzed in manual electrophoretic systems. Denaturing polyacrylamide gels are recommended for standardization purposes, given that with native gels sequence variation can also be detected making the typing prone to errors. STR electrophoretic mobility under native and denaturing conditions should also be checked since some STRs (especially AT-rich ones) have been shown to have anomalous mobility in polyacrylamide gels *(22)*.

The introduction of fluorescent-based technology and the use of DNA sequencers have revolutionized the field, allowing the typing of large multiplexes (including up to 10 systems) as well as the automation of the typing procedure. Commercially available STR multiplexes for manual electro-phoretic systems are available, but the major advantages of the use of sequenc-ers is automation and the possibility of using intelligent systems of interpretation. The use of sequence reference allelic ladders is essential for STR typing. In general, the reference allelic ladders comprise most of the alle-les of the system, but intermediate alleles are always possible even in the most simple STRs. Interpretation guidelines have been produced *(23,24)* to distin-guish these intermediate alleles and can be easily implemented in automatic sequencers. There are many multiplexcs commercially available. A very popu-lar one is the SGM Plus (Applied Biosystems), which comprises 10 loci-HUMFIBRA/FGA, HUMVWFA, HUMTH01, D18S51, D21S11, D6S477, D8S1179, D16S539, D19S433, and amelogenine. Promega (Madison, WI) multiplexes are also very popular, especially in the laboratories using manual elec-trophoretic systems or monochromatic sequencing platforms. But the extremely discriminative 15-plexes are becoming more and more popular and, among these, the Poweplex16 (Promega) and the Identifiler (Applied Biosystems) are the more commonly used by forensic labs.

In general, the combined discrimination power of STRs is enormous and the probabilities of two unrelated individuals matching by chance (pM) are lower 10^{-15} for some of these large multiplexes.

4. STRs in Sexual Chromosomes and Mitochondrial (mt)DNA

Y chromosome-specific polymorphisms have proven to be especially useful in forensic work. The applications of Y polymorphisms include deficiency pater-nity testing, when a male offspring is in question, to different applications in criminal casework. Y polymorphisms are especially interesting in the analysis of male DNA fraction in stains involving male/female mixtures, the most com-mon biological material available in sexual crimes. Especially important is the use of these markers in cases where preferential sperm DNA extractions fails (this is estimated to occur in 5–15% of forensic cases) and also in rapes com-mitted by azoospermic individuals. Although the variation in the Y chromo-some is low, the nonpseudoautosomal region still bears different kinds of polymorphisms, including biallelic markers, STRs, and minisatellites. SNPs and STRs are the most interesting. The most-used Y STRs are the trinucleotide repeat DYS392 and the tetranucleotide repeats DYS19, DYS385, DYS389-I, DYS389-II, DYS390, DYS391, and DYS393. This STRs comprises the so-called minimum Y STR haplotype *(25)*, but new STRs have recently been described *(26,27)*. Also, commercially available Y-STR plexes have been recently intro-duced.

As for mtDNA, statistical interpretation in cases of match is more compli-cated and appropriate corrections taking into account population substructure and sampling errors need to be performed. Population compilations are therefore very important and many efforts have been done regarding this *(28)*. A review and a compilation of recent works in the field can be found in reference *(29)*. STRs in the X-chromosome are actually being introduced *(30)*, and they are of interest for some deficiency paternity testing cases.

Analysis of the mtDNA control region is an efficient method for the study and comparison of bones, old and degraded DNA and, especially, the analysis of telogenic hairs.

In these cases, samples of mtDNA variation can be analyzed using a variety of strategies. The combination of PCR amplification with direct DNA sequencing usually is the ultimate choice for identification, and it has been proven to be a reliable and reproducible method in forensic casework *(31)*.

Analysis of mtDNA is a valid method to be applied in forensic genetics and it is accepted in courts all over the world. However, problems such as mutation rate, heteroplasmy, the statistical approach, make sometimes the interpetation difficult. A good review of mtDNA analysis in forensics can be found in reference *(32)*. ISFG DNA Commission recommendations and European DNA Profiling Group recommendations on the use of mtDNA, including nomenclature, prevention of contamination (aspect that it is crucial in mtDNA analysis) and statistical interpretation have been recently published *(33,34)*.

5. Future Perspectives: SNP Typing

Single nucleotide polymorphisms (SNPs) represent the most abundant form of genomic sequence variation among individuals: 3 million common SNPs with a population frequency of more than 5% have been estimated to be present in the human genome.

SNPs have a number of characteristics that make them very appropriate for forensic studies. First, they have lower mutation rates than STRs, and this is valuable for paternity testing. Second, they can be analyzed in short amplicons and, in general, short sizes are desirable because the size of the amplified product is critical for the successful amplification of degraded samples. Finally, they are very suitable for analysis using high-throughput technologies, which have become increasingly necessary because of the implementation of large criminal databases in European countries and for the need to perform large population studies that provide precise estimations of gene frequencies essential for the correct interpretation of forensic cases.

It is now clear that SNP typing on a large scale is and will be of prime importance in human genetics and particularly valuable in the identification of genes that predispose individuals to common, multifactorial disorders by using linkage disequilibrium mapping. In addition, there are crucial markers for pharmacogenetics and pharmacogenomics. These potential applications of SNP typing, together with progress in identifying large sets of SNPs, are the driving forces behind intense efforts to establish the technology for large-scale analysis of SNPs.

A great variety of chemistries and detection platforms have been proposed for SNP typing (*see* Chapter 6). There is not a single ideal method for typing SNPs, and the choice depends on both the need and the field of application, but for most of the applications (forensics included) the choice of the method must be a high-throughput technique that can be easily applied in molecular labs. '

References

1. Jeffreys, A. J., Wilson, V., and Thein, S. L. (1985) Hypervariable minisatellite regions in human DNA. *Nature* **314**, 67–73.
2. The International Human Genome Mapping Consortium. (2001) *Nature* **409**, 934.
3. Litt, M., and Luty, J. A. (1989) A hypervariable minisatellite revealed by in vitro amplification of a dinucleotide repeat within the cardiac muscle actin gene. *Am. J. Hum. Genet.* **44**, 397–401.
4. Tautz, D. (1989) Hypervariability of simple sequences as a general source for polymorphic DNA markers. *Nucleic Acid Res.* **17**, 6463–6471.
5. Nakamura, Y., Leppert, M., O'Connell, P., Wolff, R., Holm, T., Culver, M., et al. (1987) Variable number of tandem repeats (VNTR) markers for human gene mapping. *Science* **235**, 1616–1622.
6. Beckman J. S., and Weber, J. L. (1992) Survey of human and rat microsatellites. *Genomics* **12**, 627–631.
7. Jeffreys, A. J., Tamaki, K., MacLeod, A., Monckton, D. G., Neil, D. L., and Armour, J. A.L. (1994) Complex gene conversion events in germline mutation at human minisatellites. *Nat. Genet.* **6**, 136–145.
8. Di Rienzo, A., Peterson, A. C., Garza, J. C., Valdes, A. M., Slatkin, M., and Freimer, N. B. (1994) Mutational processes of simple-sequence repeat loci in human populations. *Proc. Natl. Acad. Sci. USA* **91**, 3166–3170.
9. Southern, E. M. (1975) Detection of specific sequences among DNA fragments separated by gel electrophoresis. *J. Mol. Biol.* **98**, 503–517.
10. Mullis, K., and Faloona, F. (1987) Specific synthesis of DNA in vitro via polymerase-catalyzed chain reaction, in *Methods in Enzymology* (Wu, R., ed.), Academic Press, New York, pp. 335–350.
11. Kleppe, K., Ohstuka, E., Kleppe, R., Molineux, L., and Khorana, H. G. (1971) Studies on polynucleotides. XCVI. Repair replications of short synthetic DNA's as catalyzed by DNA polymerases. *J. Mol. Biol.* **56**, 341–361.
12. Hagelberg, E., Sykes, B., and Hedges, R. (1989) Ancient bone DNA amplified. *Nature* **342**, 485.
13. Alvarez-García, A., Muñoz, I., Pestoni, C., Lareu, M. V., Rodríguez-Calvo, M. S., and Carracedo, A. (1996) Effect of environmental factors on PCR-DNA analysis from dental pulp. *Int. J. Legal Med.* **109**, 125–129.

14. Conner, B. J., Reyes, A. A., Morin, C., Itakura, K., Teplitz, R. L., and Wallace, R. B. (1983) Detection of sickle cell beta S-globin allele by hybridization with synthetic oligonucleotides. *Proc. Natl. Acad. Sci. USA* **80,** 278–282.

15. Saiki, R., Bugawan, T. L., Horn, T. G., Mullis, K. B., and Erlich, H. A. (1986) Analysis of enzymatically amplified beta-globin and HLA-DQ alpha DNA with allele-specific oligonucleotide probes. *Nature* **324,** 163.

16. Saiki, R. K., Walsh, P. S., Levenson C. H., and Erlich, H. A. (1989) Genetic analysis of amplified DNA with immobilized sequence-specific oligonucleotide probes. *Proc. Natl. Acad. Sci. USA* **86,** 6230–6234.

17. Gross, A. M., and Guerrieri, R. A. (1996) HLA DQA1 and Polymarker validations for forensic casework: standard specimens, reproducibility, and mixed specimens. *J. Forensic Sci.* **41,** 1022–1026 .

18. Budowle, B., Giusti, A. M., and Allen R. C. (1990). Analysis of PCR products (pMCT118) by polyacrylamide gel electrophoresis, in *Advances in Forensic Haemogenetics* (Polesky, H. F., and Mayr, W. R., eds), Springer, Berlin, 148–150.

19. Hauge X. Y., and Litt, M. (1993) A study of the origin of "shadow bands" seen when typing dinucleotide repeat polymorphisms by the PCR. *Hum. Mol. Genet.* **2,** 411–415.

20. Urquhart, A., Kimpton, C., Downes, T. J., and Gill, P. (1994) Variation in short tandem repeat sequences-a survey of twelve microsatellite loci for use as forensic identification markers. *Int. J. Legal Med.* **107,** 13–20.

21. Brinkmann, B., Klintschar, M., Neuhuber, F., Hühne, J., and Rolf, B. (1998) Mutation rate in human microsatellites: influence of the structure and length of the tandem repeat. *Am. J. Hum. Genet.* **62,** 1408–1415.

22. Lareu, M. V., Pestoni, C., Phillips, C., Barros, F., Synder Combe-Court, D., Lincoln, P., et al. (1998) Normal and anomalous electrophoretic behaviour of PCR-based DNA polymorphisms in polyacrylamide gels. *Electrophoresis* **19,** 1566–1573.

23. Gill, P., Sparkes, R., and Kimpton, C. (1997) Development of guidelines to designate alleles using an STR multiplex system. *Forensic Sci. Int.* **89,** 185–197.

24. Gill, P., Whitaker, J., Flaxman, C., Brown, N., and Buckleton, J. (2000) An investigation of the rigor of interpretation rules for STRs derived from less than 100 pg of DNA. *Forensic Sci. Int.* **112,** 17–40.

25. Kayser, M., Cagliá, A., Corach, D., Fretwell, N., Gehrig, C., Graziosi, G., et al. (1997) Evaluation of Y-chromosomal STRs: a multicenter study. *Int. J. Legal Med.* **110,** 125–133.

26. White, P. S., Tatum, O. L., Deaven, L. L., and Longmire, J. L. (1999) New, male-specific microsatellite markers from the human Y chromosome. *Genomics* **57,** 433–437.

27. Ayub, Q., Mohyuddin, A., Qamar, R., Mazhar, K., Zerjal, T., Mehdi, S., et al. (2000) Identification and characterization of novel human Y chromosomal microsatellites from sequences database information. *Nucl. Acids Res.* **28,** e8.

28. Roewer, L., Krawczak, M., Willuweit, S., Nagy, M., Alves, C., Amorim, A., et al. (2001) Online reference database of European Y-chromosomal short tandem repeat (STR) haplotypes. *Forensic Sci. Int.* **118,** 106–113

29. Roewer, L. (2001) Y chromosome polymorphisms. *Forensic Sci. Int.* **118**, 105.
30. Hering, S., and Szibor, R. (2000) Development of the X-linked tetrameric microsatellite marker DXS9898 for forensic purposes. *J. Forensic Sci.* **45**, 929–931.
31. Carracedo, A., D'Aloja, E., Dupuy, B., Jangblad, A., Karjalainen, M., Lambert, C., et al. (1998) Reproducibility between laboratories of mtDNA analysis: a report of the European DNA Profiling Group (EDNAP). *Forensic Sci. Int.* **97**, 165–170.
32. Holland, M. M., and Parsons, T. J. (1999) Mitochondrial DNA analysis-validation and use for forensic casework. *Forensic Sci. Rev.* **11**, 1–25.
33. Carracedo, A., Bär, W., Lincoln, P. J., Mayr, W., Morling, N., Olaisen, B., et al. (2000). DNA Commission of the International Society for Forensic Genetics: guidelines for mitochondrial DNA typing. *Forensic Sci. Int.* **110**, 79–85.
34. Tully, G., Bär, W., Brinkmann, B., Carracedo, A., Gill, P., Morling, N., Parson, W., and Schneider, P. (2001) Considerations by the European DNA Profiling (EDNAP) group on the working practices, nomenclature and interpretation of mitochodrial DNA profiles. *Forensic Sci. Int.* **124**, 83–91.

2

DNA Extraction and Quantitation of Forensic Samples Using the Phenol–Chloroform Method and Real-Time PCR

Silvano Köchl, Harald Niederstätter, and Walther Parson

Summary

Forensic laboratories are increasingly confronted with problematic samples from the scene of crime, containing only minute amounts of deoxyribonucleic acid (DNA), which may include polymerase chain reaction (PCR)-inhibiting substances. Efficient DNA extraction procedures, as well as accurate DNA quantification methods, are critical steps involved in the process of successful DNA analysis of such samples. The phenol–chloroform method is a sensitive method for the extraction of DNA from a wide variety of forensic samples, although it is known to be laborious compared with single-tube extraction methods. The relatively high DNA recovery and the quality of the extracted DNA speak for itself. For reliable and sensitive DNA quantitation, the application of real-time PCR is described. We modified a published real-time PCR assay, which allows for the combined analysis of nuclear and mitochondrial DNA, by introducing 1) improved hybridization probes with the use of minor groove binders; 2) an internal positive control (for both nuclear and mitochondrial DNA) for the detection of PCR inhibitors; and 3) different amplicon lengths for the determination of the degradation state of the DNA. The internal positive controls were constructed by site directed mutagenesis by overlap extension of the wild-type mitochondrial and nuclear DNA target with the advantage that no additional probes, which are cost-intensive, are required. The quantitation system is accomplished as a modular concept, which allows for the combined determination of the above-mentioned features (quantity/inhibition or quantity/degradation) depending on the situation,

Key Words: Real-time PCR (rtPCR); phenol–chloroform method; forensic DNA extraction.

From: *Methods in Molecular Biology, vol. 297: Forensic DNA Typing Protocols*
Edited by: A. Carracedo © Humana Press Inc., Totowa, NJ

1. Introduction

Successful deoxyribonucleic acid (DNA) profiling of forensic samples is largely dependent on the quality and the amount of DNA that is recovered from the sample in question. This is of particular importance when casework samples are to be analyzed, which frequently involve difficult specimen that contain only minute amounts of DNA and are likely to have suffered environmental stress (DNA degradation). Apart from that, the quality of a forensic trace is impacted by the nature of the substrate on which it was deposed (e.g., blood on denim). When the DNA is extracted from the source, trace compounds of the substrate may be coextracted, which can further influence the typing process. As a consequence, the efficiency and sensitivity of the extraction procedure are critical parameters that define the suitability of an extraction method for forensic samples.

The phenol–chloroform method *(1)* is a well-established forensic extraction procedure even though it is known to be laborious compared with alternative approaches and involves toxic reagents, such as phenol, which requires special safety precautions in the laboratory (laminar flow fume hood). As a matter of fact, phenol–chloroform extraction is still the method of choice for samples containing only very little amounts of DNA (e.g., hair shafts, bone samples, decomposed samples) or samples suspected to contain polymerase chain reaction (PCR)-inhibiting substances. Although this method involves intensive manual interaction—the sample is handled through at least three generations of reaction tubes—the DNA recovery of the phenol–chloroform extraction is known to be relatively high.

To control the success of the extraction step, DNA quantitation usually is performed for forensic casework material, although the usability of a sample in the forensic context is determined by the ability to generate a DNA profile after all. The information on the DNA quantity is mostly used to estimate the appropriate amount of DNA extract to be added to the PCR master mix to avoid overloading with excess of DNA. Common quantitation techniques involve photometric/fluorometric determination of the DNA amount, which are insensitive to the source of DNA, in contrast to specific DNA-based hybridization assays *(2–4)*. Both of these are less sensitive to the detection of DNA compared with the subsequent PCR assay, that is, extracts, in which quantitation failed, may still bring a useful DNA profile. A negative quantitation result does not necessarily indicate the absence of DNA—in contrast, the actual DNA amount may be masked as a result of substances included in the extract that interfere with the detection method. This is why some laboratories refrain from quantitation per se and directly apply an aliquot of the extract to PCR (mostly singleplex or small multiplexes) to estimate the quantity by analyzing the peak heights of the resulting DNA profile. Note that the latter method is not an explicit DNA quantitation method, but the estimate is based on the experience of the individual laboratory.

In contrast to the above-mentioned quantitative techniques, real-time PCR (rtPCR) is a very sensitive, stable, reproducible, and specific DNA quantitation method and leads to directly applicable results because the amount of DNA is inferred by the same process (i.e. PCR), which is then used for DNA profiling.

Here, we describe a rtPCR assay that is based on the coamplification of a nuclear DNA (nDNA) target (Retinoblastoma gene) and a mitochondrial DNA (mtDNA) target (spans over the genes for transfer ribonucleic acid lysine and ATP synthase 8) modifying the method published by Andreasson et al. *(5)*. We added the following three features to the assay. First, fluorescent probes with a minor groove binder (MGB; ref. *6*) are used, which enhance the sensitivity of the hybridization and the PCR efficiency for the amplification of longer fragments. Second, an internal positive control (IPC) is coamplified with the genome-specific target (either nDNA or mtDNA), which allows for the detection of PCR inhibitor present in a sample. This information is useful for the subsequent processing of the sample as (additional) purification or a dilution of the DNA extract may be the consequence to overcome inhibition. Third, the degradation stage of the DNA can be determined by application of different amplicon lengths used for the quantitation process. This serves as basis for further selection of amplification kits or locus-specific primer pairs and which helps with the interpretation of DNA profiles deduced from that extract.

1.1. Phenol–Chloroform Method

In general, this method involves disruption and lysis of the stain material, digestion of cell components and removal of contaminants by organic solvents. The DNA is finally recovered by alcohol and salt precipitation and subsequent rehydration. An alternative protocol involves the purification of the extracted DNA by means of column based methods instead of the alcohol precipitation *(7)*.

Cell lysis is performed using an enzyme- and detergent-based buffer (Proteinase K with sodium dodecyl sulfate). Organic extraction is performed by adding an equal volume of water-saturated, buffered phenol to the aqueous DNA sample, vigorously vortexing the mixture, and centrifugation to allow phase separation. The upper, aqueous layer is carefully removed to a new tube, avoiding the phenol interface. This step is followed by the addition of chloroform to extract residual phenol from the aqueous phase. The DNA is concentrated by ethanol precipitation in the presence of salt. After washing with 70% ethanol, the pellet DNA is dried in a speed vac and dissolved in low salt buffer. This method is suitable for the extraction of DNA from a wide range of cell types and stain materials.

If the stain material consists of a mixture of sperm and nonsperm cells, such as epithelial cells, the phenol–chloroform extraction is preceded by a step called differential extraction *(8)*. Differential extraction is a procedure in which sperms are separated from the other cells before lysis and DNA extraction. This is accomplished by selective digestion of the nonsperm cell fraction and separation of intact sperms by centrifugation. The nonsperm cell DNA is isolated under mild conditions that break only the epithelial cells but leave the sperm cells intact.

For the extraction of DNA from hairs, a buffer system containing Proteinase K and Ca^{2+} instead of ethylene diamine tetraacetic acid (EDTA) improves the efficiency of hair digestion significantly, resulting in an enhanced success rate in DNA typing *(9)*.

1.2. rtPCR Quantitation Using the TaqMan Assay

The TaqMan assay is a real-time, homogeneous PCR system in which the sample is amplified and typed simultaneously without the need for additional manipulations post-PCR. The assay uses standard PCR primers to generate an amplicon and an internal fluorescent hybridization probe *(10)*, which is specific for a sequence region within the amplicon. The assay is run on an instrument that is capable of measuring fluorescence directly through the lid of the reaction tube at each cycle of PCR—so that detection occurs online. A quencher molecule is attached to the 3' end of the probe, so that the probe does not emit fluorescence in its normal state. During PCR, the amplicon accumulates and the probe specifically binds to the product during the annealing phase. In the extension phase, Taq polymerase cleaves the probe via its 5'-exonuclease activity and thus separates the fluorochrome and quencher molecules *(11–14)*. At this point, fluorescent signal is emitted and detected. The course of the reaction can be displayed by an amplification plot (**Fig. 1A**). The initial cycles of PCR, in which only little change in fluorescence occurs, are used to define the baseline for the amplification plot. The threshold fluorescence signal is the level of detection or the point at which a reaction reaches a fluorescent intensity above background. The threshold is set in the exponential phase of the amplification for the most accurate reading. The cycle at which the sample reaches this level is called the cycle threshold (Ct; refs. *15* and *16*). The ΔRn-value (baseline-corrected endpoint reporter signal) is a measure of the amount of PCR product amplified in the course of real time PCR. When Ct values are plotted against the decade log of the initial target copy number, a straight line is obtained (**Fig. 1B**). This line can be used to identify the dynamic range of the assay and can be used to quantify the amount of initial target DNA from an unknown sample by calculating the actual template copy number from the derived Ct value (calibration with known DNA standards required; *see* **Note 1**).

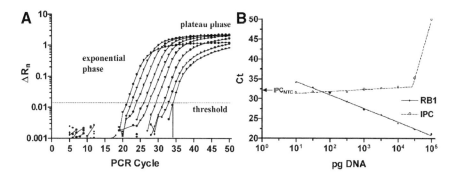

Fig. 1. (A) Amplification plots of a dilution series of the DNA standard (genomic DNA) showing the changes in fluorescence vs PCR cycle number (logarithmic view). (B) Standard curve derived from the data shown in (A); the threshold cycle Ct is defined as the fractional cycle number at which the fluorescence passes the fixed threshold. Ct values are plotted against the amount of template DNA. Also shown are Ct values of the IPC, which is included in the assay for the detection of PCR inhibitors; note that elevated Ct values of the IPC indicate the loss of amplification resulting from the competitive consumption of PCR components by elevated template concentrations (10^4–10^5).

1.2.1. MGBs

The modified probes are characterized by a MGB moiety that fits into the minor groove of double-stranded DNA, which increases the stability and specificity of probe hybridization and finally enhances the PCR efficiency for longer DNA fragments (Table 1; *see* **Note 2**). Because of the increased stability, TaqMan MGB probes are very short (approx 13 to 20 bases long) compared with standard TaqMan probes.

Furthermore, MGB probes are labeled with a nonfluorescent quencher (NFQ) in place of the previous standard TAMRA quencher dye. The NFQ, also called "dark quencher," does not emit detectable fluorescence, leading to a less complex signal with lower fluorescent background, which improves spectral discrimination and makes data interpretation easier.

1.2.2. IPC

To evaluate the performance of the rtPCR assay and to include an objective measure of potential PCR inhibition, we introduced an IPC that is amplified simultaneously in the same assay with the sample to be quantified. The IPC brings an amplification result in another dye layer and can therefore be evaluated independently from the signal of the unknown sample. The Ct value for the IPC (Ct_{IPC}) is set to 25–32 cycles (by limiting the primer concentration or

Table 1
Apparent rtPCR Efficiency Using BHQ and MGB TaqMan Probes
for Different Amplicon Lengths

Fragment lengths for RB1	BHQ	MGB
79-bp fragment	0.9896 (0.9496–1.0331)	0.9852 (0.9417–1.0332)
156-bp fragment	0.8604 (0.8257–0.8981)	0.9795 (0.9576–1.0025)
246-bp fragment	0.7222 (0.6919–0.7554)	0.8583 (0.7950–0.9318).

The rtPCR efficiency can be calculated from the slope of the standard curve by the formula E $= (10^{-1/\text{slope}}) - 1$. The numbers in brackets show 95% confidence intervals.

the copy number), to avoid troublesome competition between the amplification of the IPC and the genuine sample (*see* **Note 3**). PCR inhibitors in the DNA extract would be recorded by increased Ct values. Partial inhibition would result in Ct values between that of the negative controls (no template controls) and the total amount of cycles used for PCR (*see* **Note 4**).

The IPCs were constructed by site-directed PCR mutagenesis by overlap extension (SOE; refs. *17–19*) of the wild-type mtDNA and nuclear RB1 target. SOE results in the introduction of specific mutations in the modified template differing from the original sequence in a way that the modified template would not be amplified with the conventional primers, whereas the modified primers would only amplify the SOE product. This is true for both the nDNA and the mtDNA target. This is why the mtDNA–SOE product can be used as IPC for the quantitation of nDNA and the IPC$_{nDNA}$ as control for the quantitation of mtDNA. SOE is a fast and technically simple approach for manipulating DNA-sequences. In general, four primers are needed to introduce site-specific mutation(s) (**Fig. 2**). Two PCRs are performed, each using a perfectly complementary primer at the end of the sequence and a mismatched primer designed to introduce a mutation at a specific position. This results in overlapping fragments, in which the mutation is located in the region of the overlap (*see* **Notes 5,6**). The overlapping fragments are then annealed to each other in a second round of PCR where the entire mutated DNA fragment is amplified by means of the two complementary primers at the end of this DNA fragment.

The advantages of this procedure are that IPCs can be easily designed and kept in house, minimizing the costs of the assay. Alternative IPCs would require additional probes, which are cost-intensive.

1.2.3. Checking for DNA Degradation

The use of various fragment lengths for the rtPCR quantitation of a specific DNA target allows for the determination of DNA degradation. The latter can

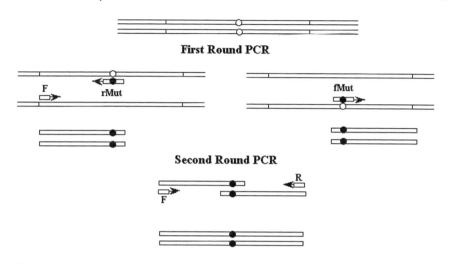

Fig. 2. First-round PCR: in two separate PCR reactions, two partially overlapping DNA fragments are amplified. The first primer pair is used to amplify the DNA that contains the mutation site together with upstream sequences. In this reaction, the reverse SOE primer (rMut) contains the mutation(s) to be introduced into the wild-type DNA-template. The second primer pair is used to amplify the DNA that contains the mutation site together with downstream sequences. In this reaction, the forward SOE primer (fMut) contains the mutation(s) to be introduced into the wild-type DNA-template. Second-round PCR: The overlapping fragments are mixed, denatured, annealed, and extended using the flanking primers F and R.

be assessed by comparing the amplification results of the different amplicons. These modifications upgrade the original rtPCR protocol to a modular concept which, depending on the combination of the individual modules, can provide information both about the quantity and the quality of DNA by using only two fluorogenic oligoprobes. In **Fig. 3**, a selection of some of these possible combinations is displayed.

2. Materials

2.1. Phenol–Chloroform Method

1. Sterile distilled water.
2. Hydrogen peroxide 30%.
3. 1 M Tris-HCl solution, pH 8.0.
4. 1 M Tris-HCl solution, pH 9.0.
5. 0.5 M EDTA disodium salt.
6. 5 M Sodium chloride.
7. Ethanol 100%.

1. simultaneous quantitation of
   mtDNA – nuclear DNA

2. DNA-quantitation and
   test for PCR-inhibition

3. DNA-quantitation and
   test for DNA-degradation

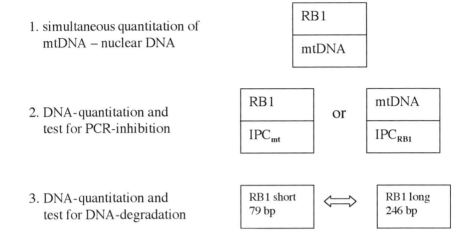

Fig. 3. Schematic representation of how the modular concept of rt PCR can be used to check besides DNA quantity for PCR inhibition or DNA degradation. Setup 1 allows simultaneous quantitation of nuclear and mtDNA as published by Andreasson et al. *(5)*. Setup 2 allows simultaneous quantitation of nuclear or mtDNA and detection of PCR inhibitors. Setup 3 allows quantitation of nuclear DNA and detection of fragmentation but needs two separate reactions.

8. Ethanol 70%.
9. Proteinase K stock solution: 20 mg/mL (dissolve 100 mg of proteinase K in 5 mL of sterile distilled water; store frozen in 1-mL aliquots).
10. 1 *M* dithiothreitol (DTT) solution.
11. Phenol solution (+ bottle of equilibration buffer for pH 8.0).
12. Chloroform:isoamylalcohol solution 24:1.
13. 3 *M* sodium acetate buffer solution, pH 5.2.
14. 10% sodium dodecyl sulfate solution.
15. Linear polyacrylamide(LPA; 5 mg/mL, Ambion).
16. 1 *M* Calcium chloride solution.
17. Extraction buffer (EB): 10 m*M* Tris-HCl, pH 8.0, 10 m*M* EDTA disodium salt, pH 8.0; 100 m*M* sodium chloride; and 2% sodium dodecyl sulfate.
18. Extraction buffer for hairs (EBH): 10 m*M* Tris-HCl, pH 8.0, 10 m*M* $CaCl_2$, 100 m*M* sodium chloride, 2% sodium dodecyl sulfate.
19. Sterile Petri dishes.

All extractions are performed in sterile 1.5-mL Sarstedt tubes with screw caps.

2.2. rtPCR Quantitation

1. ExoSapIT Amersham/Pharmacia.
2. TOPO TA Cloning Kit, Invitrogen Life Technologies.
3. TaqMan® Universal PCR Master Mix, No AmpErase® UNG.

2.3. Sequence of Primers and Fluorogenic Probes

Nuclear Target: *RB1 Gene*
Primers for cloning:
pRB1 F	5'-AGGTTGCTAACTATGAAACACTGGC-3'
pRB1 R	5'-CCATCTCAGCTACTGGAAAACATTC-3'

Primers for 79-bp amplicon: *(5)*
RB1-2672 F	5'-CCAGAAAATAAATCAGATGGTATGTAACA-3'
RB1-2750 R	5'-TGGTTTAGGAGGGTTGCTTCC-3'

Primers for 156-bp amplicon:
pRB1 F	5'-AGGTTGCTAACTATGAAACACTGGC-3'
RB1-2750 R	5'-TGGTTTAGGAGGGTTGCTTCC-3'

Primers for 246-bp amplicon:
pRB1 F	5'-AGGTTGCTAACTATGAAACACTGGC-3'
pRB1 R	5'-CCATCTCAGCTACTGGAAAACATTC-3'

BHQ probe:
RB1-2727 BHQ	5'-*FAM*-CAGCACTTCTTTTGAGCACACGGTCG-*BHQ1* - 3'

MGB probe:
RB1-2727 MGB:	5'-*FAM*-CAGCACTTCTTTTGAGCAC-*MGBNFQ*-3'

Primers for SOE:
RB1 2750 SOE F	5'-GTGCTGAACTAACCAACGCTCCGAAACGACTGAA -3'
RB1 2750 SOE R	5'-TTCAGTCGTTTCGGAGCGTTGGTTAGTTCAGCACTTC-3'
pRB1 F	5'-AGGTTGCTAACTATGAAACACTGGC-3'
pRB1 R	5'-CCATCTCAGCTACTGGAAAACATTC-3'

Primers for RB1-IPC
RB1 2750 IPC R	5'-TCGTTTCGGAGCGTTGGTTAG 3'
RB1-2672 F	5'-CCAGAAAATAAATCAGATGGTATGTAACA-3'

Mitochondrial Target: *Spans Over the Genes for Transfer Ribonucleic Acid Lysine and ATP Synthase 8*
Primers for cloning:
pMt F	5'-GGGTATACTACGGTCAATGCTCTGA-3'
pMt R	5'-CAATGAATGAAGCGAACAGATTTTC-3'

Primers for mt target: *(5)*
mt-8294 F	5'-CCACTGTAAAGCTAACTTAGCATTAACC-3'
mt-8436 R	5'-GTGATGAGGAATAGTGTAAGGAGTATGG-3'

BHQ-Probe:
mt-8345 BHQ	5'-*JOE*-CCAACACCTCTTTACAGTGAAATGCCCCA-*BHQ1* - 3'

MGB-Probe:
mt-8345 MGB	5'-*VIC* - CCA ACA CCT CTT TAC AGT GAA-*MGBDQ*-3'

Primers for SOE:
mt8294 SOE F	5'- GCCCAGTGTAGAGCTATGTTAGCATTTAGGTTTTAAGTTAA-3'
mt8294 SOE R	5'- TAAAACCTAAATGCTAACATAGCTCTACACTGGGCTCTAGAG-3'
pMt F	5'-GGGTATACTACGGTCAATGCTCTGA-3'
pMt R	5'-CAATGAATGAAGCGAACAGATTTTC-3'

Primers for mt-IPC
mt8294 IPC F	5'-CCAGTGTAGAGCTATGTTAGCATTTAGG-3'
mt-8436 R	5' - GTGATGAGGAATAGTGTAAGGAGTATGG-3'

4. Bovine serum albumin fraction V.
5. Sterile distilled water.
6. DNA standards.

3. Methods

3.1. Phenol–Chloroform Method

3.1.1. Extraction of DNA From All Types of Cells and Stain Materials Except Hairs and Sperm-Cell/Nonsperm-Cell Mixtures

1. To the sample add 500 µL of extraction buffer plus 20 µL of proteinase K (20 mg/mL).
2. Vortex and incubate at 56°C overnight with agitation in a Thermomixer.
3. Add an equal volume of buffered Phenol (pH 8.0; *see* **Notes 7, 8**), vortex, and spin for 10 min at maximum speed in a microcentrifuge.
4. Transfer the aqueous (upper) phase to a new microcentrifuge tube with 0.5 mL of chloroform (*see* **Note 9**).
5. Vortex and spin for 10 mins at maximum speed in a microcentrifuge.
6. Transfer the aqueous (upper) phase to a new microcentrifuge tube with 50 µL of 3 *M* NaAc, pH 5.2.
7. Add 0.8 mL of 100% EtOH, vortex, and precipitate at –20°C for at least 1.5 h (*see* **Notes 10, 11**).
8. Recover DNA by centrifugation for 30 min at maximum speed in a microcentrifuge and decant the supernatant.
9. To the pellet add 1 mL of 70% EtOH and spin for 20 min at maximum speed in a microcentrifuge.
10. Dry pellet in a vacuum centrifuge for 30 min (*see* **Note 12**).
11. Dissolve pellet in 50 µL of Tris buffer (10 m*M*, pH 9.0).

3.1.2. Extraction of DNA From Hairs

1. Cut hair in 1.5-mL Sarstedt tube already containing 500 mL of extraction buffer for hairs (EBH).
2. Add 20 µL of proteinase K solution (20 mg/mL) and 20 µL of DTT solution.
3. Proceed with **Subheading 3.1.1.** at **step 2**.

3.1.3. Extraction of DNA From Sperm-Cell/Nonsperm-Cell Mixtures

1. To the stain add 500 µL of extraction buffer plus 20 µL of proteinase K (20 mg/mL).
2. Vortex and incubate at 37°C for 30 min with agitation in a Thermomixer.
3. Remove stain material with tweezers sterilized in 10% H_2O_2 and spin for 5 min at maximum speed in a microcentrifuge (*see* **Note 13**).
4. Transfer supernatant (= nonsperm-cell fraction) to a new tube and proceed with **Subheading 3.1.1.**, **step 2**.
5. Add 1 mL of sterile water to the pellet, vortex and spin for 5 min at maximum speed in a microcentrifuge, and remove the supernatant.

6. Repeat **step** 5 twice.
7. Add 500 µL of extraction buffer plus 20 µL of proteinase K (20 mg/mL) plus 20 µL DTT (1 *M*) and proceed with **Subheading 3.1.1., step 2**.

3.2. rtPCR

3.2.1. Generation of IPCs by Site-Directed Mutagenesis by Overlap Extension (SOE) of the RB1 and mtDNA Target

1. Set up PCR for amplification of target sequence to be mutagenized by mixing the following reagents:

	RB-1	mtDNA
H$_2$O, sterile	12.8 µL	12.8 µL
10X PCR buffer	2 µL	2 µL
dNTP mix (2.5 m*M* each)	1.6 µL	1.6 µL
pRB1 F (10 µ*M*)	0.6 µL	–
pRB1 R (10 µ*M*)	0.6 µL	–
pMt F (10 µ*M*)	–	0.6 µL
pMt R (10 µ*M*)	–	0.6 µL
Ampli Taq Gold (5 u/µL)	0.4 µL	0.4 µL
Template DNA (5 ng/µL)	2 µL	2 µL
	20 µL	20 µL

2. Amplify using the denaturation, annealing, and extension times and temperatures listed in the table below

Cycle number	Denaturation	Annealing	Extension
Initial hold	10 min at 95°C		
30 cycles	15 s at 95°C	30 s at 61°C	45 s at 72°C
Final hold	10 min 72°C		

3. Set up first-round SOE-PCR 1 by mixing the following reagents:

	RB-1	mtDNA
H$_2$O, sterile	12.9 µL	12.9 µL
10X PCR buffer	2 µL	2 µL
dNTP mix (2.5 m*M* each)	1.6 µL	1.6 µL
pMt F (10 µ*M*)	–	1 µL
mt8294 SOE R (10 µ*M*)	–	1 µL
pRB1 F (10 µ*M*)	1 µL	–
RB1 2750 SOE R (10 µ*M*)	1 µL	–
Ampli Taq Gold (5 u/µL)	0.5 µL	0.5 µL
Amplicon RB1 (1:10.000)	1 µL	–-
Amplicon mtDNA (1:100.000)	–	1 µL
	20 µL	20 mL

4. Set up first round SOE-PCR 2 by mixing the following reagents:

	RB-1	mtDNA
H₂O, sterile	12.9 mL	12.9 mL
10X PCR buffer	2 µL	2 µL
dNTP mix (2.5 m*M* each)	1.6 µL	1.6 µL
mt8294 SOE F (10 µ*M*)	–	1 µL
pMt R (10 µ*M*)	–	1 µL
RB1 2750 SOE F (10 µ*M*)	1 µL	–
pRB1 R (10 µ*M*)	1 µL	–
Ampli Taq Gold (5 u/µL)	0.5 µL	0.5 µL
Amplicon RB1 (1:10.000)	1 µL	–
Amplicon mtDNA (1:100.000)	–	1 µL
	20 µL	20 µL

5. Amplify using the denaturation, annealing, and extension times, and temperatures listed in the table below:

Cycle number	Denaturation	Annealing	Extension
Initial hold	10 min at 95°C		
15 cycles	15 s at 95°C	30 s at 56°C	30 s at 72°C
26 cycles	15 s at 95°C	30 s at 60°C	30 s at 72°C

6. Pool equal volumes of the amplification products of SOE PCR 1 and SOE PCR 2 for the individual targets and purify the PCR products using the ExoSapIT Kit from Amersham/Pharmacia according to the manufacturer's instructions (*see* **Note 14**).

7. Set up the second-round SOE-PCR by mixing the following reagents:

Pre-Mastermix

	RB-1	mtDNA
H₂O, sterile	4.8 µL	4.8 µL
10X PCR buffer	2 µL	2 µL
dNTP mix (2.5 m*M* each)	1.6 µL	1.6 µL
pMt F (10 µ*M*)	–	0.6 µL
pMt R (10 µ*M*)	–	0.6 µL
pRB1 F (10 µ*M*)	0.6 µL	–
pRB1 R (10 µ*M*)	0.6 µL	–
50X Advantage2 PolMix	0.4 µL	0.4 µL
	10 µL	10 µL

Final Mastermix

	RB-1	mtDNA
H₂O sterile	8 µL	8 µL
Pre-Mastermix	10 µL	10 µL
Pooled and purified SOE1 amplification products	2 µL	2 µL
	20 µL	20 µL

8. Amplify using the denaturation, annealing, and extension times and temperatures listed in the table below:

Cycle number	Denaturation	Annealing	Extension
Initial hold	2 min at 95°C		
5 cycles	15 s at 95°C	45 s at 72°C	
28 cycles	15 s at 95°C	30 s at 60°C	45 s at 72°C
Final hold	30 min at 72°C		

9. Check amplicons on a gel and clone into TAvector according to the manufacturers instructions.
10. Verify the induced mutations and the correct sequences of the IPCs by sequencing.

3.2.2. rtPCR for Quantitation of nuclear DNA (+ mtIPC)

1. Set up PCR for quantitation of nuclear DNA (+ mtIPC) by mixing the following reagents:

rtPCR Pre-Mastermix

10X BSA (2.5 mg/mL)	2 µL
pRB1 F (10 µM)	0.6 µL
RB1-2750 R (10 µM)	0.6 µL
RB1-2727 MGB (10 µM)	0.4 µL
mt-8294 IPC F (10 µM)	0.28 µL
mt-8436 R (10 µM)	0.28 µL
mt-8345 MGB (10 µM)	0.4 µL
plasmid mt-IPC (40,000 copies/µL)	0.44 µL

2. rtPCR Mastermix for quantitation of nuclear DNA (+ mtIPC); 10 µL of TaqMan® Universal PCR Master Mix, 5 µL of rt-PCR Pre-Mastermix for quantitation of nuclear DNA (+mt-IPC); and up to 20 µL of H_2O and/or sample (*see* **Note 15**).
3. When the setup is complete, seal reactions, spin briefly (1 min at 1000g), place plate into the thermal cycler block, and start the run (*see* **Note 16**).
4. Interpretation guidelines for possible results, which can be obtained with the real time PCR-setup: DNA quantitation and test for PCR inhibition.

Target DNA	IPC	
+	+	Detectable signals (i.e. Ct values smaller than the number of cycles performed) both for the target DNA and the IPC means that the extract contains no inhibitors. To exclude partial inhibition, the Ct-values of the IPC obtained for the unknown samples have to be in the range of those observed in the no template controls (NTCs).
+	–	A high copy number of target DNA can lead to elevated Ct values or even a complete drop-out of the IPC resulting from the using up of the reaction components by the more abundant target.

–	+	No detectable signal for the target DNA but a detectable signal for the IPC indicates that the DNA content of the extract is below the detection limit of the rt-PCR method.
–	–	No detectable signal for the target DNA and IPC in the unknown sample, but detectable IPC signal in the no template controls, indicates the presence of PCR-inhibitor(s) in the extract. The copy number of the target can't be assessed at this stage

4. Notes

1. When plasmids (containing the nuclear or mitochondrial target) are used for the generation of standard curves, rtPCR amplification efficiencies have to be compared to genomic DNA (by comparing the slopes of the standard curves) as the circular form of plasmids may negatively affect PCR efficiency. If this is the case, the plasmids have to be linearized.

2. Besides increased sequence specificity and lower fluorescent background of MGB probes in comparison to unmodified probes, MGB probes increase the apparent PCR-efficiency for longer amplicons as displayed in **Table 1**.

3. To include an internal positive control into the real time PCR setup following rules have to be followed: 1) the IPC must not influence the PCR efficiency for the target sequence, especially at low DNA concentrations of the target sequence; and 2) Ct-values for the IPC should be stable over a wide range of copies of target DNA (The Ct-value of the IPC can be adjusted either by limiting primer concentrations or the amount of the IPC-template).

4. To demonstrate that the rtPCR setup with the IPC included is appropriate to reveal the presence of PCR inhibitors in a specific DNA extract, we performed mock DNA extractions on materials known to contain PCR inhibitors and spiked our standard curve with constant volumes of the extracts. The effect of PCR-inhibitor(s) on the rtPCR reaction parameters are shown in **Fig. 4**, considering blue denim as example.

5. The region of overlap between the two SOE primers should contain a number of bases corresponding to a Tm of approx 68–72°C.

6. The 3' ends of both SOE-primers should be at least 10 bases in length without mismatch to the original target sequence.

7. For the addition of phenol and chloroform/isoamylalcohol we use a dispenser. Before use the dispenser pipe is cleaned with 10% hydrogen peroxide solution and the first two volumes are discarded from the dispenser.

8. Phenol is a hazardous waste material that needs to be disposed properly. Phenol is highly corrosive and can cause severe burns to skin and damage clothing. Gloves, safety glasses, and a lab coat are to be worn whenever working with phenol, and all manipulations should be carried out in a fume hood.

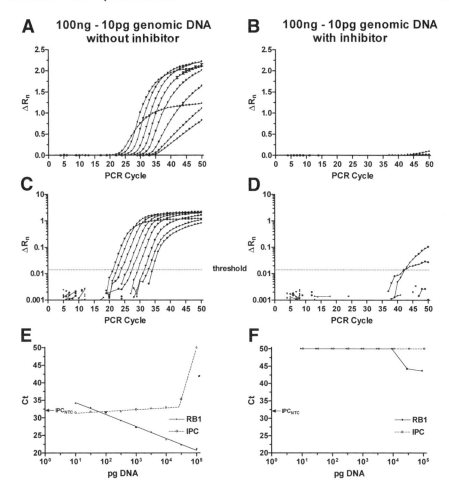

Fig. 4. (**A**) Amplification plots of a dilution series (10 pg to 100 ng) of the DNA standard–linear view. (**B**) Amplification plots of the same dilution series of the DNA standard spiked with constant amounts of the inhibitor–linear view. The addition of extract from blue denim led to complete inhibition of rtPCR at any concentration of the standard curve up to 10 ng input DNA (Ct-values equal to that of the no template controls and the total amount of cycles). (**C**) is the same as (**A**) but displayed in log view. (**D**) is the same as (**B**) but displayed in log view. (**E**) Standard curve derived from the data shown in (**A**) and (**C**); Ct values are plotted against the amount of template DNA. Also shown are Ct values of the IPC (note the elevated Ct values and the complete drop-out of the IPC at high amounts of input target DNA as a result of the consumption of the reaction components by the more abundant target). (**F**) Standard curve derived from the data shown in (**B**) and (**D**).

9. The two phases (organic phase and aqueous layer) need to be carefully separated in that the nucleic acids and proteins tend to be at the interface. Leaving too much of the aqueous layer behind will cause loss of material and aspirating too close to the interface can include protein.

10. Precipitation of the DNA at –20°C should be performed at least for 1.5 h. It is possible to place the samples at –20°C overnight at this stage.

11. For extractions from stains with small amounts of DNA, use LPA as a coprecipitant. LPA offers the advantage that it is chemically synthesized and is not derived from biological sources. Other carriers may contain small amounts of contaminating nucleic acids, which may cause problems, especially when typing mtDNA as seen in our laboratory when working with glycogen as carrier.

12. While drying the DNA pellet in the vacuum centrifuge, the screw caps of the tubes are kept in sterile Petri dishes.

13. Concerning DNA extraction from sperm-cell/nonsperm-cell mixtures, when removing the stain material with tweezers, it is important to squeeze the stain firmly to prevent loss of liquid and DNA.

14. Depending on the target sequence, the addition of nontemplate 3' overhanging residues by *Taq* DNA polymerase can lead to undesired mutations when using the SOE technique. To remove 3' overhanging residues and nonincorporated primers, purify the PCR products using the ExoSapIT Kit from Amersham/Pharmacia.

15. It is recommended to include at least three no template controls in each reaction plate in addition to extraction blocks.

16. rtPCR cocktails in a plate can be stored in the dark at room temperature for a couple of hours.

References

1. Sambrook, J., Fritsch E. F., and Maniatis, T. (1989). *Molecular Cloning: A Laboratory Manual, 2nd ed.*, Cold Spring Harbor Laboratory Press, Cold Spring Harbor, NY.

2. Waye, J. S., and Willard, H. F. (1986). Structure, organization, and sequence of alpha satellite DNA from human chromosome 17: evidence for evolution by unequal crossing-over and an ancestral pentamer repeat shared with the human X chromosome. *Mol. Cell Biol.* **6,** 3156–3165.

3. Waye, J. S., Presley, L. A., Budowle, B., Shutler, G. G., and Fourney, R. M. (1989). A simple and sensitive method for quantifying human genomic DNA in forensic specimen extracts. *BioTechniques* **7,** 852–855.

4. Walsh, P. S., Varlaro, J., and Reynolds, R. (1992). A rapid chemiluminescent method for quantitation of human DNA. *Nucleic Acids Res.* **20,** 5061–5065.

5. Andreasson, H., Gyllensten, U., and Allen, M. (2002). Real-time DNA quantification of nuclear and mitochondrial DNA in forensic analysis. *BioTechniques* **33,** 402–411.

6. Kutyavin, I. V., Afonina, I. A., Mills, A., Gorn, V. V., Lukhtanov, E. A., Belousov, E. S., et al. (2000). 3'-minor groove binder-DNA probes increase sequence specificity at PCR extension temperatures. *Nucleic Acids Res.* **28,** 655–661.

7. Hochmeister, M. N., Budowle, B., Borer, U. V., Eggmann, U., Comey, C. T., and Dirnhofer, R. (1991). Typing of deoxyribonucleic acid (DNA) extracted from compact bone from human remains. *J. Forensic Sci.* **36,** 1649–1661.
8. Gill, P., Jeffreys, A. J., and Werrett, D. J. (1985). Forensic application of DNA 'fingerprints'. *Nature* **318,** 577–579.
9. Hellmann, A., Rohleder, U., Schmitter, H., and Wittig, M. (2001). STR typing of human telogen hairs—a new approach. *Int. J. Legal Med.* **114,** 269–273.
10. Lee, L. G., Connell, C. R., and Bloch, W. (1993). Allelic discrimination by nick-translation PCR with fluorogenic probes. *Nucleic Acids Res.* **21,** 3761–3766.
11. Heid, C. A., Stevens, J., Livak, K. J., and Williams, P. M. (1996). Real time quantitative PCR. *Genome Res.* **6,** 986–994.
12. Holland, P. M., Abramson, R. D., Watson, R., and Gelfand, D. H. (1991). Detection of specific polymerase chain reaction product by utilizing the 5'–3' exonuclease activity of Thermus aquaticus DNA polymerase. *Proc. Natl. Acad. Sci. USA.* **88,** 7276–7280.
13. Livak, K. J., Flood, S. J., Marmaro, J., Giusti, W., and Deetz, K. (1995). Oligonucleotides with fluorescent dyes at opposite ends provide a quenched probe system useful for detecting PCR product and nucleic acid hybridization. *PCR Methods Appl.* **4,** 357–362.
14. Lyamichev, V., Brow, M. A., and Dahlberg, J. E. (1993). Structure-specific endonucleolytic cleavage of nucleic acids by eubacterial DNA polymerases. *Science* **260,** 778–783.
15. Gibson, U. E., Heid, C. A., and Williams, P. M. (1996). A novel method for real time quantitative RT-PCR. *Genome Res.* **6,** 995–1001.
16. Higuchi, R., Fockler, C., Dollinger, G., and Watson, R. (1993). Kinetic PCR analysis: real-time monitoring of DNA amplification reactions. *Biotechnology* **11,** 1026–1030.
17. Higuchi, R., Krummel, B., and Saiki, R. K. (1988). A general method of in vitro preparation and specific mutagenesis of DNA fragments: study of protein and DNA interactions. *Nucleic Acids Res.* **16,** 7351–7367.
18. Ho, S. N., Hunt, H. D., Horton, R. M., Pullen, J. K., and Pease, L. R. (1989). Site-directed mutagenesis by overlap extension using the polymerase chain reaction. *Gene* **77,** 51–59.
19. Horton, R. M., Cai, Z. L., Ho, S. N., and Pease, L. R. (1990). Gene splicing by overlap extension: tailor-made genes using the polymerase chain reaction. *BioTechniques* **8,** 528–535.

3

A Real-Time PCR Protocol to Determine the Number of Amelogenin (X–Y) Gene Copies From Forensic DNA Samples

Antonio Alonso and Pablo Martín

Summary

We present a fluorogenic real-time polymerase chain reaction (PCR) procedure to target a segment (106–112 base pairs [bp]) of the X–Y homologous amelogenin gene by measuring the 5' nuclease activity of the *Taq* deoxyribonucleic acid (DNA) polymerase using two (X-Fam-labeled and Y-Vic-labeled) specific Taqman MGB probes to enable simultaneous the detection of two specific PCR products (AMGY: 112-bp and AMGX: 106 bp) as they accumulate cycle by cycle during PCR. The method makes possible not only human nuclear DNA quantitation but also sex determination and has been applied to the analysis of low copy number DNA samples in forensic and ancient DNA studies. Specific quantification of human nuclear DNA is a recommended procedure in forensic casework as a way to adjust the DNA input on subsequent end-point PCR-based DNA typing approaches ensuring the optimal use of the limited amounts of nuclear DNA found in many forensic evidences. Nuclear DNA quantification also aids in the interpretation of the consistency of multiplex STR profiling data obtained from low copy number DNA samples.

Key Words: Real-time PCR; amelogenin gene; forensic genetics; ancient DNA; low copy number DNA samples; sex determination; STR profiling.

1. Introduction

We present a fluorogenic real-time polymerase chain reaction (PCR) procedure to target a segment (106–112 base pair [bp]) of the X–Y homologous amelogenin gene *(1,2)* by measuring the 5' nuclease activity of the *Taq* deoxyribonucleic acid (DNA) polymerase using two (X-Fam-labeled and Y-Vic-labeled) specific Taqman MGB probes to enable the simultaneous detection of two specific PCR products (AMGY: 112-bp and AMGX: 106 bp) as they ac-

From: *Methods in Molecular Biology, vol. 297: Forensic DNA Typing Protocols*
Edited by: A. Carracedo © Humana Press Inc., Totowa, NJ

cumulate cycle by cycle during PCR *(3)*. During each extension cycle the 5′ nuclease activity of *Taq* DNA polymerase cleaves the annealed probes separating the reporter dye molecule from the quencher, which results in increased fluorescence of the reporter dye signal. Therefore, the accumulation of specific AMGX and AMGY PCR products is detected by monitoring the increase in fluorescence levels of the AMGX-FAM or AMGY-VIC reporter dyes, respectively. The higher the initial input of the target genomic DNA, the sooner a significant increase in fluorescence is observed. The cycle at which fluorescence reaches an arbitrary threshold level during the exponential phase of the PCR is named threshold cycle (Ct). Different standard curves can be generated by plotting the log of the starting DNA template amount of a set of previously quantified male (XY) and female (XX) DNA standards against their Ct values. Therefore, an accurate estimation of the starting X and Y DNA copies from unknown samples is accomplished by comparison of the measured Ct values with the Ct values of the standard curves. The method makes possible not only DNA quantitation but also sex determination and has been applied to the analysis of low copy number DNA samples in forensic and ancient DNA studies *(3,4)*. Real-time quantitative PCR offers several advantages with respect to other current DNA-quantification methods (hybridization, refs. *5* and *6*) or end-point PCR methods, refs. *7* and *8*), including higher sensitivity and dynamic range of quantitation, unnecessary post-PCR processing, automation feasibility, and high throughput. Other interesting real-time PCR designs for both nuclear (single copy genes, ref. *9*) and repetitive Alu sequences, ref. *10*) and mitochondrial (mt)DNA *(3,9)* have been described. Specific estimation of the human DNA quantity is a recommended procedure in forensic casework *(11,12)* that will aid in deciding whether the isolated DNA is suitable for nuclear or mtDNA analysis and to adjust the DNA input to improve the performance of subsequent end-point PCR-based DNA typing specially from low copy number DNA samples.

2. Materials

2.1. Specimens

The method can be applied to any DNA sample that may contain human DNA. It has been used as described previously to determine sex and to quantify the amount of human DNA from DNA extracts isolated from blood, saliva, semen, hair, bone, and teeth samples by using proteolytic digestion followed by phenol–chloroform purification and Centricon-100 filtration *(13)*. Some samples were further purified with silica columns using the QIAamp DNA Blood Midi Kit (Qiagen). The type of DNA extraction method could have a great influence on the performance of the assay (*see* **Note 1**).

2.2. Reagents

1. Human female genomic DNA 9947A at a 0.1 ng/µL concentration (Applied Biosystems, Foster City, CA).
2. Human genomic DNA from the male cell line ATCC CCL-256.1 at a 2.5 ng/µL concentration (Reliagene Technologies, New Orleans, LA).
3. Forward primer (AMG_F) (CCC TGG GCT CTG TAA AGA ATA GTG).
4. Reverse primer (AMG_R) (ATC AGA GCT TAA ACT GGG AAG CTG).
5. Probe AMGX (6FAM-TAT CCC AGA TGT TTCTC-MGB).
6. Probe AMGY (VIC-CAT CCC AAA TAA AGT G-MGB). (*See* **Note 2** for further information on probe designs.)
7. Taqman PCR Core Reagent Kit, including Ampli*Taq*Gold DNA polymerase; dUTP, dATP, dCTP, dGTP; 1.2 mL 10X Taqman buffer A; and 2 × 1.5 mL 25m*M* $MgCl_2$ (Applied Biosystems).
8. Bovine serum albumin (BSA).
9. TE (1X).

2.3. Disposables

1. Micro Amp optical 96-well reaction plates, ABI PRISM optical adhesive covers, and compression pads (Applied Biosystems).
2. 1.5-mL sterile microcentrifuge tubes.
3. Aerosol-resistant pipet tips.

2.4. Equipment

1. A laminar flow cabinet.
2. ABI PRISM 7000 Sequence Detection System (Applied Biosystems).

2.5. Software

1. ABI Prism 7000 SDS software (Applied Biosystems)
2. Primer Express 2.0 (Applied Biosystems)
3. Microsoft Excel.

3. Methods

3.1. Experimental Design and Plate Document Setup

Before starting a real-time PCR run, the assay type should be determined and a plate document must be set up. The plate document is a representation of the 96-well reaction plate where you can enter sample names, select and modify sample types (unknowns, standards, and no-template controls), and create and ad specific detectors. The following procedure can be used to set up an absolute AMG X/Y quantification assay using the ABI Prism 7000 SDS Software.

1. Open the ABI Prism 7000 SDS Software and make the appropriate selection (absolute quantification, 96-well clear, and blank document) from the "new document"

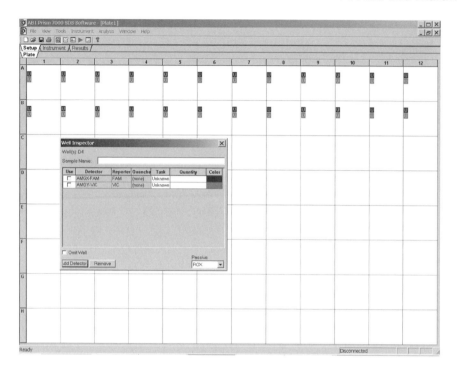

Fig. 1. The plate window (under the set-up menu) showing also (superimposed) the well inspector window used to add both detectors (MG-X-FAM and AMG-Y-VIC) to A1-B12 wells.

window. By selecting "setup," then "plate," a blank 96-well plate document window is acceded.

2. Create two new detectors by selecting "tools," "detector manager," "file," then "new" to open the new detector window where the name (AMGX-FAM and AMG-Y-VIC), an optional description, the reporter dye (FAM for the AMGX detector and VIC for the AMGY detector), the quencher dye (none for MGB probes), and the color (blue for AMGX-FAM and pink for AMG-Y-VIC) can be specified.

3. Open "well inspector" from the "view menu" to add both detectors to all the wells of the plate that are going to be in use. Use also "well inspector" to enter sample type information (unknowns, standards, and no-template controls) and the DNA quantity of the standards. A plate document where both detectors (AMGX-FAM and AMGY-VIC) were added to wells A1 to A12 and B1 to B12 by using the well inspector is shown in **Fig. 1.** For each set of samples to be quantified in one experiment, we routinely include a twofold serial dilution of the female DNA standard (from 1000 pg to 8 pg) to generate the standard AMG-X quantification curve for quantification of both male and female DNA. At least two male DNA controls (2500 pg and 250 pg) should also be included on each

experiment to monitor the performance of the AMGY-VIC detector or alternatively a standard AMG-Y quantification curve can be generated if a twofold serial dilution of a male DNA standard is included (*see* **Note 3**). Several no-template controls (including not only PCR blanks but also DNA extraction blanks) need also to be run along with the samples to monitor background contamination (*see* **Note 4**).

4. When all the information has been set up save the document and print the edited 96-well plate document that will be used as the worklist for PCR set up.

3.2. DNA Samples Preparation

To minimize the possibility of contamination, DNA samples preparation and PCR setup were conducted in a laminar flow cabinet located in a dedicated pre-PCR laboratory. All the reagents, tubes, and plastic tips (aerosol resistant) were sterilized by autoclaving them before use. Ultraviolet irradiation and treatment with 10% bleach were used to eliminate possible DNA contaminants.

3.2.1. Preparation of AMG X DNA Standards

Prepare twofold serial dilutions of the female genomic DNA from the cell line 9947A (from 1000 pg/10 μL to 8 pg/10 μL) in TE buffer as follows.

1. Label eight autoclaved microcentrifuge tubes 1 through 8.
2. Transfer 40 μL of Human female genomic DNA 9947A at a 100 pg/μL concentration (Applied Biosystems) into the tube labeled 1 (DNA standard 1).
3. Aliquot 20 μL of TE buffer into each of the seven remaining tubes labeled 2 through 8.
4. Add 20 μL of DNA standard 1 (tube 1) to the 20 μL of TE buffer in tube 2. Vortex to mix thoroughly.
5. Add 20 μL of female DNA standard 2 (tube 2) to the 20 μL of TE buffer in tube 3. Vortex to mix thoroughly.
6. Add 20 μL of female DNA standard 3 (tube 3) to the 20 μL of TE buffer in tube 4. Vortex to mix thoroughly.
7. Continue the serial dilution through tube 8.

If the dilution steps are performed correctly, the eight DNA standards tubes (1 through 8) will have the following concentrations of female DNA:

Tube	DNA quantity
Tube 1	1000 pg/10 μL
Tube 2	500 pg/10 μL
Tube 3	250 pg/10 μL
Tube 4	125 pg/10 μL
Tube 5	62.5 pg/10 μL
Tube 6	31.25 pg/10 μL
Tube 7	15.625 pg/10 μL
Tube 8	7.8125 pg/10 μL

3.2.2. Preparation of AMG Y DNA Standard Controls

Prepare at least two male genomic DNA controls of different DNA concentration (2500 pg/μL and 250 pg/μL) from the cell line CCL-256.1 (at a concentration of 2500 pg/μL) in TE buffer as follows.

1. Label two autoclaved Eppendorf tubes as MC1 and MC2 (MC: male control).
2. Aliquot 90 μL of TE buffer into each of the two tubes labeled MC.
3. Add 10 μL of male genomic DNA CCL-256.1 at a 2500 pg/μL concentration into the tube labeled MC1. Vortex to mix thoroughly.
4. Add 10 μL of male DNA MC1 to the 90 μL of TE buffer in tube MC2. Vortex to mix thoroughly.

If the dilution steps are performed correctly, the two MC DNA standards tubes will have the following concentrations of male DNA:

- MC1: 2500 pg/10 mL
- MC2: 250 pg/10 mL

3.2.3. Preparation of Forensic DNA Samples

Aliquots (1–5 μL) of DNA extracts isolated from forensic samples are adjusted to a final volume of 10 μL by using TE buffer. It is important to avoid *Taq* inhibitors on the DNA extracts using appropriate DNA purification methods to guarantee the performance of the assay from some forensic samples (*see* **Note 1**).

3.3. PCR Setup

1. Thaw the components of the Taqman PCR Core Reagent Kit
2. Determine the number of reactions to be setup. Add 1 or 2 reactions to this number to compensate for pipeting errors.
3. Multiply the volume per reaction (in microliters) by the total number of reactions to obtain the final master mix volume using **Table 1**.
4. Add the final volume of each reagent, in the order listed to a sterile microcentrifuge tube. Mix gently.
5. Place on the cabinet a sterile 96-well plate and pipette 40 μL of PCR master mix into each well
6. Pipet the DNA template (10 μL) of each sample into the respective well containing the PCR master mix according to the positions established in the 96-well document. Use the print copy of the plate document to check each position.
7. Seal the 96-well plate with an optical adhesive cover and place the compression pad (gray side down) on top of the sealed reaction plate.

3.4. PCR Running Parameters

1. Turn on the ABI Prism 7000 SDS by pressing the power button on the lower left front of the instrument and load the 96-well plate in the sample block so that well A1 is in the upper-left corner.

Table 1
PCR Master Mix Components

Components	Volume per Reaction ×	Number of reactions	Final volume
Sterile water	15 µL		
Autoclaved BSA (500 ng/mL)	10 µL		
10X Taqman buffer A	5 µL		
25 mM MgCl₂ solution	3 µL		
dATP (10 mM)	1 µL		
dCTP (10 mM)	1 µL		
dGTP (10 mM)	1 µL		
dUTP (20 mM)	1 µL		
AmpliTaqGold polymerase (5 U/mL)	0.5 µL		
Forward Primer (AMG F) (100 mM)	0.25 µL		
Reverse primer (AMG R) (100 mM)	0.25 µL		
AMG X- FAM Taqman probe (15 mM)	1 µL		
AMG Y- VIC Taqman probe (15 mM)	1 µL		
Total volume	40 µL		

2. Open the plate document previously set up and clicks the "instrument" tab to select the PCR running conditions (repetitions, temperature, and time) from the "thermal profile" panel.
3. Select the following thermal cycler conditions: An initial denaturation of 95°C for 10 min, followed by 50 cycles of 95°C for 15 s and 60°C for 1 min to anneal and extend as shown in **Fig. 2**.
4. Save the plate document.
5. Click the "start" button from the "instrument" window to launch the run. The change in fluorescence can be monitored cycle by cycle during the run by selecting "results," then "amplification plot."
6. When the run has finished disconnect the instrument from the plate document using the instrument buttons of the "instrument" window and turn off the ABI PRISM 7000 SDS.

3.5. Analysis and Interpretation Results

1. After a run is complete, the collected data can be analyzed by clicking the "Analyze" button using default or user modified "threshold" and "baseline" analysis settings (in the "analysis setting" dialog box). The results are immediately available in the "Results" tab.
2. Selecting the amplification plot tab (one of the seven secondary tabs of the "Results" tab) you can see the post-run normalized reporter signal of one or both detectors (Rn or Delta Rn) vs cycle number of all samples selected in the wells. Inspect the results obtained from the female DNA standards with the

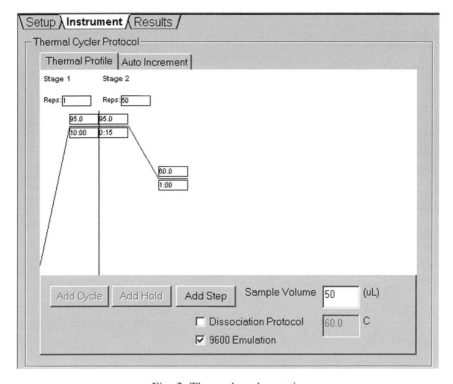

Fig. 2. Thermal cycler settings.

AMGX detector. In **Fig. 3**, a linear amplification plot of the eight twofold serial dilutions of the female genomic DNA from the cell line 9947A is displayed as detected with the AGMX-FAM detector.

3. Select the wells corresponding to the male DNA controls to check results with both AMGX-FAM and AMGY-VIC detectors. In **Fig. 4**, a linear amplification plot of one of the male genomic DNA controls is displayed as detected with both the AGMX-FAM (red curve) and AMGY-VIC (green curve) detectors.

4. Select the wells corresponding to the unknowns DNA samples to check results with both AMGX-FAM and AMGY-VIC detectors.

5. Select the Standard curve" tab to display the standard curve graph (starting DNA copy number vs Ct) for the samples designated as standards as well as some statistical data associated with the standard curve (slope, intercept, and R2). In **Fig. 5**, the AMGX standard curve generated with the female DNA 9974A standard dilutions is displayed (*see* **Note 5** to learn how to evaluate the reproducibility of DNA standards from independent experiments).

6. Select the "report" tab to display a tabular report of the data (Ct values and calculated DNA quantity using the AMGX-FAM standard curve). For those samples that were positive with both the AMGX-FAM and AMGY-VIC detectors (XY

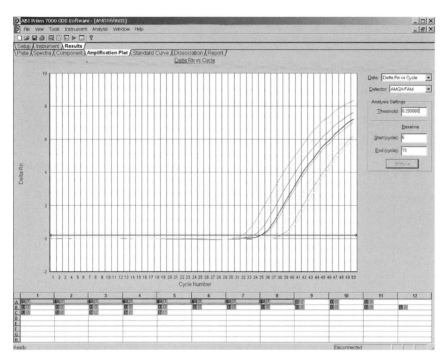

Fig. 3. Linear amplification plot of the eight twofold serial dilutions of the female genomic DNA from the cell line 9947A is displayed as detected with the AGMX-FAM detector.

males), the total DNA amount should be calculated multiplying by two the DNA quantity determined with the AMGX-FAM detector. An example of the data displayed on the report tab is shown below where the results of the female DNA standards along with the quantification results obtained from some bone DNA samples are displayed (**Fig. 6**).(*See* **Note 4** to learn more about the detection limit of this quantitative assay.)

For further information on the use of the ABI PRISM 7000 SDS, read the ABI PRISM 7000 Sequence Detection System User Guide (Applied Biosystems).

4. Notes

1. It is important to remember that the presence of *Taq* inhibitor compounds on the DNA extracts could have a great influence on the performance of this quantitative assay, producing both completely false-negative results and false DNA concentration estimations as a result of a partial *Taq* inhibition. A relatively high incidence of PCR inhibitors could be predicted when analyzing bone and ancient DNA samples and other forensic samples. The presence of *Taq* inhibitors on the DNA extracts can be prevented or at least reduced by using appropriate DNA-

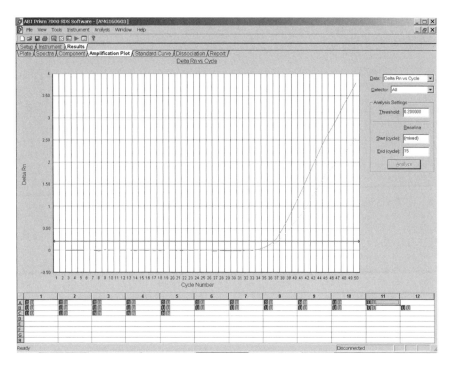

Fig. 4. Linear amplification plot of one of the male genomic DNA controls is dis-played as detected with both the AGMX-FAM (red curve) and AMGY-VIC (green curve) detectors.

purification methods. In our experience the method of organic extraction after Proteinase K digestion followed by ultrafiltration using Centricon devices (Millipore) is an efficient method to wash out a high proportion of inhibitor com-pounds from the DNA extracts. However, in some occasions (specially from old bone samples) the use of a silica-based purification method was necessary to remove the inhibitor from the DNA extract. The use of a silica column with a high binding capacity (QIAamp DNA Blood Midi Kit) (Qiagen) was essential to prevent the lost of human DNA, which is normally the minor DNA component of the DNA extracts isolated from bones that generally contains high amounts of DNA from bacteria and other microorganisms. However, the use of BSA to pre-vent *Taq* inhibition should be a standard practice on quantitative real-time PCR assays in forensic and ancient DNA studies. The development of an internal stan-dard control to determine the PCR efficiency from each individual sample could be of great help to interpret negative real-time PCR results.

2. Detection of the specific AMGX fragment (106 bp) and AMGY fragment (112 bp) was achieved using the primers pair sequences previously described (*1*) and two newly designed fluorogenic MGB probes that specifically detect the AMGX-

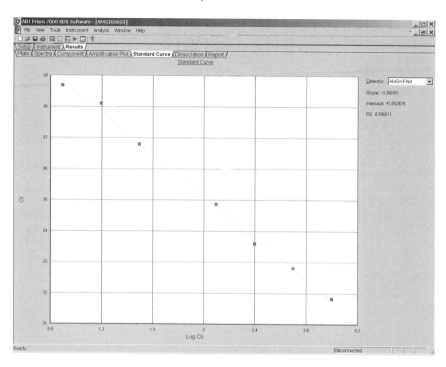

Fig. 5. AMGX standard curve generated with the female DNA 9974A standard dilutions

fragment (FAM-labeled) or the AMGY-fragment (VIC-labeled) using Primer Express 2.0 software (Applied Biosystems). The MGB probes were designed to target the 6-bp X-deletion/Y-insertion segment within the AMG second intron fragment targeted in this study using the human sequence data previously reported (Accessions no. M55418 and M55419; ref. *1*).

3. Twofold serial dilutions of a male genomic DNA (for instance by preparing serial dilutions of the male cell line CCL-256.1 DNA from 1250 pg to 40 pg of haploid AMGY gene content, as previously described; ref. *3*) can be used to generate the AMGY-VIC DNA standard curve if quantification of AMGY gene copies is required. However, total human nuclear DNA quantification was performed using the AMGX-FAM detector from both male and female DNA samples whereas the AMGY-VIC detector was generally used just as a qualitative assay to detect the presence or absence of the AMGY (112 bp) amplicon to perform sex determinations. (*See* **Note 5** to learn more about the detection limit of the assay.) At the present time we are working on a new AMGY MGB probe design to improve the detection limit of this detector that is slightly less sensitive than the AMGX-FAM detector.

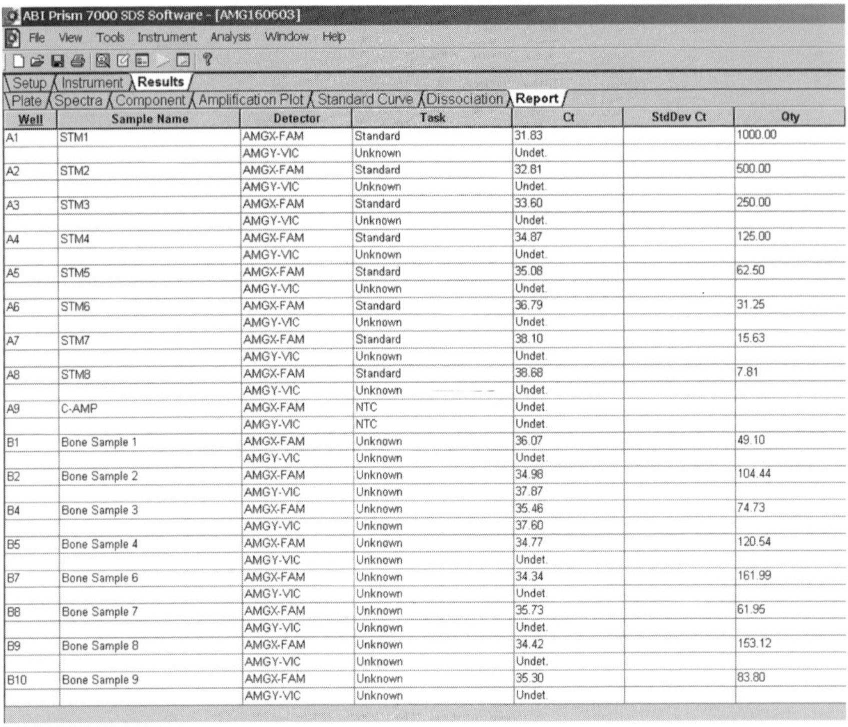

```
ABI Prism 7000 SDS Software - [AMG160603]
File  View  Tools  Instrument  Analysis  Window  Help
```
Setup / Instrument / **Results**
Plate / Spectra / Component / Amplification Plot / Standard Curve / Dissociation / **Report** /

Well	Sample Name	Detector	Task	Ct	StdDev Ct	Qty
A1	STM1	AMGX-FAM	Standard	31.83		1000.00
		AMGY-VIC	Unknown	Undet.		
A2	STM2	AMGX-FAM	Standard	32.81		500.00
		AMGY-VIC	Unknown	Undet.		
A3	STM3	AMGX-FAM	Standard	33.60		250.00
		AMGY-VIC	Unknown	Undet.		
A4	STM4	AMGX-FAM	Standard	34.87		125.00
		AMGY-VIC	Unknown	Undet.		
A5	STM5	AMGX-FAM	Standard	35.08		62.50
		AMGY-VIC	Unknown	Undet.		
A6	STM6	AMGX-FAM	Standard	36.79		31.25
		AMGY-VIC	Unknown	Undet.		
A7	STM7	AMGX-FAM	Standard	38.10		15.63
		AMGY-VIC	Unknown	Undet.		
A8	STM8	AMGX-FAM	Standard	38.68		7.81
		AMGY-VIC	Unknown	Undet.		
A9	C-AMP	AMGX-FAM	NTC	Undet.		
		AMGY-VIC	NTC	Undet.		
B1	Bone Sample 1	AMGX-FAM	Unknown	36.07		49.10
		AMGY-VIC	Unknown	Undet.		
B2	Bone Sample 2	AMGX-FAM	Unknown	34.98		104.44
		AMGY-VIC	Unknown	37.87		
B4	Bone Sample 3	AMGX-FAM	Unknown	35.46		74.73
		AMGY-VIC	Unknown	37.60		
B5	Bone Sample 4	AMGX-FAM	Unknown	34.77		120.54
		AMGY-VIC	Unknown	Undet.		
B7	Bone Sample 6	AMGX-FAM	Unknown	34.34		161.99
		AMGY-VIC	Unknown	Undet.		
B8	Bone Sample 7	AMGX-FAM	Unknown	35.73		61.95
		AMGY-VIC	Unknown	Undet.		
B9	Bone Sample 8	AMGX-FAM	Unknown	34.42		153.12
		AMGY-VIC	Unknown	Undet.		
B10	Bone Sample 9	AMGX-FAM	Unknown	35.30		83.80
		AMGY-VIC	Unknown	Undet.		

Fig. 6. An example of the data displayed on the report tab, where the results of the female DNA standards along with the quantification results obtained from some bone DNA samples are displayed.

4. The sensitivity of the AMGX-FAM design was better than the AMGY-VIC design (we are at present working on new AMGY probes designs to improve the sensibility of this detector), but in both cases determination of a single nuclear DNA genome seems to be theoretically possible if we assume 3 pg as the haploid human genome content of a single cell. However, amplification dropout have been observed for both the AMG-X and AMG-Y detectors when DNA input was less than 60 pg that corresponded to approximately 20 AMG-X copies in females and 10 AMG-X and 10 AMG-Y copies in males. Therefore, the possibility of random dropout cannot be excluded as a cause of sex determination failure when very low copy number initiates real-time PCR. However, when using highly sensitive PCR methods to deal with low copy number DNA samples, the influence of sporadic background contamination should be considered, and very stringent criteria should be followed to determine the authenticity of the DNA analysis *(4,14–16)*.

5. Each laboratory should perform validation studies to evaluate the intra-lab reproducibility of the quantification assay from independent real-time PCR experi-

ments. A standard curve should be rejected if the correlation coefficient of the trendline is < 0.95. Occasionally one or two points can be removed if a particular DNA dilution deviates significantly from the trendline produced by the rest of the data. Microsoft Excel spreadsheets can be used to generate standard curves with average Ct data from different individual experiments. Validation studies between laboratories also are needed to evaluate the potential applications of this technology in forensic studies.

References

1. Nakahori, Y., Takenaka, O., and Nakagome, Y. (1991) A human X–Y homologous region encodes 'amelogenin.' *Genomics* **9**, 264–269.
2. Sullivan, K. M., Mannucci, A., Kimpton, C. P., and Gill, P. (1993) A rapid and quantitative DNA sex test: fluorescence-based PCR analysis of X–Y homologous gene amelogenin. *BioTechniques* **15**, 637–641.
3. Alonso, A., Martín, P., Albarrán, C., García, P., García, O., Fernández de Simón, L., et al. Real-time PCR designs to estimate nuclear and mtDNA copy number in forensic and ancient DNA studies. *Forensic Sci. Int.,* in press..
4. Alonso, A., Martín, P., Albarrán, C., García, P., Primorac, D., García, O., et al. (2003) Specific quantification of human genomes from low copy number DNA samples in forensic and ancient DNA studies. *Croat. Med. J.* **44**, 273–280.
5. Walsh, P. S., Varlaro, J., and Reynolds, R. (1992) A rapid chemiluminescent method for quantitation of human DNA. *Nucleic Acids Res.* **20**, 5061–5065.
6. Waye, J. S., and Willard, H. F. (1986) Structure, organization, and sequence of alpha satellite DNA from human chromosome 17: evidence for evolution by unequal crossing-over and an ancestral pentamer repeat shared with the human X chromosome. *Mol. Cell Biol.* **6**, 3156–3165.
7. Sifis, M. E., Both, K., and Burgoyne, L. A. (2000) A more sensitive method for the quantitation of genomic DNA by Alu amplification. *J. Forensic Sci.* **47**, 589–592.
8. Fox, J. C., Cave, C. A., and Schumm, J. W. (2003) Development, characterization, and validation of a sensitive primate-specific quantification assay for forensic analysis. *BioTechniques* **34**, 314–318.
9. Andreasson, H., Gyllensten, U., and Allen, M. (2002) Real-time DNA quantification of nuclear and mitochondrial DNA in forensic analysis. *BioTechniques* **33**, 402–411.
10. Walker, J. A., Kilroy, G. E., Xing, J., Shewale, J., Sinha. S. K., and Batzer, M. A. (2003) Human DNA quantitation using Alu element-based polymerase chain reaction. *Anal. Biochem.* **315**, 122–128.
11. Recommendations of the DNA Commission of the International Society for Forensic Haemogenetics relating to the use of PCR-based polymorphisms (1992). *Forensic Sci. Int.* **55**, 1–3.
12. Quality Assurance Standards for Forensic DNA Testing Laboratories. DNA Advisory Board (1998). *Forensic Sci. Com.* **2**,. (Available at www.fbi.gov/hq/lab/fcs/current/index.htm.)

13. Alonso, A., Andelinovic, S., Martin, P., Sutlovic, D., Erceg, I., Huffine, E., et al. (2001) DNA typing from skeletal remains: evaluation of multiplex and megaplex STR systems on DNA isolated from bone and teeth samples. *Croat. Med. J.* **42,** 260–266.
14. Hofreiter, M., Serre, D., Poinar, HN., Kuch, M., and Pääbo S. (2001) Ancient DNA. *Nat. Rev.* **2,** 353–359.
15. Budowle, B., Hobson, D., Smerick, J., and Smith, J. (2001) Low copy number: consideration and caution. Proceedings from the Twelfth International Symposium on Human Identification 2001, available at www.promega.com.
16. Gill, P., Whitaker, J., Flaxman, C., Brown, N., and Buckelton, J. (2000) An investigation of the rigor of interpretation rules for STRs derived from less than 100 pg of DNA. *Forensic Sci. Int.* **112,**17–40.

4

Species Determination

The Role and Use of the Cytochrome b *Gene*

Adrian Linacre and James Chun-I Lee

Summary

Many large mammalian species are on the verge of extinction in part because of the trade in their skin, bone, horn, or body parts for supposed medicinal purposes. Identification of the species is required to determine that a crime has been committed. This chapter details a robust DNA technique using part of the cytochrome *b* gene on the mitochondrial genome that will work on poor-quality samples such as powdered horn. An appropriate deoxyribonucleic acid (DNA) extraction technique is required to obtain at least 10 ng of DNA. Amplification of part of the cytochrome *b* gene using universal primers produces a fragment of approx 486 bp in size. Direct sequencing of the PCR products allows comparison of the DNA sequence at this locus to those already described on the EMBL DNA database.

Key Words: CITES; DNA; mitochondria; cytochrome *b*; species; forensic.

1. Introduction

The trade in endangered species is an acute problem in many parts of the world that affects many rare animal species. The Convention on International Trade in Endangered Species of Wild Flora and Fauna (CITES) lists a growing and depressing number of species on the verge of extinction in the wild. Many of these animal species are still traded illegally, often for their skins or for the supposed medicinal qualities. It is the role of laboratories to determine the species of origin from powdered remains, skins, bones, and horns.

There are methods of species determination using protein analysis, but these have largely been superseded by deoxyribonucleic acid (DNA) typing. The choice of DNA locus is key to the success of the test, and there are certain criteria that must be met. It is necessary to use a locus that is sufficiently con-

From: *Methods in Molecular Biology, vol. 297: Forensic DNA Typing Protocols*
Edited by: A. Carracedo © Humana Press Inc., Totowa, NJ

served such that all members of the same species have a very similar DNA sequence; the locus must be sufficiently polymorphic such that members of different, but closely related species, can be distinguished; the locus must be on a fragment of DNA that can be amplified from poor-quality samples; and it must be possible to analyze the locus from a wide range of species using the same protocol. The cytochrome *b* gene on the mitochondrial genome has been found to successfully meet all the above criteria.

The cytochrome *b* gene is part of a complex of genes involved with oxidative phosphorylation *(1)*. The complete DNA sequence of this gene has been determined for a wide number of animal species *(2–6)* and has been found to exhibit sufficient interspecies polymorphisms with few intraspecies polymorphisms. The complete cytochrome *b* gene is approximately 1140 bp. It may not always be possible to amplify such a large fragment from powdered remains. The method outlined in this chapter uses a part of the gene locus that has been found to be highly informative *(7)*. The primers are designed to amplify a 486-bp product of which 402 bp are used for sequence comparison. The structure of the cytochrome *b* gene is shown in **Fig. 1**.

2. Materials

1. QIAamp DNA Mini kit.
2. L14724 (7.5 µ*M*) 5'-CGAAGCTTGATATGAAAAACCATCGTTG-3'.
3. H15149 (7.5 µ*M*) 5'AAACTGCAGCCCCTCAGAATGATATTTGTCCTCA-3'.
4. AmpliTaq Gold DNA Polymerase (Applied Biosystems, Foster City, CA; 5 U/ 0.5 µL)
5. AmpliTaq Gold PCR Buffer (Applied Biosystems; 10X).
6. dNTPs (10 m*M* each of dATP, dCTP, dGTP, and dTTP).
7. DNA Terminator Sequencing Kit (ABI PRISM™ BigDye™ Cycle Sequencing Kit, Applied Biosystems)
8. Quick Spin Columns (Boehringer-Mannheim, Mannheim, Germany).
9. Template Suppression Reagent (Applied Biosystems).
10. Thermal cycler.
11. PRISM 310 Genetic Analyzer (Applied Biosystems).
12. Vacuum evacuator.
13. MicroAmp reaction tubes .

3. Methods

3.1. PCR for Amplification of Part of the Cytochrome b Gene (see Note 3)

1. Aliquot approx 10 ng of good quality DNA into a sterile 0.2-mL tube (*see* **Note 1**).
2. Add 1 µL of each primer (final 0.15 µ*M* of each; *see* **Note 2**).
3. Add 5 µL of PCR buffer.
4. Add 5 µL dNTPs.

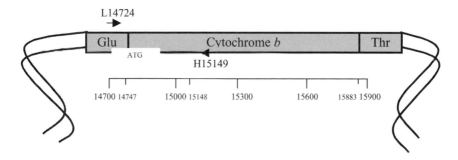

Fig. 1 The primer positions of L14724 and H15149 on mitochondrial DNA. Numbering is according to the human mtDNA sequence and primer design is according to the suggestions in refs. *1* and *2*.

5. Add 0.5 µL of AmpliTaq Gold.
6. Add water to 50 µL.
7. Amplify using the following conditions: 95°C for 11 min, followed by 35 cycles of 95°C for 45 s, 50°C for 45 s and 72°C for 90 s, followed by 72°C for 30 min (*see* **Note 4**).

3.2. Confirmation of PCR

Samples can be separated on an agarose gel to confirm the success of the amplification (**Fig. 2**). A 2% agarose gel should be cast in 1X TAE with 1 µg/mL ethidium bromide. A small size gel is normally sufficient requiring 50 mL of agarose mix. Heat the agarose in a microwave to dissolve the agarose completely and allow to cool to 55°C before casting the gel. Once the gel has solidified, run 5 µL of each sample along with a size marker for 20 min at approx 80 volts before visualizing the bands on a uv transilluminator (245 nm). The polymerase chain reaction (PCR) products should be approx 486 bp in length.

3.3. Sequencing of PCR Products

The PCR products can be directly sequenced (**Fig. 3**). Because the size is 486 bp, the complete sequence can be determined in one reaction providing that the PCR product is sufficiently pure. The method of DNA sequencing is a standard dyelabeled terminator method. A commercial kit is used (ABI PRISM™ BigDye™ Terminator) because this method has been found to be successful. The optimum amount of template DNA is approx 50 ng, although DNA concentrations of between 10 and 80 ng will still produce good quality sequence data. The primers used in the DNA sequence reaction are the same as those used in the amplification.

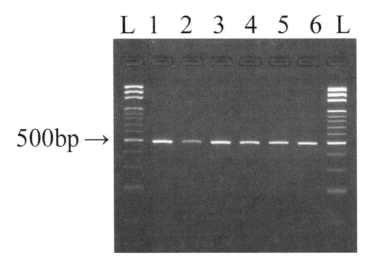

Fig. 2. An agarose image of PCR products after amplification of part of the cyto-chrome *b* gene. Lane L is the 100-bp ladder; lanes 1–6 are PCR products from human, macaque, Asian elephant, mouse, White Rhino, and pig, respectively.

The DNA sequence of both strands should be determined and compared to ensure that there are no differences as a result of the sequencing reaction.

3.3.1. Cycle Sequencing Method

1. Aliquot 10 μL of template solution containing 20 ng into two separate tubes (*see* **Note 5**).
2. Add 8 μL of sequencing reaction mix to the tube.
3. Add 2 μL of primer L14724 to one tube and primer H15149 to the other. The final concentration of each primer should be 0.25 μ*M*.
4. Seal the tubes and place on a thermal cycler
5. Perform cycle sequencing reactions using the following conditions: 96°C for 1 min, followed by 25 cycles of 96°C for 10 s, 50°C for 5 s, and 60°C for 4 min, followed by a rapid thermal ramp to 4°C and hold until ready to purify.

3.3.2. Separation of Sequenced Fragments

1. The extract from the DNA sequencing reaction must be treated to remove the unincorporated primers. A number of methods are available to do this, and most use a simple spin column.
2. Place the samples in a vacuum evacuator and allow the samples to dry (*see* **Note 6**).
3. Re-suspend the dried pellet in 25 μL of template suppression reagent.
4. The samples are now ready for separation (*see* **Note 7**).

```
                              1                                                    50
          H. sapiens 1    ......cca. .a..c...at ta....c... ......c.a. .t...c....
          H. sapiens 2    ......cca. .a..c...at ta....c... ......t.a. .t...c...
          M. cyclopis 1   ....tcca. .a..c..... .a.....a.c .......ca. .c..tc....
          M. cyclopis 2   ....ttcca. .a..c..... .a.....a.c ........a. .t..tcg...
             E. maximus   ......c... cc........ t.....c..g t.t.....c. .c.....a..
           L. africana    ......g... .......... t.....ct.. c.t.....c. .c..t..a..
       M. domesticus 1    .....a.... .a......a. a......t.. t.t........ .t...c....
       M. domesticus 2    .....a.... .a......a. a......t.. t.t........ .t...c....
             C. simum     .....t.... .c..t..... .......... ..c....... .c...c....
           D. bicornis    .....t.... .c..t..... .......... ..c....... .c..tc....
           S. scrofa 1    .......... .c........ a.......... .......... .c.....g.
           S. scrofa 2    .......... .c........ a.......... .......... .c.....g.
          B. namadicus 1  .....t.... ......g.. .......... ........g .......tg.
          B. namadicus 2  .....t.... ......g.. .......... ........g .......tg.
     C. nippon taiouanus 1 ........t. .c.....a. ......g... ........g .......g.
     C. nippon taiouanus 2 ........t. .c.....a. ......g... ........g .......g.
     M. reevesi micrucus 1 .....a..t. .c.....a. .......... ........g .......g.
     M. reevesi micrucus 2 .....a..t. .c.....a. .......... ........g .......g.
              O. aries 1  ....t..... .c.....a. .......... ........g .......g.
              O. aries 2  ....t..... .c.....a. .......... ........g .......g.
     C. crispus swinhoei 1 .......... .......a. .......... ........g ....t...g.
     C. crispus swinhoei 2 .......... .......a. .......... ........g ....t...g.
         C. familiaris 1  .......... .......a. .......... gcc......g .t..t....
         C. familiaris 2  .......... .......a. .......... gcc......g .t..t....
 M. pentadactyla Linnaeus 1 ....t.... .......a. a.....c... c.c.....cg .....g....
 M. pentadactyla Linnaeus 2 ....t.... .......a. a.....c... c.c.....cg .....g....
      P. laruata taiuana 1 .......... .......... t........c gct....... .c..tg.a..
      P. laruata taiuana 2 .......... .......... t........c gct....... .c..tg.a..
             P. tigris 1  .......... .......... a.....c..t ..c....... .t...c....
             P. tigris 2  .......... .......... a.....c..t ..c....... .t...c....
 F. bengalensis chinensis 1 ........ .......... a.....c..t ..c.....c. .c...c....
 F. bengalensis chinensis 2 ........ .......... a.....c..t ..c.....c. .c...c....
             F. catus 1   .......... .......... a.....c..t ..c....... .t..tc....
             F. catus 2   .......... .......... a.....c..t ..c....... .t..tc....
             Consensus    ATGACCAACA TTCGAAAATC CCACCCACTA ATAAAAATTA TAAACAACTC
```

Fig. 3. Alignment of the first 50 bp of the PCR products from the cytochrome *b* gene from 19 different mammalian species. The sequence alignment was by the PileUp program of the GCG computer package and the consensus sequence was determined using the Pretty program. "." indicates the same base as the consensus sequence.

3.4. Analysis of Results

1. The size of the sequence products should be 486 bp (*see* **Note 8**).
2. Remove the primer sequences on either end of the sequence data.
3. Remove sequence from the 5' end of the L14724 primer to mitochondrial position 14746 so that the sequence starts at the start of the cytochrome *b* gene (position 14747; *see* **Note 9**). This should result in sequence lengths of 402 bp if the original product was 486 bp.
4. Align the sequence data from each of the two primers used to determine a consensus DNA sequence for the gene sequence. The two DNA sequences should not show significant differences.
5. Export the consensus DNA sequence data to the GCG Computer Package (*see* **Note 10**).

4. Notes

1. DNA should be extracted, purified, and quantified using a standard method. The use of chelating agents such as Chelex® is simple and safe but will not always produce DNA that is free from inhibitors. QIAamp (Qiagene) is a proven method for extracting DNA from a wide range of tissue types. DNA also can be extracted from bone using the salt chloroform method *(8)*. A control DNA can be used at the same time as unknown DNA. A good control DNA is from a domestic or farmed animal unlikely to be the same species as the unknown. Cow (*Bos namadicus*) or mouse (*Mus domesticus*) DNA is ideal and normally available.

2. The primers used in this method amplify a 486-bp fragment. This primer set has been found to be useful in the amplification of products from highly degraded samples. The full cytochrome *b* gene locus can be amplified from good quality samples using the primer sets described in ref. *1*.

3. If more than three samples are being prepared, it is better to create a master mix. For each sample, add 1.1 µL of each primer, 5.5 µL of buffer, 5.5 µL of dNTPs, 0.5 µL of enzyme, and make with a marginal excess of dH_2O to a volume of 50 µL per sample. Aliquot the appropriate volume into separate tubes then add 10 ng of template DNA.

4. The cycling parameters have been specified using the Applied Biosystems 9600. It is possible that the parameters will need to be altered if another thermalcycler is used.

5. The quantity of DNA template required to generate optimal sequence data is 50 ng. This should be diluted into a volume of 10 µL. Adequate sequence data can be obtained from concentrations as low as 20 ng and as high as 100 ng. It is advised to dilute, or concentrate, the sample to between 20 and 100 ng in a volume of 10 µL.

6. A vacuum pump is the normal method for drying the sequence products, but if unavailable it is possible to place the open reaction tubes used to collect the purified sequence products in a heating block with water filling the holes of the heating block. Leave the heating block at 95°C to remove the fluid.

7. There are two main methods of separating sequenced DNA fragments; polyacrylamide gel electrophoresis using a 377 DNA Sequencer (Applied Biosystems), or by capillary electrophoresis using a PRISM Genetic Analyser (Applied Biosystems). The authors prefer the simplicity of capillary electrophoresis and use either the 310 or 3100 versions.

8. Most mammalian species will produce a fragment of 486 bp using the primers listed in this chapter. An exception includes Lion (*Panthera leo*) where there is a 17-base and 4-base deletion resulting in a fragment size of 464 bp.

9. The human consensus sequence starts at position 14747 with the sequence 5'-ATGACCCCAAT-3'. Edit the sequence to the 5' side of this particular DNA sequence.

10. There are alternative computer programs available, but this program has been found to be the most cited and used method for sequence comparison.

References

1. Irwin, D. M., Kocher, T. D., and Wilson A. C. (1991) Evolution of the cytochrome *b* gene of mammals. *J. Mol. Evol.* **32,** 128–144.
2. Kocher T. D., Thomas, W. K., Meyer, A., Edwards, S. V., Paabo, S., Villablanca, et al. (1989) Dynamics of mitochondrial DNA evolution in mammals: amplification and sequencing with conserved primers. *Proc. Natl. Acad. Sci USA* **86,** 6196–6200.
3. Lau, C. H., Drinkwater, R. D., Yusoff, K., Tan, S. G., Hetzel, D. J. S., and Barker J. S. F. (1998) Genetic diversity of Asian water buffalo (*Bubalus bubalis*): mitochondrial DNA D-loop and cytochrome *b* gene variation. *Anim. Genet.* **29,** 253–264.
4. Cook C. E., Wang, Y., and Sensabaugh G. (1999) A mitochondrial control region and cytochrome *b* phylogeny of sika deer (*Cervus nippon*) and report of tandem repeats in the control region. *Mol. Phyologenet. Evol.* **12,** 47–56.
5. Su, B., Wang, Y-W., Lan, H., Wang, W., and Zhang, Y. (1999) Phylogenetic studies of complete cytochrome *b* genes in musk deer (*Genus Moschus*) using museum samples. *Mol. Phyologenet. Evol.* **12,** 241–249.
6. Kuwayama, R., and Ozawa, T. (2000) Phylogenetic relationships among European red deer, wapiti and sika deer inferred from mitochondrial DNA sequences. *Mol. Phyologenet. Evol.* **15,** 115–123.
7. Hsieh, H-M, Chiang H-L, Tsai L-C, Lai S-Y, Huang N-E, Linacre A. M. T., et al. (2001) Cytochrome *b* gene for species identification of the conservation animals. *Foren. Sci. Int.* **122,** 7–18.
8. Mullenbach, R., Lagoda P. J. L., and Welter C. (1989). An efficient salt/chloroform extraction of DNA from blood and tissues. *Trends Genet.* **5,** 391.

5

Constructing STR Multiplex Assays

John M. Butler

Summary

Multiplex polymerase chain reaction (PCR) refers to the simultaneous amplification of multiple regions of deoxyribonucleic acid (DNA) using PCR. Commercial short tandem repeat (STR) assays that can coamplify as many as 16 different loci have become widely used in forensic DNA typing. This chapter will focus on some of the aspects of constructing robust STR multiplex assays, including careful design and quality control of PCR primers. Examples from the development of a cat STR 12plex and a human Y chromosome STR 20plex are used to illustrate the importance of various parts of the protocol. Primer design parameters and Internet-accessible resources are discussed, as are solutions to problems with residual dye artifacts that result from impure primers.

Key Words: Multiplex PCR; short tandem repeat; STR; forensic DNA; quality control; PCR primer design; primer compatibility.

1. Introduction

Short tandem repeat (STR) markers are abundant throughout most genomes and sufficiently polymorphic to serve as effective genetic markers *(1)*. Researchers in a number of fields use STRs for a variety of reasons, including gene mapping, disease diagnostics, evolutionary biology, and human identification. The ability to study multiple STR markers in parallel with multicolor fluorescence detection technologies has revolutionized the amount of information that can be collected in a timely fashion. The relatively small sizes for the tandem 2- to 6-bp repeat regions make them accessible to amplification using the polymerase chain reaction (PCR). Multiplex PCR, where multiple regions are simultaneously amplified in a single reaction, has greatly benefited forensic deoxyribonucleic acid (DNA) typing because less DNA material is required to obtain results from multiple loci. In addition, the amount of labor required to

From: *Methods in Molecular Biology, vol. 297: Forensic DNA Typing Protocols*
Edited by: A. Carracedo © Humana Press Inc., Totowa, NJ

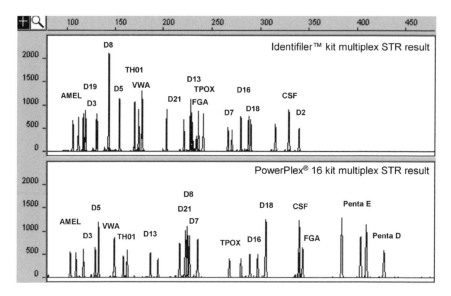

Fig. 1. Example of results from two commercial multiplex STR kits each capable of simultaneous amplification of 16 different loci. The top panel depicts Identifiler (Applied Biosystems) kit results on a DNA sample whereas the bottom panel contains PowerPlex 16 (Promega Corporation) kit results on the same sample. The loci names are listed above the corresponding peaks.

obtain results at all of the markers is reduced because loci are being typed in parallel rather than sequentially.

Commercial STR assays that can coamplify as many as 16 different loci *(2,3)* have become widely used in forensic DNA typing (**Fig. 1**). These kits have been embraced largely because they simplify sample processing, they promote uniformity across the community and enable database compatibility, and they remove the burden of reagent quality control from the individual laboratories. Although almost all forensic DNA laboratories use commercial kits, it is beneficial to understand the challenges with multiplex PCR assay development. In addition, there may be some situations where it would be helpful to have in-house assays to assess the usefulness of various markers before finalizing a set for database or casework purposes (e.g., Y-chromosome STR loci). A laboratory may have a set of markers that they are interested in examining that are of no interest or perceived commercial value to a company and thus would have little hope of being included in a commercial assay.

Several different strategies have been taken in the literature for PCR multiplex development *(4,5)*. In many cases, extensive PCR-optimization experiments are conducted with multiplex development that may seem daunting to

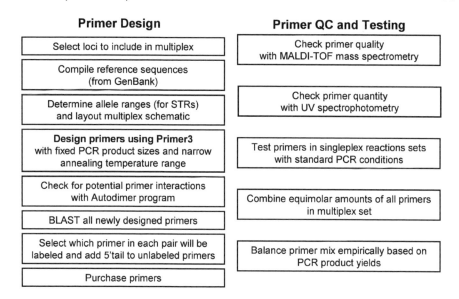

Primer Design

Select loci to include in multiplex

Compile reference sequences (from GenBank)

Determine allele ranges (for STRs) and layout multiplex schematic

Design primers using Primer3 with fixed PCR product sizes and narrow annealing temperature range

Check for potential primer interactions with Autodimer program

BLAST all newly designed primers

Select which primer in each pair will be labeled and add 5'tail to unlabeled primers

Purchase primers

Primer QC and Testing

Check primer quality with MALDI-TOF mass spectrometry

Check primer quantity with UV spectrophotometry

Test primers in singleplex reactions sets with standard PCR conditions

Combine equimolar amounts of all primers in multiplex set

Balance primer mix empirically based on PCR product yields

Fig. 2. Steps for development of STR multiplexes described in this chapter.

some laboratories *(5)*. Because compatible primers are the key to successful multiplex PCR, careful primer design and appropriate quality control measurements are essential to insure that the PCR primers will work under uniform PCR conditions and will not adversely interact with one another *(6–8)*. Upfront informatics plays an important role, as does empirical experimentation.

An overview of the steps used in a careful primer design and testing approach is illustrated in **Fig. 2**. Primer design can be performed with a variety of computer programs that will be described in the **Subheadings 2 and 3**. The creation of a two-dimensional plot that illustrates spatial and spectral aspects of STR allele ranges (**Fig. 3**) makes it easier to conceptualize desired PCR product sizes (*see* **Note 1**). After the purchase of dye-labeled and unlabeled PCR primers, quality control of each individual primer is performed before combining them for multiplex assay testing (*see* **Note 2**). Selecting fluorescent dye combinations can be important to ensure compatibility with detection instrumentation and to provide the smallest amount of spectral overlap and potential bleed through between dye colors (*see* **Note 3**).

The approach described here has been used to construct a Y-STR 10plex *(8)* and a cat STR 12plex *(9)* with three different dye labels and a Y-chromosome STR 20plex using four dye labels *(10,11)*. In addition, a number of multiplex single nucleotide polymorphism detection assays have been performed with this approach *(12)*. Examples from the cat STR 12plex and Y-STR 20plex will be illustrated.

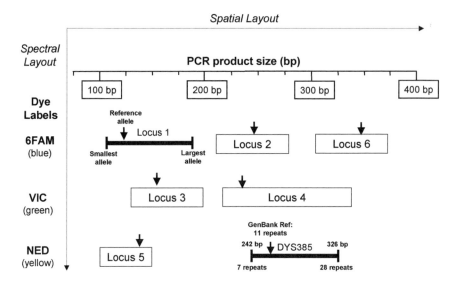

Fig. 3. Multiplex STR design layout using spatial (PCR product size) and spectral (dye label color) dimensions. PCR product size ranges for the various loci can be easily seen with this approach along with the size of the reference allele used for PCR primer design.

2. Materials

1. A number of internet-accessible computer programs and databases can be used for PCR primer design including Primer3 and GenBank. The programs used in the approach described here are listed in **Table 1**.
2. An in-house program written in Visual Basic 6.0 has been developed that can check potential primer–primer interactions in a pairwise and batch mode fashion *(6,13)*.
3. Numerous commercial sources exist for oligonucleotide synthesis. For these studies, unlabeled oligonucleotides were purchased from Qiagen Operon (Alameda, CA). Fluorescently labeled PCR primers were obtained from Applied Biosystems (Foster City, CA) with 6FAM (blue), VIC (green), NED (yellow), or PET (red) dyes attached.
4. Primers are received lyophilized. The unlabeled primers are brought to 100 μmol/ L or 200 μmol/L stocks with appropriate volumes of deionized water. The dye labeled primers are brought to 100 or 200 μmol/L concentrations with TE buffer (10 mmol/L Tris, 1 mmol/L ethylenediamine tetraacetic acid; *see* **Note 4**). The primer stocks are stored in the dark at 4°C. Frequent freeze-thaw cycles can accelerate break down of the dye attachment to the oligonucleotide.
5. The first quality control test performed is usually mass spectrometry to ensure that the primer was properly synthesized. Poor-quality primers that contain numerous synthesis by-products (e.g., **Fig. 4**) are returned to the manufacturer for resynthesis prior to proceeding with primer testing.

Table 1
Internet Sites Useful for PCR Primer Design Process

GenBank
http://www.ncbi.nlm.nih.gov/Genbank/

GenBank contains DNA sequence entries that may serve as reference sequences for primer design. A particular sequence may be located within GenBank by performing a BLAST search with a portion of the sequence for a locus, such as a published PCR primer.

Primer3
http://www-genome.wi.mit.edu/cgi-bin/primer/primer3_www.cgi

Primer3 permits rapid and flexible PCR primer design for one reference sequence at a time. A reference sequence is pasted into an Internet browser window and the user indicates primer design parameters. A set of possible primer pairs is returned over the World Wide Web in a matter of seconds. The default primer Tm values of 57–63°C generally select primers that work quite well with a PCR annealing temperature of 55°C.

BLAST
http://www.ncbi.nlm.nih.gov/BLAST/

BLAST (Basic Local Alignment Search Tool) enables a rapid search of GenBank or other DNA sequence databases to determine if similar sequences to the query are present. If the query is a PCR primer, then similar sequences could indicate possible mispriming sites. If a high amount of similarity is seen with an undesired sequence or sequences, then the PCR primer should be redesigned to avoid the potential mispriming sites that would reduce the efficiency of PCR amplification.

BLAT
http://genome.ucsc.edu/cgi-bin/hgBlat

BLAT (BLAST Like Alignment Tool) performs homology searches. BLAT on DNA sequences is designed to quickly find sequences of 95% and greater similarity of length 40 bases or more. BLAT does not work well for querying with PCR primers rather it is useful for mapping large portions of a locus into the human genome reference sequence.

BCM Search Launcher: Multiple Sequence Alignments
http://searchlauncher.bcm.tmc.edu/multi-align/multi-align.html

A user can input multiple DNA sequences in FASTA format and obtain back an alignment of those sequences. This information can be useful in evaluating multiple sequence entries from GenBank in a search for possible single nucleotide polymorphisms that may disrupt PCR primer annealing.

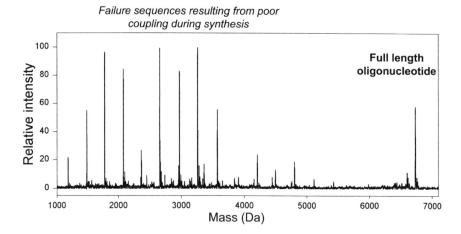

Fig. 4. Mass spectrum of a poor quality primer that contains numerous failure sequences and is therefore undesirable in a multiplex PCR reaction. This result was generated with approx 10 pmol of unpurified oligonucleotide using conditions described previously *(7)*.

6. Additional quality control tests that may be performed include ultraviolet (UV) spectrophometry at 260 nm to evaluate the quantity of the received oligonucleotide (*see* **Note 5**) and high-performance liquid chromatography (HPLC) to assess purity of labeled primers (and remove impurities from incomplete dye attachment).

7. For initial testing purposes, the forward and reverse primers for a locus are mixed at a concentration of 1 µmol/L to create singleplex and multiplex working primer solutions. Empirical adjustment of primer concentrations is later performed in an effort to balance PCR product yields.

8. Other reagents typically included in PCR (*see* **Note 6**) include a DNA polymerase (*see* **Note 7**), 250–300 µmol/L dNTPs, 1.5–5 mmol/L $MgCl_2$, 1X DNA polymerase buffer, and 0.16 mg/mL bovine serum albumin (BSA; Sigma).

9. Equipment required includes: 1) Pipet with tips capable of accurately dispensing volumes as low as 1 µL; 2) a thermal cycler, such as GeneAmp 9700 (Applied Biosystems); and 3) capillary electrophoresis instrument with multi-color detection capabilities, such as single capillary ABI 310 Genetic Analyzer or 16-capillary ABI 3100 Genetic Analyzer (Applied Biosystems).

10. Optional equipment for quality control of primers includes (*see* **Note 1**): 1) A matrix-assisted laser desorption ionization time-of-flight (MALDI-TOF) instrument, such as BIFLEX III (Bruker Daltonics); 2) a UV spectrophotometer, such as Cary 100 (Varian Instruments); and 3) HPLC, such as Varian Helix (Varian Instruments).

11. Software for STR data analysis: GeneScan/Genotyper (Applied Biosystems).

3. Methods

This section will go through the steps in multiplex PCR assay development that are illustrated in **Fig. 2**.

3.1. Primer Design

1. Select loci to include in the multiplex. It is best to select all loci up front as the assay development is being initiated. Although it is possible to add loci after earlier loci are put together, primer design options become less flexible as space on the two-dimensional assay design layout fills up.

2. Compile reference sequences and determine reference allele size (repeat number). For example, GenBank accession AC022486, which serves as the reference sequence for the DYS385 locus, contains 11 GAAA repeats (*see* **Note 8**). Performing an initial BLAST or BLAT search with a particular locus may uncover sequences entries from multiple clones in GenBank or in the human genome itself. If multiple entries are observed, sequence alignments can be helpful to create a consensus reference sequence (*see* **Note 9**).

3. Determine allele ranges for each STR locus. If extensive population studies have been performed for a particular STR locus, then full allele ranges are probably reasonably well known and PCR products from multiple loci can be placed closer together in the same dye color without fear of overlapping sizes. Typically, it is wise to leave room for one or two possible undiscovered alleles on each end of the STR locus range. This strategy would mean that the smallest allele for one tetranucleotide locus could be 10–18 bp larger than the largest allele of the neighboring locus in the same dye color.

4. Layout multiplex schematic with candidate positions for each locus (*see* **Fig. 3**). Estimate spacing between loci and calculate required size for each PCR product from its reference sequence.

5. Design primers using Primer3 with fixed PCR product sizes and narrow annealing temperature range: 1) Select desired PCR annealing temp and design primers to be approx 2–5°C above PCR annealing temperature where possible (*see* **Note 10**). Try to keep the calculated primer annealing temperatures within ±5°C. At this stage of the primer design process, do not worry about potential cross-reactions from primers used to amplify other loci. 2) Some flanking regions are less desirable than others for primer design due to palindromic sequences or long polynucleotide stretches. Those loci with unstable flanking regions usually will become the larger loci in an assay, as more flexibility is required in terms of primer placement. Likewise, STR loci with long repeat stretches will by necessity have larger PCR product sizes than loci with a smaller number of repeats.

6. Check for potential primer interactions across the various STR loci that will be included in the multiplex assay (*see* **Note 11**).

7. BLAST all newly designed primers to search for potential mispriming sites that may occur in other parts of the human genome beyond the intended target region.

8. Select a primer in each pair to be fluorescently labeled. It is often convenient to select the forward primer for each locus to maintain consistency when purchasing the primers.

9. Add a 5' tail to unlabeled primers to promote full adenylation (i.e., nontemplate addition) during PCR (*see* **Note 12**).

10. Place an order for PCR primers. Until the primer combinations have been demonstrated to work well in a multiplex format, it is advisable to purchase the smallest possible quantity of each primer in order to decrease development costs.

3.2. Primer Quality Control and Testing

1. Check primer quality with MALDI-TOF mass spectrometry.
2. Check primer quantity with UV spectrophotometer (*see* **Note 5**).
3. Mix primers in locus-specific pairs at 1 µmol/L concentration.
4. Test primer pairs in singleplex reactions with standard PCR conditions to ensure that the correct size product(s) is generated.
5. Combine equimolar amounts (e.g., 1 µmol/L) of primers in multiplex set.
6. Test initial equimolar primer mix with standard PCR conditions (*8,10*).
7. Balance primer mix empirically based on PCR product yields.
8. Test adjusted primer mix on the same quantity of multiple DNA templates to ensure consistency across samples (*see* **Notes 13** and **14**).
9. Perform sensitivity studies with serial dilutions of DNA templates.
10. Create allelic ladders with common alleles. Alternatively typing may be performed without allelic ladders using precise sizing and sequence information from a single sample (*11*).
11. Write Genotyper macro for allele calling.

4. Notes

1. The creation of spatial and spectral two-dimensional layouts (**Fig. 3**) is beneficial in examining potential PCR product sizes for the loci intended to be present in a multiplex PCR assay. Most multiplex STR assays will involve PCR products in the size range of 75–400 bp and use three different dye labels. With polymorphic STR markers, it is important to have a good idea of overall allele ranges before designing the assay to avoid putting loci too close together that are next to one another in the same dye color. Typically leaving room for one or two new alleles at each end of the expected allele range is prudent. It is also important to remember that the reference sequence allele (represented by the vertical arrows along the horizontal locus allele range bars in **Fig. 3**), which is used for primer design, only represents one of the possible alleles and could be anywhere along the expected allele range.

2. Full characterization and quality control of PCR primers involves a UV spectrophometry measurement to determine concentration, an HPLC run to evaluate purity, a MALDI-TOF mass spectrometry analysis to confirm correct sequence and purity, and a capillary electrophoresis run to determine the level of residual dye artifacts ("dye blobs"). Dye artifacts are only a problem with capillary elec-

trophoresis systems as they are co-injected during electrokinetic injection. Dye artifacts originating from impure primers usually have minimal impact on DNA separations in gel systems.

3. A number of fluorescent dye combination choices exist. Selection of dye labels used in a multiplex PCR assay impacts vendor options. Publicly available dyes such as fluorescein and tetramethyl rhodamine are less expensive and more widely available. However, they may not work as well as proprietary fluorescent dye labels in terms of brightness and spectral resolution. In our laboratory, we have chosen to use Applied Biosystems dyes as they work best with the ABI instruments we have in terms of color separation and sensitivity. Thus, our multiplexes contain 6FAM (blue), VIC (green), NED (yellow), and PET (red) for dye labels. Regardless of which dye combinations are selected for a multiplex assay, it is essential to use an appropriate color separation matrix to avoid pull-up between dye colors.

4. Storage of dye labeled primers in a slightly basic solution, such as TE at pH 8.0, rather than deionized water, which is typically pH 5.0, can reduce degradation of the primer. If resuspended at pH < 7.0, the fluorescent dye molecular can begin to degrade more rapidly and give rise to more residual dye artifacts ("blobs").

5. A concentration determination of PCR primers using a UV spectrophotometer in one's own laboratory may reveal that oligonucleotides are not always quantified uniformly within and between manufacturers. If primers are being purchased from multiple vendors, then conducting a UV spectrometer quantification check in one's own laboratory is useful in order to properly match primer pair concentrations. A UV spectrometer check will also help maintain consistency if multiple batches of a primer are used over time. Maintaining consistent relative primer concentrations is especially important with multiplex PCR assays where a dozen or more primers are expected to work together in a single tube at empirically defined concentrations.

6. PCR volumes tested with multiplexes constructed in our laboratory have ranged from 5 to 25 μL. Tubes or trays used in thermal cycling must be well sealed for low volume reactions to prevent any evaporation. The rubber gasket supplied with GeneAmp 9700 cyclers for 96-well plates works well.

7. A hot start enzyme like AmpliTaq Gold DNA Polymerase (Applied Biosystems) that activates at a high temperature is beneficial with multiplex PCR as it minimizes extension from primer-primer interactions that can form at lower temperatures than the assay annealing temperature and produce competing primer dimers.

8. Sequence entries in GenBank are often from the complementary strand. Thus, these reference sequences need to be made reverse and complement (r&c) in order to conform to familiar STR repeat and primer position nomenclatures. For example, the GenBank accession AC022486 for DYS385 contains 11 TTTC repeats that can be converted to the more familiar GAAA repeat structure reported by Schneider et al. *(14)*.

9. A consensus reference sequence can be created by aligning multiple GenBank entries in an effort to identify possible primer binding site polymorphisms

between the various STR alleles reported in GenBank. Alignments may be performed via the BCM Search Launcher program (**Table 1**) once candidate reference sequences have been put into a FASTA format. Sequence differences in flanking regions around the STR repeat can be flagged as possible polymorphisms and these regions should be avoided during primer design.

10. Although it is usually best to have primers with calculated annealing temperatures above the PCR annealing temperature, this is not always necessary. Sometimes it is not possible to design a primer with a higher melting temperature (Tm) because of the lack of available sequence information or sequence issues (e.g., palindromes or polynucleotide stretches). For example, in the cat STR 12plex, one of the primers has a calculated Tm of 50°C because of limited sequence information yet it works fine with a PCR annealing temperature of 59°C (data not shown). Thus, a lower than desired primer Tm does not mean that the primer pair will not work well in a multiplex PCR environment and empirical testing is always required to prove the value of each primer.

11. A computer program has been written within our group at NIST that enables automated screening of potential primer–primer interactions via batch analysis. This Autodimer program has been written in Visual Basic and described in previous publications (*6,8*). It is publicly available through the STRBase web site (http://www.cstl.nist.gov/biotech/strbase).

12. Use of a single G or a 7-base tail GTGTCTT on the 5' end of the unlabeled primer within a locus-specific primer pair can promote full adenylation of PCR products amplified from that locus. **Figure 5** demonstrates how the partially adenylated doublet peaks for a STR locus from a heterozygous individual are converted to fully adenylated ones using the 7-base tail with identical PCR conditions.

13. Residual dye molecules exist for most fluorescent dye labeled primers that have not been extensively purified or stored properly (*see* **Note 4**). These dye blobs can interfere with allele calls in some size ranges but can be removed with Edge Bioscience spin columns after PCR amplification (*15*), as shown in **Fig. 6**.

14. The addition of bovine serum albumin (BSA) improves PCR amplification in multiplex reactions as shown in **Fig. 7**, most likely because BSA helps reduce inhibition of the polymerase by the residual dye molecules present from the multiple primers in the PCR reaction.

Acknowledgments

This multiplex PCR assay design process has been made easier with the development of an autodimer program, written by Dr. Peter Vallone in our laboratory, to screen for potential primer–primer interactions. The work of Richard Schoske on the Y-STR multiplexes and Margaret Kline for the PowerPlex 16 and Identifiler data also is gratefully acknowledged. Certain commercial equipment, instruments, and materials are identified to specify experimental procedures as completely as possible. In no case does such identification imply a recommendation or endorsement by the National Institute of

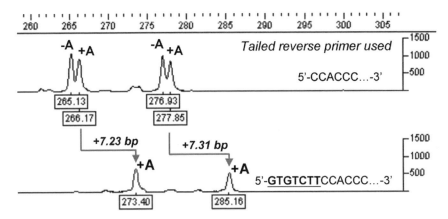

Fig. 5. Full adenylation improves with the addition of a 5' tail to the unlabeled primer. In the top panel, both alleles at this heterozygous locus exhibit doublets from -A and +A peaks that are approx 1 bp apart. The bottom panel shows the same DNA sample amplified at the same locus with 5'-tailed primers that promote full adenylation of both alleles. The PCR product sizes for this STR locus are approx 7 bp larger with the 7-base GTGTCTT 5'-tail in the bottom panel.

Standards and Technology nor does it imply that any of the materials, instruments or equipment identified are necessarily the best available for the purpose. This work was funded in part by the National Institute of Justice through an interagency agreement with the NIST Office of Law Enforcement Standards.

References

1. Butler, J. M. (2001) *Forensic DNA Typing: Biology and Technology behinds STR Markers.* Academic Press, London.
2. Krenke, B. E., Tereba, A., Anderson, S. J., Buel, E., Culhane, S., Finis, C. J., et al. (2002) Validation of a 16-locus fluorescent multiplex system. *J. Forensic Sci.* **47,** 773–785.
3. Applied Biosystems (2001) AmpFlSTR Identifiler PCR Amplification Kit User's Manual, Foster City, CA, P/N 4323291.
4. Shuber, A. P., Grondin, V. J., and Klinger, K. W. (1995) A simplified procedure for developing multiplex PCRs. *Genome Res.* **5,** 488–493.
5. Henegariu, O., Heerema, N. A., Dlouhy, S. R., Vance, G. H., and Vogt, P. H. (1997) Multiplex PCR: critical parameters and step-by-step protocol. *BioTechniques* **23,** 504–511.
6. Butler, J. M., Ruitberg, C. M., and Vallone, P. M. (2001) Capillary electrophoresis as a tool for optimization of multiplex PCR reactions. *Fresenius J. Anal. Chem.* **369,** 200–205.

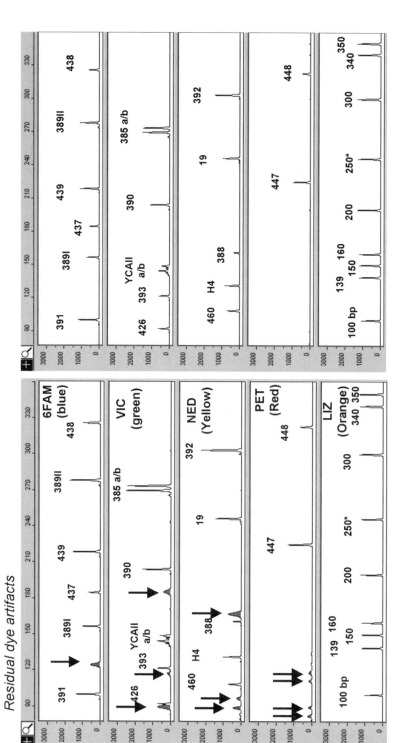

Fig. 6. Residual dye removal with Edge spin columns (*see ref. 13*). Arrows in the left panel indicate positions of dye blobs that exist for each primer dye label used in the NIST Y-STR 20plex assay (*10*). The right panel shows the same PCR product after purification with an Edge column.

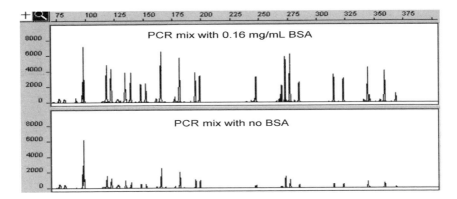

Fig. 7. Benefits of BSA addition to cat STR 12plex assay *(9)*. DNA sample concentration and PCR components are identical between the two panels except that the top panel contains 0.16 mg/mL BSA.

7. Butler, J. M., Devaney, J. M., Marino, M. A., and Vallone, P. M. (2001) Quality control of PCR primers used in multiplex STR amplifications. *Forensic Sci. Int.* **119,** 87–96.
8. Schoske, R., Vallone, P. M., Ruitberg, C. M., and Butler, J. M. (2003) Multiplex PCR design strategy used for the simultaneous amplification of 10 Y chromosome short tandem repeat (STR) loci. *Anal. Bioanal. Chem.* **375,** 333–343.
9. Butler, J. M., David, V. A., O'Brien, S. J., and Menotti-Raymond, M. (2002) The MeowPlex: a new DNA test using tetranucleotide STR markers for the domestic cat. *Profiles in DNA*, Promega Corporation, Volume 5, No. 2, pp. 7–10. Available at: http://www.promega.com/profiles/502/ProfilesInDNA_502_07.pdf; accessed 18 May 2004.
10. Butler, J. M., Schoske, R., Vallone, P. M., Kline, M. C., Redd, A. J., and Hammer, M. F. (2002) A novel multiplex for simultaneous amplification of 20 Y chromosome STR markers. *Forensic Sci. Int.* **129,** 10–24.
11. Schoske, R. (2003) The design, optimization and testing of Y chromosome short tandem repeat megaplexes. PhD dissertation, American University.
12. Vallone, P. M. and Butler, J. M. (2004) Y-SNP typing of U.S. African American and Caucasean samples using allele-specific hybridization and primer extension. *J. Forensic Sci.* **49,** 723–732.
13. Vallone, P. M. and Butler, J. M. (2004) AutoDimer: a screening tool for primer–dimer and hairpin structures. *Biotechniques*, in press.
14. Schneider, P. M., Meuser, S., Waiyawuth, W., Seo, Y., and Rittner, C. (1998) Tandem repeat structure of the duplicated Y-chromosomal STR locus DYS385 and frequency studies in the German and three Asian populations. *Forensic Sci. Int.* **97,** 61–70.
15. Butler, J. M., Shen, Y., and McCord, B. R. (2003) The development of reduced size STR amplicons as tools for analysis of degraded DNA. *J. Forensic Sci.* **48,** 1054–1064.

6

Y Chromosome STR Typing

Leonor Gusmão and Cíntia Alves

Summary

Because of their unique transmission properties and male specificity, markers located on the nonrecombining region of the Y chromosome (NRY) have become an important tool in forensic investigation. In the past few years, more than 50 polymorphic Y chromosome-specific short tandem repeats (STRs) have been described and a set of 9 loci were selected, considered as the minimal haplotype included in the forensic databases, Y-STR Haplotype Reference Databases, the largest now available online (http://www.yhrd.org). Here, we describe a multiplex amplification strategy developed for ABI platforms to amplify the nine loci included in the minimal haplotype (DYS19, DYS385a/b, DYS389I, DYS389II, DYS390, DYS391, DYS392, DYS393) as well as a second set of markers (DYS437, DYS438, DYS439, DYS460, DYS461, GATA A10, GATA C4, and GATA H4) used to improve the minimal haplotype diversity and, hence, the discrimination power. Together, these 17 Y-STRs can be used to define highly discriminative haplotypes, providing a powerful tool in male lineage identification.

Key Words: Y chromosome STRs; Multiplex PCR; DYS19; DYS385; DYS389I; DYS389II; DYS390; DYS391; DYS392; DYS393; DYS437; DYS438; DYS439; DYS460; DYS461; GATA A10; GATA C4; GATA H4.

1. Introduction

Because of their levels of diversity and typing simplicity, the short tandem repears (STRs) are the most used markers in the forensics field. In particular, they can be studied using very simple and reliable polymerase chain reaction (PCR) techniques, and they can be typed in low quantity or degraded deoxyribonucleic acid (DNA) samples.

Y chromosome-specific markers, located on the nonrecombining portion, or NRY, are transmitted from father to son unchanged (unless a mutation occurs) and, therefore, can be used to construct highly informative haplotypes. Through

From: *Methods in Molecular Biology, vol. 297: Forensic DNA Typing Protocols*
Edited by: A. Carracedo © Humana Press Inc., Totowa, NJ

the years, Y-STRs have become particularly useful in forensic DNA analysis, paternity testing, and in male-lineage studies.

1.1. Y Chromosome-Specific STRs in Forensic Applications

Y-STR analysis is particularly useful for the discrimination of stains in a forensic investigation when a male suspect is involved. This is the case in most violent crimes, including sexual offences. Mixtures of body fluids from different individuals are frequent in forensic casework, and the Y chromosome analysis can be particularly helpful in detecting a male DNA fraction in stains involving male/female mixtures. With Y-specific analysis, only the male component is detected, and this allows a direct determination of the Y haplotype without the need for differential extraction *(1–3)*.

The use of Y-STR markers in paternity cases is limited to those situations in which a male descendent is in question. However, a result based exclusively on Y-chromosome STRs does not exclude as father any relative male in the same patrilineage. The possibility of using Y-STR markers is especially important in deficiency cases. In these situations, namely when the alleged father is deceased, it is possible to access his complete Y chromosome information using, as a test, any relative male in the patrilineage.

1.2. Y Chromosome-Specific STR Loci

From the Y chromosome polymorphic STRs described until now, DYS19, DYS385, DYS389I, DYS389II, DYS390, DYS391, DYS392, DYS393, and YCAII are those from which more data have been accumulated, being the most used in forensic genetics. With the help of collaborative efforts made in the construction of large databases (www.yhrd.org), these markers are the best studied for amplification performance and specificity, multiplex amplification strategies, sequence structure, and nomenclature, as well as worldwide allele-frequency distributions. DYS434, DYS435, DYS436, DYS437, DYS438, DYS439, DYS460, DYS461, GATA A10, GATA C4, and GATA H4 were reported by Ayub et al. *(4)* and White et al. *(5)*, and, although they are not so widely used in the forensic field as the previous, some sequencing, population distribution and multiplex amplification data have started to accumulate. More Y-STRs were recently described *(6–9)*, and many more are expected to be published in the near future.

The application of Y chromosome markers in forensic investigations requires the selection of polymorphic loci, the study of parameters of forensic interest (including amplification performance and specificity, sequence variation and nomenclature and determination of mutation rates), the development of typing methods to improve amplification of low quantity and degraded samples, as well as the construction of large databases.

1.3. PCR Performance and Specificity

The inclusion of Y STRs in forensic routine requires previous studies concerning PCR performance and Y specificity. The PCR amplification of an STR can be, in some cases, improved by the redesign of previously described primers to reduce nonspecific amplification or to reduce the size of the amplified fragments, as the case of DYS389 *(10)* and DYS385 primers *(11)*. Y-chromosome specificity can be tested with the amplification of female DNA, acting as negative amplification controls. An example of non-Y specificity is the amplification of female DNA samples when using the first described primers for DYS391 *(12)* and DYS393 *(13)*. The screening of point mutations in the flanking regions of the STRs currently used in forensics is important to avoid null alleles by primer mismatching. Point mutations have been described in the flanking regions of DYS391, DYS437, and DYS438 *(14)*.

1.4. Y-STR Nomenclature

The use of a consensus nomenclature is crucial to allow for second opinions, proficiency testing, exchange of data, and databasing. Although for some STRs, with simple repeat structure, it is easy to find a consensus nomenclature, for others, with a complex structure, it becomes more difficult. For example, for the first described STRs, nomenclature changes were made for DYS19, DYS390, and DYS389 to include nonrepetitive motives or motives that were found to be variable with the accumulation of new sequence data. To prevent nomenclature changes, according to the International Society of Forensic Genetics guidelines "alleles should be named taking into account both variant and nonvariant repeats" *(15)*. However, the use of recently described STRs introduced additional nomenclature problems and, although only a few population studies were so far published for these STRs, for some of them different nomenclatures are being used *(16)*.

1.5. Population Genetics and Databasing

The use of Y STRs as inclusion evidence involves the definition of population genetic profiles, with the elaboration of a large number of population databases. The construction of Y-specific STR databases is more complex than those for unlinked autosomal markers because the informative content of Y-specific STRs results from the possibility of constructing highly discriminative haplotypes. The suitability of the Y-STR databases for practical use in the forensics field will be greatly increased with the typing of each individual to as many loci as possible instead of typing a great number of individuals for a small number of Y-STRs *(17)*.

The development of Y-STR haplotype reference databases is important, not only for haplotype frequency estimation and subsequent application for match probability calculations in forensic studies, but also for performing comparative population analysis.

1.6. Y-STR Multiplex Amplification

Multiplex amplification techniques can be used to increase the information content of the Y-STR haplotype typing approach and also to reduce the need for large sample quantities in forensic cases *(18)*. A great effort was made by some groups to develop STR multiplex systems including a large number of markers *(8,9,19–21)*.

There are already some multiplex systems commercially available, namely, from Reliagene (Y-PLEX™ 6 enables simultaneous amplification of DYS393, DYS19, DYS389II, DYS390, DYS391, and DYS385; Y-PLEX™ 5 amplifies DYS389I, DYS389II, DYS439, DYS438, and DYS392; and Y-PLEX™ 12 amplifies all loci in Y-PLEX™ 6 and Y-PLEX™ 5 plus the Amelogenin locus) and from Promega Corporation (PowerPlex® Y System enables simultaneous amplification of DYS19, DYS385, DYS389I, DYS389II, DYS390, DYS391, DYS392, DYS393, DYS437, DYS438, and DYS439).

Two multiplex PCR-amplification methods are here described that allow the typing of 17 polymorphic Y chromosome-specific STRs. The first multiplex (YSTRM1) was optimized to efficiently amplify, in the same PCR, the nine Y-STR loci: DYS19; DYS385a/b; DYS389I; DYS389II; DYS390; DYS391; DYS392; DYS393 (minimal haplotype). A second multiplex (YSTRM2) allows the simultaneous amplification of eight additional Y-STR loci: DYS437; DYS438; DYS439; DYS460; DYS461; GATA A10; GATA C4; and GATA H4.

2. Materials

1. PCR reagents: deoxynucleotide triphosphate solution (dNTPs, a mixture of dATP, dCTP, dGTP, and dTTP in the same concentration); magnesium chloride ($MgCl_2$); AmpliTaq Gold® DNA polymerase and Gold buffer (AB Applied Biosystems); labeled and nonlabeled oligonucleotide primers (primer sequences and labels are described in **Subheading 3**). The amplification reagents should be stored at –20°C. The labeled primer solutions are sensitive to light and must be stored in the dark.
2. Analysis of the amplified product can be performed in an ABI PRISM® 310 Genetic Analyser. The following material is required (according to the instrument manufacturer's instructions): sample tubes and septa (AB Applied Biosystems, Foster City, CA); TAMRA 500 internal size standard (AB Applied Biosystems); dry heating block or thermal cycler; 310 capillaries, 47 cm × 50 μm (AB Applied Biosystems); Performance Optimizer Polymer 4, POP-4 (AB Applied Biosystems); deionized formamide; and ice.

To prevent cross-contaminations, it is recommended one use disposable gloves and aerosol-resistant pipet tips. Pre- and post-PCR samples, reagents, and instruments should be used and stored separately. Formamide is potentially hazard (irritant and teratogen) and should be handled accordingly.

3. Methods

PCR amplification protocols were optimized in a PCR System 2400 Thermal Cycler (AB Applied Biosystems) and detection tested on an ABI PRISM® 310 Genetic Analyser. Protocols may need to be optimized for different instruments.

3.1. Loci Information

The loci included in the YSTRM1 multiplex are the better-studied Y chromosome-specific STR markers and, until now, the were most used in the forensics field. Together, these nine loci represent the so-called "minimal haplotype" included in the Y-STR Haplotype Reference Databases (YHRDs), the largest forensic databases available online (available at: http://www.yhrd.org). The 8 loci included in the YSTRM2 multiplex are the most polymorphic loci of the 12 described by Ayub et al. *(4)* and White et al. *(5)*.

The GenBank accession numbers, repeat motifs, size of PCR products, and the subsequent repeat units for the Y-STR loci amplified with YSTRM1 and YSTRM2 primers are summarized in **Table 1**.

DYS392 is a trinucleotide repeat, DYS438 is a pentanucleotide repeat, and the remaining loci are tetranucleotide repeats. Both DYS389 and DYS385 primers amplify two loci. Because the annealing site of the DYS389 forward primer is duplicated, two different size PCR fragments are amplified; the largest fragment (DYS389 II) includes the smaller one (DYS389 I), both of which are polymorphic. The DYS385 primers amplify a tetranucleotide repeat sequence that is duplicated on the Y chromosome and the two PCR-amplified fragments are in the same size range and cannot be assigned to either of the two loci. Therefore, data concerning this marker are always reported as allele classes defined by the combination of both loci alleles.

Although not widespread in forensics, because of the low increase in haplotype diversity, amplification strategies have already been described for the separate amplification of both alleles at DYS389 (http://www.medfac.leiden univ.nl/fldo) and DYS385 loci *(22)*.

In the same way as for DYS434 and DYS437 *(19)*, DYS460 is adjacent to DYS461 and, therefore, when these two STRs are amplified together a third fragment is amplified by DYS460 forward and DYS461 reverse primers, including both loci (**Fig. 1**).

Table 1
Y-STR Consensus Structure, GenBank Accession Numbers, and Allele Ranges

Marker	GenBank accession no.	Repeat motif	Allele size[a]	Allele range
DYS19 (DYS394)	X77751	$(TAGA)_3TAGG(TAGA)_n$	143–179	10–19
DYS385	Z93950	$(AAGG)_{6-7}(GAAA)_n$	240–312,324	7–25, 28
DYS389 I	G09600	$(TCTG)_3(TCTA)_n$	235–267	9–17
DYS389 II	G09600	$(TCTG)_n(TCTA)_n N_{28}(TCTG)_3(TCTA)_n$	343–387	23–34
DYS390	G09611	$(TCTG)_n(TCTA)_n(TCTG)_{0-1}(TCTA)_{0-4}$	188–232	17–28
DYS391	G09613	$(TCTG)_3(TCTA)_n$	128–160	6–14
DYS392	G09867	$(TAT)_n$	181–217	6–18
DYS393	G09601	$(AGAT)_n$	104–140	8–17
DYS437	AC002992	$(TCTA)_m(TCTG)_n(TCTA)_4$	180–196	13–17
DYS438	AC002531	$(TTTTC)_1(TTTTA)_{0,1}(TTTTC)_n$	201–241	6–14
DYS439	AC002992	$(GATA)_n$	232–260	8–15
DYS460 (GATA A7.1)	G42675	$(ATAG)_n$	105–133	6–13
DYS461 (GATA A7.2)	G42671	$(TAGA)_n(CAGA)_1$	144–172	8–15
GATA A10	G42674	$(TCCA)_2(TATC)_n$	150–178	11–18
GATA C4	G42673	$(TCTA)_2[(TCTA)_2(TGTA)_2]_{2,3}(TCTA)_n$	238, 246–274	17,19–26
GATA H4	G42676	$(AGAT)_4CTAT(AGAT)_2(AGGT)_3(AGAT)_n N_{24}$ $(ATAG)_4(ATAC)_1(ATAG)_2$	268–292	24–30

The allele sizes are those obtained when using the primers described in this work. In bold are the segments that are not included in the allele nomenclature.

[a]These sizes are the real size of the alleles obtained by sequence analysis.

DYS460 Forward Primer-caagaagaat tatctaggaa agtcaagaca gtagcaagca caagaatacc

agaggaatct gacacctctg ac(atag)$_n$ ataatagaca aataca<u>taat aaatgat</u>*agg cagaggatag*

*atgatatgga t*agacagata tatctaatag gtagatgata gataataggt agatagaaga tagg(taga)$_n$(caga)$_1$

taagagagaa acagaaatat agtgacacag ca-**DYS461 Reverse Primer**

Fig. 1. DYS460 and DYS461 sequences and annealing sites. DYS460 reverse primer annealing sequence is underlined and DYS461 forward primer annealing sequence is in grey italic.

3.2. PCR Amplification

Different technical methods were investigated with the aim of developing the two multiplex amplification systems for the simultaneous amplification of YSTRM1 and YSTRM2 loci.

The best YSTRM1 amplification results were obtained when using between 1 and 10 ng of male template DNA in a 25-µL reaction volume containing 2 mM MgCl$_2$, 200 µM of each dNTP, 1X Gold Buffer (AB Applied Biosystems) and 1 Unit of AmpliTaq Gold® DNA polymerase (AB Applied Biosystems).

The best YSTRM2 amplification results were obtained when using between 1 and 10 ng of male template DNA in a 25-µL reaction volume containing 1.5 mM MgCl$_2$, 200 µM of each dNTP, 1X Gold Buffer (AB Applied Biosystems) and 1 Unit of AmpliTaq Gold® DNA polymerase (AB Applied Biosystems).

3.2.1. Primer Mix Setup

Primer sequences and labels are given in **Table 2**. For those systems with overlapping allele size ranges, amplified in the same multiplex, the primers were labeled with different dyes (see allele size ranges in **Table 1**) to allow for unambiguous typing of all the markers (**Fig. 2**).

Various primer concentrations were tested and the best co-amplification results were obtained when using the concentrations indicated in **Table 3**. A primer mix can be prepared for a large number of reactions (**Table 3**) and stored at –20°C until needed to set up a PCR. This has the advantage of reducing pipetting errors for small volumes and allows better homogeneity between samples.

3.2.2. Amplification Procedure

To set up the amplification, prepare a PCR master mix for all samples by determining the number of reactions and adding one or two reactions to this

Table 2
Primer Sequences, References, and Labels

Primers	Label	Primer sequence (5'–3')	Ref.
YSTRM1			
DYS19-F	6-FAM	CTA CTG AGT TTC TGT TAT AGT	*21*
DYS19-R		GGG TTA AGG AGA GTG TCA CT A	
DYS385-F	HEX	AGC ATG GGT GAC AGA GCT A	*10*
DYS385-R		CCA ATT ACA TAG TCC TCC TTT C	
DYS389 -F	TET	CCA ACT CTC ATC TGT ATT ATC TAT	*23*
DYS389-R		TCT TAT CTC CAC CCA CCA GA	
DYS390-F	6-FAM	TAT ATT TTA CAC ATT TTT GGG CC	*23*
DYS390-R		TGA CAG TAA AAT GAA CAC ATT GC	
DYS391-F	TET	CTA TTC ATT CAA TCA TAC ACC CA	*12*
DYS391-R		CTG GGA ATA AAA TCT CCC TGG TTG CAA G	
DYS392-F	HEX	AAA AGC CAA GAA GGA AAA CAA A	*21*
DYS392-R		AGA CCC AGT TGA TGC AAT GT	
DYS393-F	HEX	GTG GTC TTC TAC TTG TGT CAA TAC	*23*
DYS393-R		AAC TCA AGT CCA AAA AAT GAG G	
YSTRM2			
DYS437-F	TET	GAC TAT GGG CGT GAG TGC AT	*4*
DYS437-R		AGA CCC TGT CAT TCA CAG ATG A	
DYS438-F	6-FAM	TGG GGA ATA GTT GAA CGG TAA	*4*
DYS438-R		GTG GCA GAC GCC TAT AAT CC	
DYS439-F	TET	TCC TGA ATG GTA CTT CCT AGG TTT	*4*
DYS439-R		GCC TGG CTT GGA ATT CTT TT	
DYS460-F	6-FAM	AGC AAG CAC AAG AAT ACC AGA G	*21*
DYS460-R		TCT ATC CTC TGC CTA TCA TTT ATT A	
DYS461-F	TET	AGG CAG AGG ATA GAT GAT ATG GAT	*21*
DYS461-R		TGA TGC TGT GTC ACT ATA TTT CTG	
GATA A10-F	HEX	CCT GCC ATC TCT ATT TAT CTT GCA TAT A	*5*
GATA A10-R		ATA AAT GGA GAT AGT GGG TGG ATT	
GATA C4-F	HEX	AGT GTC TCA CTT CAA GCA CCA AGC AC	*5*
GATA C4-R		GCA GCA AAA TTC ACA GTT GGA AAA ATG T	
GATA H4-F	TET	GTT ATG CTG AGG AGA ATT TCC AA	*21*
GATA H4-R		CCT CTG ATG GTG AAG TAA TGG AAT TAG A	

number to compensate for pipetting errors. In **Table 4**, volumes are indicated for all the PCR reagents per reaction according to the stock concentration. If stock solutions with different concentrations are used, the volumes must be adjusted to keep the same concentration of the reagents in the final reaction solution. Buffer and $MgCl_2$ volumes are indicated for a buffer without $MgCl_2$.

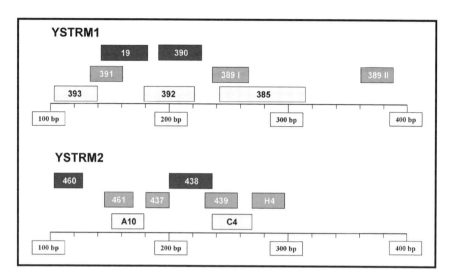

Fig. 2. YSTRM1 and YSTRM2 allele size ranges and labels.

If the buffer already contains $MgCl_2$ (usually at a concentration of 15 mM), the volume must be adjusted to reach a final concentration of 2 mM (YSTRM1) or 1.5 mM (YSTRM2). Note that the total reaction volume should be 25 μL and that changes in any reagent volume (primer mix, $MgCl_2$, AmpliTaq Gold, or Template DNA) should be compensated by changing the volume of water. The inclusion of a "negative control" (PCR mix plus water instead of DNA template) is important for detection of possible PCR contamination by external DNA.

3.2.3. Thermal Cycling Conditions

The thermal cycling conditions were optimized in a GeneAmp PCR system 2400 thermocycler (AB Applied Biosystems). The use of other instruments may require some adjustments on denaturing, annealing, and extension steps. The number of cycles can be also adjusted for different input DNA. In forensic DNA samples, it is not recommended to increase the total number of cycles for more than 35–40 cycles.

YSTRM1 thermal cycling conditions are preincubation for 11 min at 95°C and 1 min at 96°C; followed by 10 cycles of 30 s at 94°C, 30 s at 58°C, 45 s at 70°C (ramp 23%); plus 22 cycles of 30 s at 90°C, 30 s at 56°C, 45 s at 70°C (ramp 23%); and a final incubation step of 60°C for 60 min.

YSTRM2 thermal cycling conditions are preincubation for 11 min at 95°C and 1 min at 96°C; followed by 10 cycles of 30 s at 94°C, 30 s at 60°C, 45 s at

Table 3
Primer Concentrations and Preparation of the PCR Primer Mix.

Primers	Final concentration in PCR	Volume in 25-μL PCR mix	Primer mix (100 reactions)
YSTRM1			
DYS19	0.5 μ*M*	2.5 μL	250 μL
DYS385	0.25 μ*M*	1.25 μL	125 μL
DYS389	0.19 μ*M*	0.95 μL	95 μL
DYS390	0.2 μ*M*	1 μL	100 μL
DYS391	0.036 μ*M*	0.18 μL	18 μL
DYS392	0.27 μ*M*	1.35 μL	135 μL
DYS393	0.024 μ*M*	0.12 μL	12 μL
YSTRM2			
DYS437	0.04 μ*M*	0.2 μL	20 μL
DYS438	0.8 μ*M*	4 μL	400 μL
DYS439	0.2 μ*M*	1 μL	100 μL
DYS460	0.22 μ*M*	1.1 μL	110 μL
DYS461	0.12 μ*M*	0.6 μL	60 μL
GATA A10	0.12 μ*M*	0.6 μL	60 μL
GATA C4	0.12 μ*M*	0.6 μL	60 μL
GATA H4	0.18 μ*M*	0.9 μL	90 μL

The primer volumes were calculated for primer stock solutions with a 5 m*M* concentration

Note: The primer pair mixture and all the labeled primer solutions are light sensitive and must be stored in the dark.

70°C (ramp 23%); plus 22 cycles of 30 s at 90°C, 30 s at 58°C, 45 s at 70°C (ramp 23%); and a final incubation step of 60°C for 60 min.

3.3. Analysis of Amplified Fragments

The detection analysis used for both multiplexes was optimized on an ABI PRISM® 310 Genetic Analyser (AB Applied Biosystems). The results obtained for both multiplexes are displayed in **Fig. 3** (YSTRM1) and **Fig. 4** (YSTRM2). When using other ABI platforms for YSTRM1 and YSTRM2 analysis, use the instrument's user's manual for appropriate adjustments on sample preparation and electrophoresis conditions.

3.3.1. Sample Preparation

For sample preparation, it is recommended that one make a loading mixture for all the samples to be analyzed (14.4 μL of deionized formamide and 0.6 μL

Table 4
PCR Amplification Mix

	Stock concentration	Volume per sample
YSTRM1		
Water		4.1 μL
Gold Buffer	10X	2.5 μL
MgCl$_2$	25 μ*M*	2 μL
dNTPs	10 μ*M*	0.5 μL
Primer mix		14.7 μL
TaqGold	5 units/μL	0.2 μL
		↓
Reaction mix		24 μL
Template DNA	1–10 ng/μL	1 μL
YSTRM2		
Water		1.3 μL
Gold Buffer	10X	2.5 μL
MgCl$_2$	25 μ*M*	1.5 μL
dNTPs	10 μ*M*	0.5 μL
Primer mix		18 μL
TaqGold	5 units/μL	0.2 μL
		↓
Reaction mix		24 μL
Template DNA	1–10 ng/μL	1 μL
Total reaction volume		25 μL

Note: To prevent cross-contamination, it is recommended that one gloves and aerosol-resistant pipet tips.

of TAMRA 500 internal size standard per sample). In the preparation of the loading mixture, make the calculations for one or two additional samples to compensate for pipetting errors. Dispense 15 μL of the loading mixture into each ABI310 tubes and add 1 μL of the PCR product. Before loading, denature the samples by heating them at 95°C for 3 min and placing them in ice for at least 5 min.

3.3.2. Analysis Conditions

Samples are analyzed by electrophoresis using Performance Optimized Polymer 4 (POP-4; AB Applied Biosystems) and filter set C using the following conditions: Module "GS STR POP-4 (1 mL) C"; Inj. secs: 5; inj kV: 15.0;

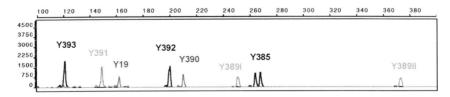

Fig. 3. Electrophoregram of a sample typed with the YSTRM1 multiplex.

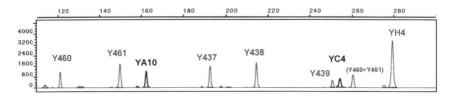

Fig. 4. Electrophoregram of a sample typed with the YSTRM2 multiplex.

run kV: 15.0; run °C: 60 and; tun time: 24 min. Data are analyzed using a matrix (Set C) generated using 6-FAM, TET, HEX, and TAMRA matrix standards. Matrix standardization protocols are available on the ABI PRISM® 310 Genetic Analyser User's Manual. Fragment sizes are determined automatically using the GeneScan® Analysis Software, version 3.1, and samples should be typed by comparison with sequenced allelic ladders.

3.4. Allelic Ladders

The use of sequenced allelic ladders is very successful for comparison purposes in forensic and other studies, and it is thus recommended by the DNA Commission of the International Society of Forensic Genetics *(24)*. The general strategy for ladder construction is primarily to isolate and sequence different size STR alleles found in a first screening of a population sample. After identifying the different alleles by sequence analysis, the samples can be mixed and amplified together to produce a ladder. The volume of each individual sample in the mixture must be adjusted to produce a well-balanced ladder. For multiplex analysis, the best strategy is to produce single ladders for each locus and mixed them together to make up the multiplex ladder.

For all the markers included in both YSTRM1 and YSTRM2, ladders can be amplified in a 50-μL final reaction volume comprising 1.5 mM MgCl$_2$, buffer, 2 U Taq DNA Polymerase, and 200 μlM of each deoxyribonucleoside triphosphate (dNTP). Primer concentrations between 0.2 μM and 0.5 μM are recommended, depending on the locus and the number of alleles included in the ladder. Amplifications can be performed in 35 cycles of 30 s at 94°C, 30 s at 58°C, and 1 min at 72°C (for a GeneAmp PCR system 2400 thermocycler; AB Applied Biosystems). As previously mentioned, some adjustments can be required in different apparatus. Single-locus ladders can be reamplified using 1 µL (in a 50-µL final reaction volume) of between 1:1000 and 1:10.000 dilutions of the original ladder.

4. Additional Problems

Apart from those already mentioned, some other problems can arise during the YSTRM1 and YSTRM2 set up, as follows:

1. Because of variation involving instruments and primer solutions (including different dyes) between different laboratories, most of the time it is necessary to adjust primer concentrations to have a well-balanced amplification of all the loci included in the multiplexes. When a new primer stock fails to amplify in multiplex, before increasing the concentration, the quality of the primer should be checked by a singleplex amplification of the concerned STR.
2. Peak heights between 1000 and 2000 relative fluorescent units are ideal. If peak heights are too high for some loci, reduce the PCR primer concentration of those loci. If this happens to all the loci included in the multiplex, use less DNA or reduce the number of PCR cycles.
3. An amplified fragment may show a second peak (–1 bp) because of to the incomplete 3' adenine base addition. This artifact can be reduced with the increase of the PCR final extension step or by switching the dye label to the other primer.
4. An excess of DNA during PCR will improve the amplification of smaller sized loci and a reduced amplification of the larger alleles is observed.
5. A small amount of DNA in the PCR reaction can inhibit the amplification of some loci, namely, DYS19, DYS392 (YSTRM1), and DYS438 (YSTRM2), which are the most sensitive markers to PCR variations.
6. Amplification of stutter products (with one repeat less) can appear because of the enzyme slippage during the amplification. For both multiplexes described here, no significant stutter peaks were observed. However, special attention should be given in successive reamplification of the ladders. Usually, with ladder reamplification, the larger alleles amplify less efficiently with the simultaneous increase of stutter amplification. This effect has been sometimes responsible for a one repeat less drift in the correct allele typing. Therefore, after reamplification, the ladder should be tested by comparison with the original one or by using sequenced control samples.
   The Y-specific STR typing by PCR amplification and fragment size determination follows the same principles as autosomal STR typing. Therefore, recommendations concerning STR typing should be followed, including samples, apparatus, and reagent handling (*see* Chapter 5 on STR typing). User's manuals for commercial STR multiplex amplification kits can also be useful for consulting additional topics on troubleshooting.

Acknowledgments

This work was partially supported by Fundação para a Ciência e a Tecnologia (POCTI, Programa Operacional Ciência, Tecnologia e Inovação).

References

 1. Prinz, M., Boll, K., Baum, H., and Shaler, B. (1997) Multiplexing of Y chromosome specific STRs and performance for mixed samples. *Forensic Sci. Int.* **85,** 209–218.
 2. Prinz, M., Ishii, A., Coleman, A., Baum, H. J., and Shaler, R. C. (2001) Validation and casework application of a Y chromosome specific STR multiplex. *Forensic Sci. Int.* **120,** 177–188.
 3. Sibille, I., Duverneuil, C., Lorin, G., Guerrouache, K., Teissiere, F., Durigon, M., and de Mazancourt, P. (2002) Y-STR DNA amplification as biological evidence in sexually assaulted female victim with no cytological detection of spermatozoa. *Forensic Sci. Int.* **125,** 212–216.
 4. Ayub, Q., Mohyuddin, A., Qamar, R., Mazhar, K., Zerjal, T., Mehdi, S., and Tyler-Smith, C. (2000) Identification and characterization of novel human Y-chromosomal microsatellites from sequence database information. *Nucleic Acids Res.* **28,** e8.
 5. White, P., Tatum, O., Deaven, L., and Longmire, J. (1999) New, male-specific microsatellite markers from the human Y chromosome. *Genomics* **57,** 433–437.
 6. Iida, R., Tsubota, E., and Matsuki, T. (2001) Identification and characterization of two novel human polymorphic STRs on the Y chromosome. *Int. J. Legal Med.* **115,** 54–56.
 7. Iida, R., Tsubota, E., Sawazaki, K., Masuyama, M., Matsuki, T., Yasuda, T., and Kishi, K. (2002) Characterization and haplotype analysis of the polymorphic Y-STRs, DYS443, DYS444 and DYS445 in a Japanese population. *Int. J. Legal Med.* **116,** 191–194.
 8. Bosch, E., Lee, A. C., Calafell, F., Arroyo, E., Henneman, P., De Knijff, P., and Jobling, M. A. (2002) High resolution Y chromosome typing: 19 STRs amplified in three multiplex reactions. *Forensic Sci. Int.* **125,** 42–51.
 9. Redd, A. J., Agellon, A. B., Kearney, V. A., Contreras, V. A., Karafet, T., Park, H., et al. (2002) Forensic value of 14 novel STRs on the human Y chromosome. *Forensic Sci. Int.* **130,** 97–111.
10. Schneider, P. M., Meuser, S., Waiyawuth, W., Seo, Y., and Rittner, C. (1998) Tandem repeat structure of the duplicated Y-chromosomal STR locus DYS385 and frequency studies in the German and three Asian populations. *Forensic Sci. Int.* **97,** 61–70.
11. Schultes, T., Hummel, S., and Herrmann, B. (1999) Amplification of Y-chromosomal STRs from ancient skeletal material. *Hum. Genet.* **104,** 164–166.
12. Gusmão, L., González-Neira, A., Sánchez-Diz, P., Lareu, M. V., Amorim, A., and Carracedo, A. (2000) Alternative primers for DYS391 typing: advantages of their application to forensic genetics. *Forensic Sci. Int.* **112,** 49–57.

13. Dupuy, B. M., Gedde-Dahl, T., and Olaisen, B. (2002) DXYS267: DYS393 and its X chromosome counterpart. *Forensic Sci. Int.* **112,** 111–121.
14. Gusmão, L., Alves, C., Costa, S., Amorim, A., Brion, M., González-Neira, A., and Carracedo, A. (2002) Point mutations in the flanking regions of the Y-chromosome specific STRs DYS391, DYS437 and DYS438. *Int. J. Leg Med.* **116,** 322–326.
15. Gill, P., Brenner, C., Brinkmann, B., Budowle, B., Carracedo, A., Jobling, M. A., et al. (2001) DNA Commission of the International Society of Forensic Genetics: recommendations on forensic analysis using Y-chromosome STRs. *Forensic Sci. Int.* **114,** 305–309.
16. Gusmão, L., González-Neira, A., Alves, C., Lareu, M., Costa, S., Amorim, A., et al. Carracedo, A. (2002) Chimpanzee homologous of human Y specific STRs. A comparative study and a proposal for nomenclature. *Forensic Sci. Int.* **126,** 129–136.
17. Pascali, V. L., Dobosz, M., and Brinkmann, B. (1998) Coordinating Y-chromosomal STR research for the courts. *Int. J. Legal Med.* **112,** 1.
18. Carracedo, A., Beckmann, A., Bengs, A., Brinkmann, B., Caglia, A., Capelli, C., et al. (2001) Results of a collaborative study of the EDNAP group regarding the reproducibility and robustness of the Y-chromosome STRs DYS19, DYS389 I and II, DYS390 and DYS393 in a PCR pentaplex format. *Forensic Sci. Int.* **119,** 28–41.
19. Gonzaléz-Neira, A., Elmoznino, M., Lareu, M.V., Sánchez-Diz, P., Gusmão, L., Prinz, M., and Carracedo, A. (2001) Sequence structure of 12 novel Y chromosome microsatellites and PCR amplification strategies. *Forensic Sci. Int.* **122,** 19–26.
20. Butler, J. M., Schoske, R., Vallone, P. M., Kline, M. C., Redd, A. J., and Hammer, M. F. (2002) A novel multiplex for simultaneous amplification of 20 Y chromosome STR markers. *Forensic Sci. Int.* **129,** 10–24.
21. Beleza, S., Alves, C., González-Neira, A., Lareu, M., Amorim, A., Carracedo, A., and Gusmão, L. (2003) Extending STR markers in Y chromosome haplotypes. *Int. J. Leg. Med.* **117,** 27–33.
22. Kittler, R., Erler, A., Brauer, S., Stoneking, M., and Kayser, M. (2003) Apparent intrachromosomal exchange on the human Y chromosome explained by population history. *Eur. J. Hum. Genet.* **11,** 304–314.
23. Bär, W., Brinkmann, B., Budowle, B., Carracedo, A., Gill, P., Lincoln, P., et al. (1997) DNA recommendations—Further report of the DNA Commission of ISFH regarding the use of short tandem repeat systems. *Int. J. Legal Med.* **110,** 175–176.
24. Kayser, M., Cagliá, A., Corach, D., Fretwell, N., Gehrig, C., Graziosi, G., et al. (1997) Evaluation of Y-chromosome STRs: a multicenter study. *Int. J. Legal Med.* **110,** 125–133.

7

Using Online Databases for Developing SNP Markers of Forensic Interest

Christopher Phillips

Summary

In this chapter we review and compare the online single nucleotide polymorphism databases that are now available as research tools. We give an outline of the search strategies that can be used to ensure the most appropriate loci for forensic applications are chosen.

Key Words: Forensic science; forensic DNA analysis; SNP; genotyping; variation; polymorphism; online databases; linkage disequilibrium; haplotype; haplotype block; genome.

1. Introduction

The widespread use of deoxyribonucleic acid (DNA) polymorphisms in forensic analysis really started in earnest with the adoption of amplifiable short tandem repeat (STR) loci in the mid-1990s. At that time, an initial report of the identification of a repeat-based polymorphism—with observed variation and flanking sequence—was needed to develop a new marker. Fortunately, from the few-hundred tetranucleotide loci identified in the first 4 yr, a sufficient number were adopted to form the robust and sensitive multiplex tests used in every laboratory today. Since 2001, when the draft human genome was published, another class of DNA variation, single nucleotide polymorphisms (SNPs), has been available to exploit for forensic analysis *(1)*. These polymorphisms are considerably more abundant than STRs, and the majority are already very well characterized. In the same way that the complex and extensive sequencing data generated by the human genome mapping project (HGMP) has become widely available to everyone through the contemporary advances in computing power and informatics, now data for more than 4 million Human

From: *Methods in Molecular Biology, vol. 297: Forensic DNA Typing Protocols*
Edited by: A. Carracedo © Humana Press Inc., Totowa, NJ

SNP loci are freely accessible via databases directly arising from the HGMP. The purpose of this chapter is to detail the methods that can be used to select suitable loci from the most extensive of the SNP databases and the different ways to obtain the information required to use these markers in genotyping assays.

Several other genetics-orientated online databases are now proving to be essential tools in forensic analysis and the most useful of these are also briefly outlined. Many forensic researchers will already be familiar with accessing the National Centre for Biological Information (NCBI) Basic Local Alignment Search Tool (BLAST) and with the NCBI bibliographical databases of MEDLINE and PubMed. BLAST has the advantage of providing an introduction to the concept of accessing a database with an online query submission and retrieving output that is annotated with additional information (in this example, normally a short sequence submission obtains the output of a graphic showing the alignments, an ordered list of matching sequences with statistical annotation, plus hyper links to the appropriate genome databases). MEDLINE and PubMed both give useful introductions to the use of Boolean terms to focus a database query so that the output is a manageable size—an essential strategy given the huge scale of most genomic data.

2. Materials

The following list, in order of importance, describes the principal SNP databases, followed by certain databases that are useful for forensic genetics applications in general. Note that the database size: the number of SNP entries given in each case applies to late 2003.

2.1. NCBI dbSNP
(http://www.ncbi.nlm.nih.gov/entrez/query.fcgi?db=snp)

In any search for information on SNP markers, this should be the first place to begin collecting data. As well as being the principle repository of SNP data generated from the public HGMP, the NCBI host site is also the most important collection of nucleotide, gene, protein, published article, and inherited disorder databases currently available—all fully crossreferenced within the site. dbSNP is regularly updated in synchrony with genome rebuilds, ensuring the highest quality of locus mapping and scrutiny (*see* **Note 1**). One significant benefit of dbSNP being part of the NCBI information resource is the ability to search the database using a standardized query system with a unified approach termed Entrez. This system is used throughout NCBI, allowing the integration of data from several databases and a common approach to constructing queries. Important additional features of dbSNP are detailed in **Notes 2–5**.

2.2. The SNP Consortium (http://snp.cshl.org/)

This database is run by Cold Spring Harbor Laboratory on behalf of the private/public partnership of 17 organizations' forming The SNP Consortium (TSC). It comprises 1.8 million loci, all of which are listed in dbSNP—both databases are fully crossreferenced by hyperlinks, but note that TSC uses a different SNP locus ID numbering system (*see* **Note 6**).

2.3. ABI Assays-on-Demand Database (http://myscience.appliedbiosystems.com/cdsEntry/Form/ assay_search_basic.jsp)

This database is a selective subset of SNP markers taken from the complete Celera SNP database (http://www.celeradiscoverysystem.com/), which comprises 4.1 million markers discovered from the private HGMP initiative. As with TSC, the SNPs have been chosen from the Celera set specifically to provide a gene-centric SNP linkage map as part of the assay design service for the Taqman SNP typing system provided by ABI. The database can be queried with several criteria within certain limitations for the subset of data provided (*see* **Notes 7–9**).

2.4. Ensembl (http://www.ensembl.org/Homo_sapiens/)

An extensive genome database and browser run by EBI and The Sanger Centre. This database parallels the NCBI content to a large extent and has a similar search system and graphical browser. The Sanger Centre web site provides an alternative BLAST site (http://www.sanger.ac.uk/cgi-bin/blast/ submitblast/hgp) and sequence alignment tool with SSAHA (http:// www.sanger.ac.uk/Software/analysis/SSAHA/).

2.5. HGVBase (formerly HGBase; http://hgvbase.cgb.ki.se/)

HGVbase is a database of 2.86 million human genome variants (late 2003) that includes, but is not limited to, SNPs, deletion/insertion polymorphisms (DIPs), and STRs. Low-frequency variants and new mutations are also listed along with approx 40% of dbSNP loci recurated for the database. A useful page provided by the site is a full listing of 45 online SNP-related databases (http://hgvbase.cgb.ki.se/cgi-bin/main.pl?page=databases_.htm).

2.6. Other Databases of Use for Forensic Research

2.6.1. NCBI BLAST http://www.ncbi.nlm.nih.gov/blast/

BLAST is a tool for calculating sequence similarity rather than a database *(2)*, but for developing forensic SNP assays, it will be the most common application querying the NCBI nucleotide databases collectively termed GenBank.

There are two main reasons for using nucleotide BLAST: finding a location for a submitted sequence (the query being: does this sequence exist in a database?) and checking for coincidental sequence similarity for a submitted sequence, usually a design for a polymerase chain reaction (PCR) primer or detection probe (the query being: what is the degree of specificity or uniqueness of this sequence?). The alignment comparisons required for each of the above queries are provided by MegaBLAST and standard BLAST (blastn), respectively (*see* **Note 10**). The two statistics that annotate the returns from blastn: the bit score and E-value are explained in notes (*see* **Note 11***)*.

2.6.2. NCBI UniSTS
(http://www.ncbi.nlm.nih.gov/entrez/query.fcgi?db=unists)

UniSTS is a database collating information about linkage markers, or sequence tagged sites (STS). For each marker, UniSTS displays the primer sequences, product size, and mapping information, as well as cross-references to LocusLink, dbSNP, and Entrez Map Viewer. It gives the most extensive data for STRs of any database and can be queried directly with a D number (e.g., D21S11) an accession number or even a common name (e.g., FGA).

2.6.3. NCBI LocusLink (http://www.ncbi.nlm.nih.gov/LocusLink/)

LocusLink is the most important point of reference for all data relating to genetic loci. It provides a single query interface to curated sequence and gives descriptive information about all the current known genes in 10 organisms. The very extensive genetic information provided is crossreferenced to other relevant NCBI sections for official nomenclature, aliases, sequence accessions, phenotypes, EC numbers, MIM (Mendelian inheritance in man) numbers, UniGene clusters, homology, and map locations. This is an essential database for checking the characteristics (and therefore the significance of any linkage) of genes in close proximity to candidate SNP markers.

2.6.4. The Dusseldorf STR Database
(http://www.uni-duesseldorf.de/WWW/MedFak/Serology/database.htm)

This is an extensive STR allele frequency database with lists of supporting publications.

2.6.5. The Marshfield Centre for Medical Genetics
(http://research.marshfieldclinic.org/genetics/Map_Markers/maps/
IndexMapFrames.html)

This site collates mapping information for a range of polymorphisms and is one of the most useful marker databases for locating the positions of STRs (*see* **Note 12**).

2.6.6. Mitomap (http://www.mitomap.org/)

Described as "a compendium of polymorphisms and mutations of human mitochondrial DNA," this is the best mitochondrial genome resource encompassing a full range of databases, all of which can be independently queried.

2.6.7. ALFRED (http://alfred.med.yale.edu/alfred/index.asp)

This ALlele FREquency Database now has 856 polymorphisms, 377 populations, and 17,569 frequency tables and includes several of the standard forensic loci currently in use. Submissions are encouraged to further extend the scope of the database.

2.6.8. Y-STR and EMPOP Databases (http://ystr.charite.de/index_gr.html and http://www.empop.org/basis/index.php3)

The Y chromosome STR marker and mtDNA sequence polymorphism databases are referred to in detail in other sections of this book.

3. Methods
3.1. Selection Criteria for Forensic SNP Markers

Developing SNPs for forensic analysis requires that the markers used possess certain characteristics that address the specialized needs of the field. It is widely agreed that there is a need for a large set of SNPs to provide levels of discrimination comparable to the existing panel of STR markers. A recommendation of between 50 and 80 markers made in one study *(3)* suggests a need to consider linkage (because multiple SNPs are required per chromosome) and robustness in multiplex PCR as selection criteria. An upper limit to the number of loci that can be realistically multiplexed requires that SNPs should have a reasonably high variability. Therefore three factors emerge as potential selection criteria: linkage, flanking sequence quality, and level of polymorphism.

3.1.1. Linkage

Detailed analysis of the human genome and the patterns of association between genes and neighboring polymorphic markers has revealed a nonrandom distribution of linkage disequilibrium (LD). Current studies examining LD distribution have found that chromosome segments or blocks exist where the markers and genes are in almost complete LD across relatively large distances *(4–6)*. Such blocks are not consistent with the established model of genetic distance measured by a uniform recombination rate, and it is generally agreed that they represent areas of extremely low recombination interspersed with mostly, smaller chromosome segments, often with recombination rates much higher than average that are called recombination hotspots *(7)*. The international hapmap project aims to map haplotype blocks and analyze block variability in different population groups (www.hapmap.org). Because data from hapmap is not yet available, an alternative approach is to use a minimum distance between markers based on the observations of average haplotype block size found so far. Two studies obtained similar observations from different chromosomes: Daly et al. *(8)* reported blocks ranging in size between 3 and 92 kb on 5q, whereas De La Vega et al. *(9,10)* reported a wider range of block size in chromosomes 6, 21, and 22 (5 to 300 kb) but with an average block size of 26 kb and 18 kb in Europeans and Africans, respectively. However, in the latter study more than 95% of blocks in Europeans and 97% in Africans were in the range of 1 to 100 kb. The biggest block found so far is 804 kb *(4)*, but it is safe to conclude that blocks longer than 100 kb are rare and represent only 2–3% of the blocks found on chromosomes 6, 21, and 22 *(9)*. If a minimum distance of 100 kb is used to separate a SNP and a nearby gene, very few selected markers are likely to be in LD beyond this distance. Many of the principles underlying haplotype block mapping do not have universal support; for a thorough review, see Wall and Pritchard *(11)*.

3.1.2. Flanking Sequence Quality

The sequence around a SNP directly affects the ability to design a robust and extensive multiplex genotyping assay. Flanking sequence must be free from: extremes in %GC, additional substitution sites in close proximity (clustering SNPs), consecutive identical bases (polybase sequence), potential for secondary structures (e.g. hairpins arising from GCGC or GGCC type base motifs), and segments of short tandem repeats (*see* **Note 13**).

3.1.3. Polymorphism Levels

The traditional forensic measurement of polymorphism: discrimination index (Dp) does not fall significantly between a minimum allele frequency of 0.5 and 0.3. As shown by the red lines in **Fig. 1**, the Dp only drops in this allele frequency range by 6.5% of the highest value (from 0.62 to 0.58). This suggests 0.3 could be a reasonable lower limit of minimum allele frequency that will be inclusive enough to provide a large pool of candidates. An additional feature of SNP variability is a consistent difference in polymorphism level between populations. Approximately 20–30% of SNPs show a minimum allele frequency below 0.1 in at least one of the three TSC study populations. Whether this presents a problem in selecting markers depends on the eventual cumulative Dp of the SNP set in each population and on the demographics of the region served by each lab. Some markers show such extensive stratification in allele frequency distributions that this characteristic can be used by itself to predict the population of origin of an unknown sample *(12)*.

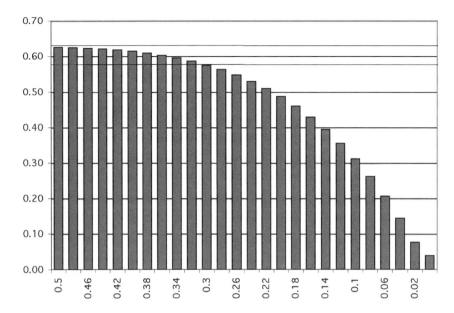

Fig. 1. Dp values for different minimum allele frequencies.

3.2. Using Entrez and the NCBI Cross Database Search Facility

Entrez (http://www.ncbi.nlm.nih.gov:80/gquery/gquery.fcgi) is a unified search engine for the NCBI suite that can be applied individually or to a total of 13 different databases simultaneously. For example, inserting the term TH01 in the cross query page returns numerous hits returned as numbers against the corresponding databases: 155 literature citations in PubMed, 1 nucleotide sequence hit in GenBank, 1 protein sequence hit in Protein, and 1 marker hit in UniSTS. One obvious advantage is the ability to view how effective the search has been in numbers of hits before progressing with detailed follow-up work. Note that an effective search should be one that returns a realistic number of hits, for example, SNP used as the query term returns 6.9 million hits from dbSNP alone.

Clicking on any of the database returns will detail the hits as individual pages (*see* **Note 14**). Using Boolean terms can help to reduce the number of hits to manageable sizes, for instance, entering TH01 AND STR reduces the PubMed hits to 115. However, the UniSTS hit for TH01 disappears at the same time. To fully exploit the power of Entrez for cross-database searching, it is important to be familiar with the query terms (also termed fields) used in each of the 13 databases. Because marker type (STR, SNP, restriction fragment length polymorphism, DIP) is not a query term and the operator AND is exclusive, the hit for TH01 was not returned because the UniSTS database entry does not use polymorphism type as a recorded characteristic of the marker. Full descriptions of each field, plus examples of their use with Boolean operators, can be obtained from the Entrez help page (*see* **Notes 15** and **16**) from which each database is individually hyper linked (http://web.ncbi.nlm.nih.gov/entrez/query/static/help/helpdoc.html).

When searching for candidate SNP markers for forensic applications, there is the problem of nearly 7 million individual SNP database entries and the need to adapt the search strategy to the selection criteria outlined in **Subheading 3.1.** In addition, the SNP database needs to be queried individually using the Entrez system, rather than querying all the NCBI sites jointly. The fields available that are most useful for searching EntrezSNP for forensic SNPs are detailed separately in **Subheading 3.4.** below.

3.3. Boolean Terms

Boolean terms define the rules used in all computer database searching by using the principles of logic developed by the mathematician Boole. In the context of a database search, these principles refer to the relationship between search terms, given by the three logical operators: OR, AND, NOT. Each is described briefly:

> AND (often termed intersection) is exclusive—only returning database entries that contain the provided terms.
> OR (often termed union) is inclusive—returning database entries that contain at least one of the provided terms.
> NOT (often termed difference) excludes from the returns, all database entries with the provided terms.

Three operator modifiers are additionally used in many Entrez queries, such as ranging: or setting a range for a value used to define a search (e.g., SNP heterozygosity), parentheses, or grouping search criteria together to provide an order for the search process and wild card: using a star in place of missing text to allow a partial entry to be used as a query term (e.g., BRC* finds BRCA1 and BRCA2). Entrez uses Boolean operators in uppercase between each search term. An example search of the publications database PubMed illustrating the principles of Entrez queries is given in **Note 17**. Entrez queries are generally quicker and more focused, using qualifying labels for search items called search field tags. PubMed has its own particular set of tags with clearly defined applications. Although users must learn their correct use, they will make each search much more specific to an individual research need.

3.4. Searching With EntrezSNP

EntrezSNP (http://www.ncbi.nlm.nih.gov:80/entrez/query.fcgi?db=snp) is the system used to access the largest NCBI database, and it consequently has the most extensive system of search field tags. All 28 are outlined in the

Table 1
EntrezSNP Search Field Tags of Importance for Forensic SNP Marker Searches

Description	Tag / Qualifier	Search field used	Example
Observed alleles with	[ALLELE]	IUPAC allele code (**Table 2**)	R[ALLELE] find SNPs a or g substitutions
Chromosome	[CHR]	number / X, Y	21[CHR] OR 22[CHR] find SNPs on chromosomes 21 and 22
Base position	[BPOS]	ranged number (used with AND & [CHR]	18000:28000[BPOS] AND Y[CHR] find SNPs in 10kb section of Y-chromosome
Heterozygosity	[HET]	ranged number	30:50[HET] find SNPs with heterozygosity value in range 30–50%

EntrezSNP home page, and the more important of these tags for forensic SNP selection are detailed below in **Table 1**.

Other tags are fixed for forensic SNP searching. First, the tag "organism": [ORGN] or [TAX_ID] prefixed with search field "human" ensures the list does not include the increasing number of SNPs now being collated from other genomes. Next, map weight (the number of times a SNP maps to the genome) using the term 1[WEIGHT] ensures all SNPs returned are unique. Finally, all SNPs should be validated by repeat genotyping using: by frequency[VALIDATION]. The actual final list of tags that are incorporated into any search will depend on the SNP assay to be developed, the order of importance of the search criteria for candidate loci, and the way the SNP will be used in an analysis. SNPs will be mainly selected for discrimination assays, but also it may be desirable to find SNP markers for specialized forensic applications, such as the analysis of mixtures, phenotypic traits, or population of origin, all of which require more detailed and carefully constructed search strategies *(12–14)*. The requirements of the kind of SNP assay to be used are discussed in detail in another chapter but mainly concern the type of allele substitution or the flanking sequence. Allele type can be selected with the term [ALLELE] prefixed with the IUPAC codes listed in **Table 2** as search fields.

To selecting SNPs with the appropriate flanking sequence, one needs to carefully scrutinize the list of loci produced by a search because it is not possible to select particular flanking sequence features. The graphical annotation that summarizes the properties of each SNP returned from EntrezSNP is shown by an example in **Fig. 2**. For a discrimination set, the criteria discussed earlier can

Table 2
**IUPAC Codes Used With the [ALLELE] Tag Denoting
SNP Base Substitutions**

Code	Substitution	Code	Substitution
M	A or C	V	A or C or G
R	A or G	H	A or C or T
W	A or T	D	A or G or T
S	C or G	B	C or G or T
Y	C or T	N	A or C or G or T
K	G or T		(or indeterminate base)

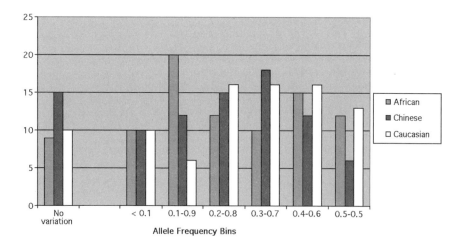

Fig. 2. Allele-frequency distributions in 100 randomly selected SNP loci in three populations.

dictate the search terms to a certain extent but assessing linkage disequilibrium using EntrezSNP is made difficult by the absence of information on other genome features. Specific chromosome regions can be applied using the ranged search field tag [BPOS], but checking linkage when searching for SNPs by map browsing (**Subheading 3.6.**) is always an easier process. However, it is possible to order a SNP list with a critical characteristic to obtain a shortened list of candidates that can then be scrutinized for other important characteristics in Map Viewer (*see* **Note 18**).

3.5. Genome Browsing Using NCBI Map Viewer

The NCBI Map Viewer is a browser tool that supports the search and display of genomic information by chromosomal position. The viewer interface provides a graphical overview of several databases in combination with user controlled map arrangements. Exploring a chromosome segment as a map is most intuitive way to find candidate SNPs for forensic use and, at the same time, to scrutinize the position and characteristics of other important neighboring genome features: sequence, genes, and clustering SNPs. Furthermore, the features of each SNP can be obtained easily via a series of hyperlinks embedded into the map view and the SNP report page.

The Map Viewer home page gives a taxonomic tree of 19 species in total, but it is possible to go directly to the human chromosome view of scaled individual ideograms (http://www.ncbi.nlm.nih.gov/mapview/map_search.cgi?taxid=9606). Clicking on the number below a chromosome produces the main Map Viewer page with the whole chromosome in four default representations: Ideogram, Contig, HS UniG, and Genes—mapping chromosome banding, genome assembly segments, mRNA alignments, and known/putative genes, respectively. The Genes map is in red and the rightmost of the four, denoting that it is the master map and so the theme of the hyperlink connections to the detailed information on the right (in this case, LocusLink and OMIM plus six additional gene-orientated databases). The number, order, and annotation of the maps displayed is arranged by following the upper right maps & options link. The choice of maps for SNP exploration from the 42 available is fairly straightforward because the variation map alone provides all the information and hyperlinks needed (*see* **Note 19**). Once the page is properly arranged, the variation map shows the relative position of SNPs to other mapped features and lines trace from the map to hyperlinked RefSNP ID numbers that produce a report page for each SNP. Next to the rs number are symbols for map, gene, heterozygosity (het) validation, genotypes, and linkout, which denote certain locus properties—these are detailed in **Fig. 3**. For forensic analysis, markers need to be unique and real (given by a green flag under map and between one to three gold stars under validation respectively; *see* **Note 20**). In addition to the map and validation items, the heterozygosity scale for the SNP can be checked for sufficient polymorphic content before going to the cluster report page. Setting a minimum heterozygosity ensures only the most informative loci are followed up in detail. A minimum allele frequency distribution of 0.3 corresponds to a heterozygosity value of 42%; therefore, a range between 40 and 50% provides a quick check for sufficient locus variability in Map Viewer.

Chromosome walking, by scrolling down the map of each chromosome, can be a slow and lengthy process, but it provides the easiest and most reliable

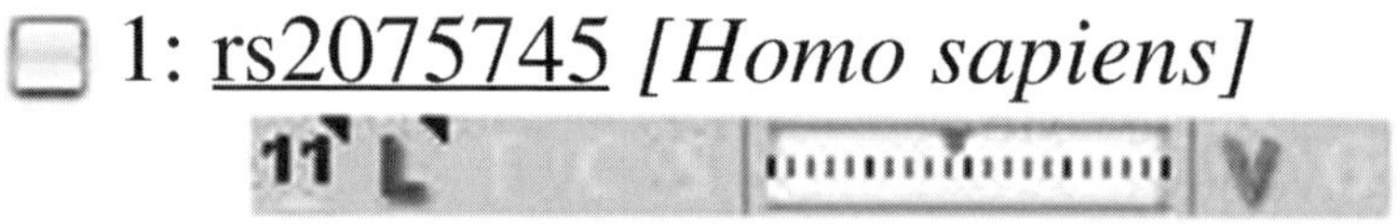

☐ 1: <u>rs2075745</u> *[Homo sapiens]*

Fig. 3. An example return from EntrezSNP showing annotation. The rs number hyper links to the RefSNP cluster report, this SNP locus occurs on chromosome 11 once (underline to chromosome number), is sited in a locus (L), has 46% heterozygosity (graduated scale), and has been validated by genotyping (V).

means to discover suitable SNPs (*see* **Note 21**). The candidate loci pinpointed can be quickly scrutinized using the map symbols. They can then be readily checked in each report page for the locus characteristics important in forensic analysis: sufficient polymorphic content—with variability in most population groups, good flanking sequence quality, and an absence of other closely clustering SNPs. Linkage can also be assessed in Map Viewer by holding the mouse over a gene "edge" to obtain the chromosome co-ordinates of the gene on the SNP side. A more precise figure is given in LocusLink (hyperlinked from the gene symbol annotating the gene).

3.6. Scrutiny of Data From a RefSNP Cluster Report Page

NCBI compiles a cluster report page for all SNP loci with a refSNP number. On this page, below the summary box, more detailed locus characteristics are summarized in seven sections: submission, fasta, resource, locus, map, variation, and validation.

3.6.1. Variation

In the submission section, each of the submitter reports can be examined individually, and this can be useful for checking the extent of genotyping performed and the populations studied in estimating the allele frequencies. This is an important step because the variation section only provides an average allele frequency for each allele, and this can disguise substantial differences in allele frequency distributions between populations in some cases. When TSC is a submitting group, it is useful to be able to follow the hyperlink to the equivalent TSC SNP report page directly and obtain allele frequency figures because this is invariably the most detailed publicly available genotyping data.

Checking the information in the variation section of the NCBI report page provides a quickly assessed summary of polymorphism level, ensuring it is sufficiently high in the first place. This section provides the all-important average heterozygosity and allele frequency figures plus the assay sample size, the number of populations studied and the total number of individuals with geno-

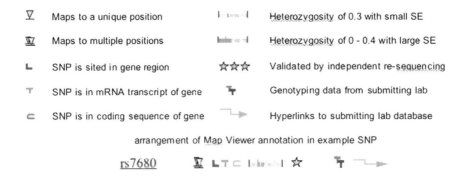

Fig. 4. NCBI Map Viewer variation map annotation symbols.

type data. Forensic candidates require the most reliable data possible plus a reasonable balance between populations, but inevitably a few loci are mainly polymorphic in Africans while others are mainly polymorphic in Europeans or Chinese. As a generalized rule of thumb roughly 30% of SNPs show more than 30% variation in polymorphic content between two or more populations.

3.6.2. Sequence Quality

The fasta section details the flanking sequence around the SNP substitution site—the amount of sequence given can vary between tens and hundreds of bases. Furthermore, the substitution site can often be positioned close to the start or end of the given sequence. This can make recovery of sufficient flanking sequence on one side an awkward process that necessitates alignment of summary sequence from the fasta section with extended sequence obtained from NCBI Sequence Viewer (see next section). Fasta sequence is arranged in 10 base blocks and in two ways: in upper case/lower case and in black/green. Upper case denotes normal, unique, genomic sequence, while lower case is used for sequence identified by RepeatMasker (http://repeatmasker.genome. washington.edu/cgi.bin/RepeatMasker) as low-complexity or repetitive element sequence. The color green is used for sequences identified by the submitter during the SNP assay process. The color black is used for flanking sequence, identified and extracted from the nucleotide databases by NCBI as part of the quality analysis of the SNP submission before incorporation into dbSNP. The fasta sequence should be carefully checked for lowercase text denoting genomic repeat elements that cannot be safely used to develop assays guaranteed to be specific only to the selected SNP. At this point, the flanking sequence also should be scrutinized for additional characteristics that might compromise the assay design process: polybase sequence, higher than average %GC (human

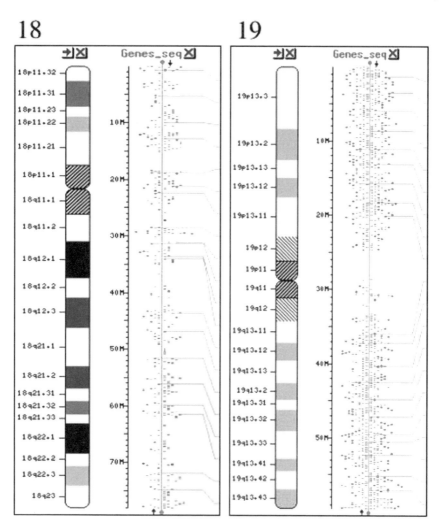

Fig. 5. Gene density plots for two chromosomes of comparable size: 18 and 19.

average: 41% ± 5%), and potential secondary structures. Examples of observed problem sequences are given in **Fig. 5**. These characteristics, the latter in particular, can be difficult to spot by visual examination, and the sequence may need to be imported into software specifically designed to reveal secondary structures such as Primer Express or Primer3 (http://www-genome.wi.mit.edu/cgi-bin/primer/primer3_www.cgi).

3.6.3. Clustering SNPs

Clustering SNP positions are not marked in the fasta section and it is necessary to go to Sequence Viewer (http://www.ncbi.nlm.nih.gov/entrez/query.fcgi?db=Nucleotide) to check for substitutions closely neighboring the chosen RefSNP site. Sequence Viewer: a graphical browser for the NCBI nucleotide database is accessed from the maps section by clicking the rs number. The default view gives 2000 bases as six 10-base blocks per line and the position of the first base of each line given on the left, in blue. Unfortunately, this is the contig not the chromosome position, so it will not provide a matching chromosome co-ordinate figure (as given in dbSNP) for the locus. Furthermore, the SNPs are marked underneath the nucleotide positions (with a brown square, substitutions, and RefSNP number) rather than embedded in the sequence, so extracting a portion of sequence by copy/paste or as a fasta dump will lose all the marked SNP positions. All this requires difficult visual scrutiny of the flanking sequence in Sequence Viewer, recording of the exact position of all visible SNPs in the 100-bp upstream/downstream segments and, finally, annotating the edited sequence in Excel or a text processing program like Notepad. The easiest process is to shorten the sequence shown in Sequence Viewer to 201bp, convert to fasta format and mark all the additional substitutions in a single line in Excel. This may seem like a long-winded method, but often very good SNP candidates have primer design constraints dictated by SNPs in close proximity that may be easily avoided in the assay design process by shifting closer to the SNP site on one side and expanding the flanking sequence on the other side (*see* **Note 22**).

3.7. RefSNP rs1490413: A Worked Example

In this illustration a candidate SNP: rs1490413 is discovered by Map Viewer examination of a portion of chromosome 1 immediately underneath the telomere of the p-arm. The SNP just qualifies for consideration for forensic use on linkage grounds: being 98kb downstream of the gene LOC200104 (reported in LocusLink as a putative, ab initio, gene model - similar to elongation factor Δ1). **Figure 6** summarizes the route map of data collection used to select this SNP moving from part 1 to part 6 in successive stages. First, the map view shown in **Fig. 6**, 1 illustrates the absence of markers on the gene map next to this SNP site and a combination of symbols, indicating that it satisfies a range of selection criteria. Moving from left to right from the RefSNP ID number: rs1490413 maps once on the genome, has a heterozygosity value of 50% with little variation in the allele frequency estimates (a thin pink line in the middle of the scale—compare with rs1117913 four positions below) and has the highest level of validation.

Short Tandem Repeats   **rs379091**
GTCTCAAAATAATAATAATAATAAT**D**ATAATAATAATAATAATAATAATTA

High %GC   **rs1574185**

GCCTGGTTGGGGGGTGTGTGTGGG**B**GGGGGGACGGTGTGGAGGGCCTG

Low %GC (plus polybase and indeterminate base)   **rs1574185**
GGTCTAATTTTTTTTCTTTTCTTTT**H**TTTTTTTNTGCAAAAAGATGTCTTTT

Polybase   **rs1574185**
AAAGTAAGAATTCAAGATGGTATTT**W**AAAAAAAAAACCTCATATCTTTTTTC

Fig. 6. Examples of SNP flanking sequence showing various problems features.

In the SNP cluster report the variation summary (**Fig. 6**, 2) indicates a good level of heterozygosity (interestingly, a value higher than theoretically possible for a binary SNP because the indeterminate results recorded as N were treated as a third allele in the averaging process) and shows four populations were studied. Going to the submission report for one of the two submitted detections of this SNP (ss2316529 and ss11365709) gives a set of details—in this case, summarized in a similar way to NCBI on a report page from TSC. As more comprehensive breakdown of the genotyping results from the submitter shown in **Fig. 6**, 4, which is obtained by clicking the ss number (used by NCBI to identify a specific assay for the SNP). The populations and sample sizes are listed with genotype counts and chi-square analysis of goodness of fit to Hardy Wienberg equilibrium. Clicking each population ID gives a more specific description, an increasingly important improvement in detail in NCBI since mid 2003. As an example, the detailed description of West Africa is: "Sub-Saharan Nations bordering Atlantic and north of Congo River, plus Central/ Southern Atlantic Island Nations." Information from the submitters analysis of polymorphism can be extremely detailed—it is possible to list all the individual typing results—and then, for instance, use sample CEPH1331.01 as an A/G heterozygote control for this SNP.

Finally, the last two parts of **Fig. 6** illustrate different formats for the analysis of flanking sequence quality and degree of clustering. The fasta sequence is all upper case/green, denoting it is unique, genomic sequence detected intact by the submission assay. The Nucleotide Viewer sequence matches the fasta data (i.e., is the same strand) and shows seven clustering SNPs sufficiently distant to be safely ignored in the assay design process.

The Map Viewer plot in **Fig. 6**, 1 shows another SNP: rs1845634 two positions above, with near identical characteristics. In fact, closer inspection of the cluster report details reveals that the flanking region is a predominantly low complexity sequence and the 50% heterozygosity value has been artificially inflated by the variation summary averaging process, being well below a minimum heterozygosity value for forensic applications in two population samples (approx 32% in Europeans and Africans).

4. Notes

1. As an open database, dbSNP receives submissions from active labs in the field and collates the data into a merged reference set. Because different laboratories will routinely report identical SNPs, the submissions are clustered into reference SNPs (termed refSNPs by NCBI). The distinction between submitted SNPs and reference SNPs is made by prefixing ID numbers with ss and rs, respectively.

2. Despite the name, dbSNP also includes STRs and DIPs (which are alternatively termed Indels). dbSNP takes submissions for SNPs discovered in all species with a fully or partially sequenced genome (totaling 23 in late 2003); the vast majority, however, are human and mouse.

3. The admission criteria of NCBI are very effective at detecting nonunique SNPs, with a checking process for all submissions that analyses a minimum 100-bp flanking sequence to position the SNP uniquely in the genome or not. The proportion of nonunique SNPs remains very small (approx 5%), and it appears to have much more in common with the pericentromeric areas; therefore, searches are best directed to the other regions of each chromosome.

4. Users can subscribe to a mailing list providing updates on the regular changes in extent and arrangement of dbSNP (http://www.ncbi.nlm.nih.gov/mailman/listinfo/dbsnp-announce).

5. Outlines of the structure and routine use of the NCBI sites are detailed in a pdf handbook (http://www.ncbi.nlm.nih.gov/books/bv.fcgi?call=bv.View..Show TOC&rid=handbook.TOC&depth=2), which can be downloaded by chapter. Of particular relevance are chapters 5 (dbSNP), 15 (Entrez), 16 (BLAST), and 20 (Map Viewer).

6. TSC SNPs have been chosen specifically for their proximity to genes because the main purpose of TSC is to construct a high-density SNP linkage map. The significant feature is the detailed genotype frequency data for 96,000 loci—most of these for three population groups. This will eventually rise to 300,000 loci. The full dataset can be searched by gene or chromosome region and data for each SNP can be downloaded in text-file format. There is a mailing list for news and update notifications (e-mail: tscsnp-announce-request@snp.cshl.org).

7. The Celera database (CDS) requires an annual subscription but the assays-on-demand subset (AOD) can be freely accessed. AOD data consists of the CDS ID number and the dbSNP ID number (when the marker is a refSNP). In addition, AOD lists accurate allele frequency estimates from 46 individuals in two to four population groups (African, European, plus less extensive Chinese and Japanese frequencies). AOD provides the best data for scrutinizing SNPs with stratified allele frequency distributions between the population groups but flanking sequence

data and map positions are not provided on the public AOD site for Celera-only SNPs.

8. Searches of the AOD database are handled by a page with query fields for 18 different characteristics and a fixed 10-kb flanking region around genes. It is possible to structure the query using set fields for the SNP type (untranslated region, coding, intronic) and allele frequency in each of the four populations in the range 0 of 0.5 in 0.01 increments. This latter field is useful for finding SNPs in particular frequency ranges in particular populations, but uses the union query operator OR, giving very large outputs.

9. CDS is a valuable database for forensic research principally because of the extra coverage it provides: approx 2.6 million of the 4.8 listed SNPs are unique to Celera, the other loci being the better validated public SNPs and new SNPs discovered from comparative sequence passes between public and Celera contigs. One of the criterion for inclusion of SNPs in CDS is a minimum level of polymorphism, so a larger proportion of loci will be useful for forensic applications on the basis of variability alone.

10. MegaBLAST is designed for long sequences and for a certain degree of mismatch, whereas blastn is designed to give a list of sequences in order of similarity. Note that a third option: "Search for short and near exact matches" is recommended for sequence specificity checks with less than 20 bases. A very good guide to program choice is provided by NCBI (http://www.ncbi.nlm.nih.gov/BLAST/producttable.shtml). Although the NCBI BLAST site is the most commonly used sequence alignment tool several other BLAST sites exist (e.g., The Sanger HGMP BLAST tool. This site can e-mail results to avoid long waits with NCBI BLAST at busy periods).

11. BLAST returns a three-part report: the header with query sequence information and a summarizing graphical overview, single-line matching sequence descriptions and, lastly, the matching alignments themselves. The graphical overview shows the query sequence as a numbered red bar, and below this the database hits as colored bars aligned to the query. The colors and proximity to the query represent the alignment scores from red (highest) through to black (lowest) and uppermost to lowest bars. The single-line descriptions give both a bit score indicating goodness of fit of each matched sequence and an expect value (E-value). The bit score is calculated from a formula that takes into account all the matching nucleotides and gaps, the higher the score the better the alignment (http://www.ncbi.nlm.nih.gov/BLAST/tutorial/Altschul-1.html). The E-value gives an idea of the statistical significance of the alignment, reflecting both the size of the database used to prepare the alignments and the score system used. The lower the E-value the more significant the hit. For example a value of 0.05 equates to 5 in 100 or 1 in 20 signifying the probability of this match by chance alone. This latter statistic requires careful interpretation in the context of the sequence comparison being performed.

12. To find the position of STRs using The Marshfield Clinic linkage map database go to "Search for Markers." Enter a D number or common name (e.g., D12S391)

and using the marker description provided (e.g., GATA11H08) obtain a precise map position with NCBI Map Viewer (http://www.ncbi.nlm.nih.gov/mapview/maps.cgi) by filling the search box and clicking find, then clicking the chromosome number in the genome map view to give the detailed chromosome map view and hyper links to the marker characteristics in UniSTS. This can be done directly using the UniSTS query system (http://www.ncbi.nlm.nih.gov/entrez/query.fcgi?db=unists) but the Marshfield site allows easier comparisons with additional STR markers and provides more latitude with nonstandard names, such as VWA or TPOX.

13. Flanking sequence features can compromise the primer (and assay probe) design process by excluding sections of sequence as potential binding sites. Poor sequence will also hinder PCR quality because primers will be difficult to balance in a multiplex with those from problem-free sequence. With the aim of finding primers that perform best in generalized PCR environments, a high-quality sequence will provide the widest range of candidate primers that can work well without specialized conditions, such as higher annealing temperatures. Choice of candidate primers is already reduced in forensic assays by the need to keep the amplicon size small. An absence of clustering SNPs is a particularly important characteristic because any variable site in close proximity will exclude 20–24 primer candidates for the available flanking sequence of a SNP (conditional on average primer length and substitution sites more than 20 bases distant from the SNP of interest).

14. Closer examination of the hits obtained for the example used: TH01 shows that Entrez can be, at once, both too powerful and too loosely defined. If the search query is not carefully constructed or the hits returned are not followed up in the correct database, the required information can be difficult to track down. The sequence hit returned for TH01 is for a plant species: *Rosa chinensis*, the protein hit is for cow (*Bos taurus*) thyroglobulin precursor (TH = thyroid hormone), and one literature citation is for an article on allopolyploidy in wheat (TH01 being an inbred line ID used in an experimental cross but a term only used once in the middle of the article text). The hit for UniSTS returns more appropriate information (from a forensic genetics viewpoint) giving STS marker 240639 which is HUMTH01 providing primer sequences (one the same as that used in the initial forensic development of this STR) plus the precise marker co-ordinates for chromosome 11 (2156529-2156690 bp) and a genome map view—all the data required for the development of this marker from scratch today.

15. The query system for SNPs is called EntrezSNP to distinguish it from the database name dbSNP and from generalized Entrez use. Hyperlinks to the other databases remain intact throughout the SNP report pages that are returned using EntrezSNP, so the benefits of the cross database functionality of using Entrez as a whole are not lost.

16. Two useful tools are provided in EntrezSNP by clipboard and history. The clipboard is a workspace for holding up to 500 items manually selected from search returns, the contents are cleared after 8 h of inactivity. History lists the database

search activity (again cleared after eight hours inactivity) as numbers prefixed by a hash (#). These can be combined using Boolean operators (e.g., placing #1 AND #2 in the search box provides an intersection of the first two searches of the current session)

17. As an example, to find an article that describes the forensic application of DNA fingerprinting that also includes the authors (A. Jeffreys and P. Gill), a search could begin with the term DNA fingerprinting. This returns 5944 hits: a list of all the publications that include some aspect of this topic in the reported work. Adding the term "forensic" using the operator AND returns 868 hits and because the terms used in combination remain in the search box each time, it is easy to then add: AND Jeffreys to obtain a list of 13, followed by: AND Gill. Note that when "Gill" is placed as the final search term, no articles are returned, even though the 1985 *Nature* article we were actually interested in finding appears on the previous list with Jeffreys alone. This is because any search of PubMed using unqualified terms as a query (i.e., without a qualifier or search field tag) will only match key text words within each article to the query (in the case of Jeffreys this includes citations within the text). To find articles by Jeffreys and Gill, we need to use the author search field tag: [au]. So adding AND Gill [au] returns a single article—the correct target of the search. Another tag [dp],or date of publication, provides an example of ranging: a range that is set using a colon (:) between defined limits. Therefore, to get a list of articles from P Gill in the 1990s, we could use Gill P [au] AND 1990:1999 [dp]. To avoid a list of articles from several different authors named P Gill, it is possible to use a flexible and powerful PubMed tag: text word [tw]—in this case, using forensic [tw] reduces the list from 281 to 36. Finally, parentheses can be used to group search terms together into a set of choices for the query. Entrez processes all Boolean operators in a left-to-right sequence, so the order in which a search statement is processed can be directed by enclosing individual concepts in parentheses. Terms placed inside parentheses are processed first as a unit and then incorporated into the overall search strategy. For example, the search statement: genotyping AND (MALDI-TOF OR microarrays) is processed by ORing the terms in parentheses first and then ANDing the resulting set with genotyping. Without the parentheses, all articles on microarrays would be returned. As is the norm with most online databases, PubMed defaults to AND if a space is used between query terms (so SNP, for example, returns 6157 hits, whereas SNP genotyping returns 497).

18. Ordering an EntrezSNP list of returns involves use of a drop down list of six possible criteria of which heterozygosity, success rate, and chromosome base position are the most useful. Generally, ordered heterozygosity will allow the easiest selection of loci providing the highest polymorphic content in most populations. The list is in reverse order, so it is necessary to go to the last page and work backwards.

19. Using several maps in tandem can provide helpful reference points for precise positioning of the segment of the chromosome being explored. For this reason, it can be useful to place an ideogram map and a gene map alongside the variation

View all haplotype sets with overlapping SNP's:

Handle|hapset_name: PERLEGEN|B000661

ss#	rs#	Chr. Pos	Contig Allele	PERLEGEN|B000661			
				1	2	3	4
ss4004417	rs2827886	23431594	G	.	.	T	.
ss4004418	rs2827887	23431756	A	.	.	T	.
ss4004419	rs2827888	23432532	T	.	.	C	.
ss4004420	rs2827889	23433814	A	.	.	G	.
ss4004421	rs2827890	23433828	A	.	G	.	.
ss4004422	rs2827891	23434232	C	N	.	A	.
ss4004423	rs2827892	23434517	T	A	.	A	.

Fig. 7. A seven-SNP, four-haplotype allele distribution in haplotype block B000661, chromosome 21 as displayed in dbSNP.

map. In the map options window it is possible to toggle a chromosome co-ordinates ruler against any map to further aid navigation using co-ordinates. Two other maps could be helpful in exploring SNP linkage issues when browsing. One is the Marshfield genetic map: a comprehensive linkage map incorporating 8000 polymorphic markers with a total sex-averaged genetic distance of 3500 cM. *(15)*. This provides a framework of genetic distance based on recombination rates that can be used to check that two candidate SNP markers are sufficiently distant to avoid linkage. The second map: dbSNP Haplotype is an annotation of genome regions in high linkage disequilibrium. The current data is patchy and mostly focused on chromosome 21 (illustrated in **Fig. 7**). When the HapMap Project data release is completed in 2004–2005, all chromosome maps will have linkage measurements indicating regions of strong or weak LD.

20. Full marker validation by independent resequencing or by multiple reports of the same substitution is important for forensic assay development because large-scale resources would be needed to revalidate unconfirmed SNPs. There are a growing number of markers in dbSNP that have been resequenced and genotyped in more than one population: giving high levels of confidence for the allele frequency reports provided in dbSNP. With so many SNPs now validated to the highest level, choosing only loci with three gold stars in Map Viewer does not seriously limit the pool of candidate markers.

21. Map Viewer can be used to find suitable SNPs either by concentrating a search on a region of a chromosome, known to have low gene densities (so called "gene deserts") or by simple chromosome walking—moving in set intervals along the chromosome. Although finding gene deserts is straightforward enough, there are several distinct problems with this approach. Firstly, because SNP discovery has concentrated on genes and the flanking regions around them, areas with low gene density normally coincide with low SNP density because of acquisition bias. Second, it is necessary to decide on simple rules for avoiding linkage of SNPs to other markers. Unfortunately, traditional genetic distance measurements, such as a centiMorgan scale, are not a completely reliable guide to linkage because, as previously discussed, LD is highly variable throughout the genome. Until haplotype block maps become widely available a minimum distance of 100 kb between markers can be used. Thirdly, variation in gene density within the human genome means some chromosomes are difficult to search with a standardized minimum spacing. Chromosome 19 in particular has a very high gene density (figure z) and in this case obtaining sufficient markers with a minimum of 100 kb between SNP and gene is difficult. Finally, many gene map positions are assumed to exist. Identifying genes in the absence of a described protein product is very difficult and putative sites are widespread. Until the human genome is fully annotated, putative sites may require the same minimum distance spacing as known genes when selecting SNPs.

22. A commonly encountered problem is the disparity in the direction of the displayed sequence in Sequence Viewer and in dbSNP. Always crosscheck the immediate flanking region of the SNP in both databases and if necessary flip the strand to reverse in Sequence Viewer before tracking any clustering SNP positions. The length of sequence examined depends to some extent on the assay design but forensic PCR requires that approx 100–120 bp of flanking region each side is needed to allow sufficient flexibility in primer design.

Acknowledgments

The selection and study of SNP markers from online genetic databases, described in this chapter, formed part of research work supported by the grant (estancias de doctores y tecnologos extranjeros en Espana) from the Ministerio de Educación y Ciencia (SB2000-0236), Madrid.

References

1. Sachidanandam, R., et al. (2001) A map of human genome sequence variation containing 1.42 million single nucleotide polymorphisms. *Nature* **409,** 928–33.
2. Gill, P. (2001). An assessment of the utility of single nucleotide polymorphisms (SNPs) for forensic purposes. *Int. J. Legal Med.* **114,** 204–210.
3. Altschul, S. F., Gish, W., Miller, W., Myers, E. W., and Lipman, D. J. (1990) Basic local alignment search tool. *J. Mol. Biol.* **215,** 403–410.
4. Dawson, E., et al. (2002) A first generation linkage disequilibrium map of chromosome 22. *Nature* **418,** 544–548.

5. Pati, N., et al. (2001) Blocks of limited haplotype diversity revealed by high resolution scanning of human chromosome 21. *Science* **25,** 1719–1723.
6. Gabriel, S. B., et al. (2002) The structure of haplotype blocks in the human genome. *Science* **296,** 2225–2229.
7. Phillips, M. S., et al. (2003) Chromosome-wide distribution of haplotype blocks and the role of recombination hotspots. *Nat. Genet.* **33,** 382–387.
8. Daly, M., Rioux, J. D., Schaffer, D. F., Hudson, T. J., and Lander, E. S. (2001) High resolution haplotype structure in the human genome. *Nat. Genet.* **29,** 229–232.
9. De La Vega, F. M., et al. (2003) A whole genome gene-centric linkage disequilibrium SNP Map. XIX Congress of Genetics July 6–11, Melbourne, Australia; 2003.
10. De La Vega, F. M., et al. (2003) Selection of single nucleotide polymorphisms for a whole-genome linkage disequilibrium mapping set. CSH Genome Sequencing & Biology Meeting, May 7–11, Cold Spring Harbor, NY, 2003.
11. Wall, J. D., and Pritchard, J. K. (2003) Haplotype blocks and linkage disequilibrium in the human genome. *Nat. Rev. Genet.* **4,** 587–597.
12. Phillips, C., Lareu, M., Salas, A., Fondevila, M., Berniel, G., Carracedo, A., et al. Population specific single nucleotide polymorphism, in *Progress in Forensic Genetics 10* (Doutremepuich, C., and Morling, N., eds.), Elsevier, Amsterdam.
13. Phillips, C., Lareu, M., Salas, A., and Carracedo, A.. (2004) Nonbinary single nucleotide polymorphism markers, in *Progress in Forensic Genetics 10* (Doutremepuich, C., and Morling, N., eds.), Elsevier, Amsterdam.
14. Brion, M., Blanco-Verea, A., Lareu, M., and Carracedo, A. 29 Y-chromosome SNP analysis in European populations, in *Progress in Forensic Genetics 10* (Doutremepuich, C., and Morling, N., eds.), Elsevier, Amsterdam.
15. Broman, K. W., Murray, J. C., Sheffield, V. C., White, R. L., and Weber, J. L. (1999) Comprehensive human genetic maps: Individual and sex-specific variation in recombination. *Am. J. Hum. Genet.* **63,** 861–869.

8

SNP Typing in Forensic Genetics

A Review

Beatriz Sobrino and Angel Carracedo

Summary

Single nucleotide polymorphisms (SNPs) are emerging as new markers of interest to the forensic community because of their abundance in the human genome, their low mutation rate, the opportunity they present of analyzing smaller fragments of deoxyribonucleic acid (DNA) than with short tandem repeats—important in degraded DNA samples—and the possibility of automating the analysis with high-throughput technologies. Many new technologies for genotyping SNPs have been developed in the past few years. We describe the principles of the allelic discrimination reactions and the technologies used for each of them. The aim of this chapter is to help in the understanding of the methodologies used in SNP genotyping and in the selection of the most appropriate techniques for forensic purposes.

Key Words: Single nucleotide polymorphism (SNP); SNP genotyping; DNA typing; forensic genetics.

1. Introduction

Single nucleotide polymorphisms (SNPs) are single-base variations at a unique physical location. Comparison of genomic deoxyribonucleic acid (DNA) sequences in different individuals reveals positions at which two, or in some cases, more than two bases, can occur. SNPs are highly abundant and are estimated to occur at 1 in every 1000 bases in the human genome *(1,2)*. They therefore represent the most common class of human polymorphism.

Depending on where a SNP occurs, the polymorphism can have different consequences at the phenotypic level. SNPs in the coding regions of genes that alter the function or structure of the encoded proteins can have clinical conse-

From: *Methods in Molecular Biology, vol. 297: Forensic DNA Typing Protocols*
Edited by: A. Carracedo © Humana Press Inc., Totowa, NJ

quences and are important in medicine for genetic diagnosis, genetic counseling, or pharmacogenetics. However, most SNPs are located in noncoding regions of the genome and have no detectable impact on the phenotype of an individual. These noncoding SNPs are useful as markers in population genetics and evolutionary studies *(3,4)* and for forensic analysis *(5)*.

The reason for the current great interest in SNPs is the prediction that they could be used as markers to identify genes that predispose individuals to complex disorders by using linkage disequilibrium. In addition, in the field of forensic genetics, SNPs have generated increasing interest, and a large proportion of current research activity is now being focused on SNP typing.

Whether SNPs will replace STRs as the primary method of choice for forensic purposes is a matter of conjecture at present. However, SNPs have a number of characteristics that make them very suitable for forensic studies. First, they have lower mutation rates than STRs, and this is valuable for paternity testing. Second, they can be analyzed from short amplicons and, in general, this is desirable, because the size of the amplified product is critical for the successful amplification of degraded samples. Finally, they are particularly suitable for analysis using high-throughput technologies, which have become increasingly important for the successful implementation of large criminal DNA databases. High-throughput techniques also make it easier to perform the large-population studies required for precise estimates of allele frequencies essential for the correct interpretation of cases involving haplotype analysis, such as Y-chromosome and mitochondrial typing.

In addition to this, there is no doubt about the usefulness of SNPs for some specialized forensic applications, in particular, mitochondrial DNA (currently used for bone, teeth, hair shaft); Y-chromosome DNA (used to analyze the male component from mixed stains and to possibly elucidate geographical origin of a sample); and commonplace physical characteristics (skin, hair, eye color) that could be developed in the future for investigative purposes.

There is not one single ideal method for typing SNPs, and the choice depends on both the requirements of the investigation and the field of application. In forensic analysis, the method must be easily applied in the majority of laboratories, with the highest level of accuracy, with a sensitivity sufficient for the analysis of low copy number or degraded DNA, and finally with good multiplexing capacity.

But how many SNPs are needed for a forensic test? It has been shown *(5,6)* that, on average, and considering SNPs with frequencies close to 0.5 for each allele, five SNPs are equivalent to one STR; therefore, a total of between 50 and 75 SNPs equates to the current STR multiplexes used in forensic casework.

The selection of SNPs for forensic analysis is not an easy task. Recently, the European Consortium: SNPforID (Growth Program GRD1-2002-71802) has selected a core group of candidate SNPs based on the validation status, polymorphism, sequence quality, SNP typing technologies, and linkage.

Linkage is one of the most important issues and needs to be carefully addressed because although recent studies indicate that linkage disequilibrium (LD) is structured into discrete blocks in the human genome *(7)*, the variability, range, and distribution of LD in different populations is not yet fully understood.

Strategies for the selection of Y chromosome SNPs *(8)*, nonbinary autosomal SNPs *(9)*, and SNPs suggesting the geographical origin of samples *(10)* have all been recently proposed for forensic purposes.

2. DNA Typing Methodologies

Intense efforts to establish technologies for the large-scale analysis of SNPs are being conducted to identify both the genes that underlie complex diseases and to realize the full potential of pharmacogenomics in elucidating variable responses to drugs. New genotyping methods, chemistries, and platforms are continuously being proposed, and it is often difficult to keep up to date and to make informed decisions on the best-available options. To understand each of the methods, it is important to distinguish between reaction principles, assay formats, and detection methods. Reaction products can be detected with more than one method, and the same detection method can analyze products obtained with different reaction principles or assay formats (**Table 1**).

The majority of SNP genotyping assays can be assigned to one of four groups based on molecular mechanism: allele specific hybridization, primer extension, oligonucleotide ligation, and invasive cleavage. There are several detection methods for analyzing the products of each type of reaction.

2.1. Allele-Specific Hybridization

Allele-specific hybridization, also known as ASO (allele specific oligonucleotide hybridization), is based on distinguishing between two DNA targets differing at one nucleotide position by hybridization *(11)*. Two allele-specific probes are designed, usually with the polymorphic base in a central position in the probe sequence. Under optimized assay conditions, only the perfectly matched probe-target hybrids are stable, and hybrids with one-base mismatch are unstable (**Fig. 1**).

ASO probes with reverse dot-blot formats were used to detect the first polymerase chain reaction (PCR)-based polymorphisms introduced in the forensic field, and they are still used in some laboratories, although they have now

Table 1
Detection Method Used for Each Allelic Discrimination Reaction

Allelic discrimination reaction	Detection method
Hybridization	FRET
	FP
	Microarrays (Fluorescence)
Primer Extension	Electrophoresis
	Mass spectrometry
	Microarrays (Fluorescence)
	FRET
	FP
	Luminescence
Ligation	Electrophoresis
	FRET
Invasive cleavage	Mass spectrometry
	FRET
	FP

FRET, fluorescence resonance energy transfer; FP, fluorescence polarization.

largely been substituted by STR analysis. To take full advantage of new ASO probe formats for SNP typing, it is necessary to use detection methods that provide high accuracy, high sensitivity, and high throughput.

2.1.1. Homogeneous Hybridization Using FRET

Fluorescence resonance energy transfer (FRET) occurs when two fluorescent dyes are in close proximity to one another and the emission spectrum of one fluorophore overlaps the excitation spectrum of the other fluorophore *(12)*. These genotyping methods combine allele discrimination using ASO probes with real-time PCR reactions and quantification. Therefore, in addition to the probes for genotyping, two PCR primers are required. The increase in fluorescence can be measured in real-time during the PCR or when the PCR has finished. There are several variations based on the same principle.

2.1.1.1. LIGHTCYCLER (ROCHE)

Two specially designed sequence specific oligonucleotides labeled with fluorescent dyes are applied for this detection method. Probe 1 carries a fluorescein label at its 3' end and probe 2 carries another label (LC Red 640 or 705) at the 5' end. The sequences of the two oligonucleotides are selected such that

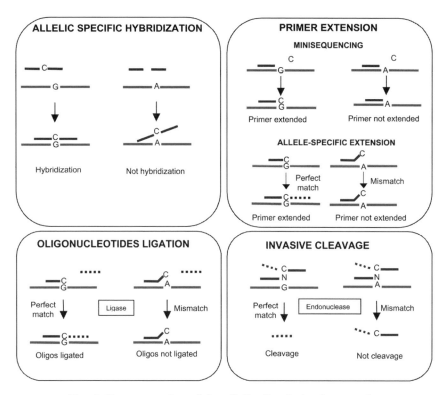

Fig. 1. Representation of the allelic discrimination reactions.

they hybridize adjacent to one another on the DNA target. When the oligonucleotides are hybridized, the two fluorescence dyes are positioned in close proximity to each other. The first dye (fluorescein) is excited and emits green fluorescent light and with the two dyes in close proximity, the emitted energy excites the adjacent LC Red 640 or 705, which subsequently emits fluorescent light (**Fig. 2A**). This energy transfer, referred to as FRET, is highly dependent on the spacing between the two dye molecules. The energy transferred at a high enough efficiency only if both molecules are within a distance of one to five nucleotides. The intensity of the light emitted by the dye LC Red 640 is filtered and measured by the optics in the LightCycler instrument. The increasing amount of measured fluorescence is proportional to the increasing amount of DNA generated during the ongoing PCR process. Because LC Red 640 or 705 only emit a signal when both oligonucleotides are hybridized, the fluorescence measurement is performed after the annealing step.

Two hybridization probes complementary to a specific region of the amplified sequence are designed. One of the probes is arranged with the polymorphic base in a central position and the other must be adjacent to allow for FRET.

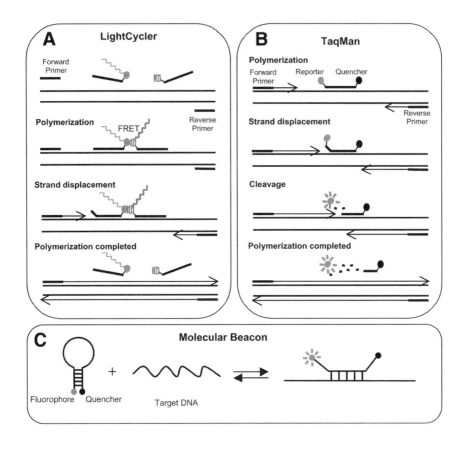

Fig. 2. Representation of different SNP genotyping methods by real-time PCR and FRET detection. (**A**) LightCytcler; (**B**) TaqMan; (**C**) Molecular Beacon.

It is well known that a single mismatch can significantly reduce the melting temperature of the oligonucleotide and that this reduction primarily depends on the length of the oligonucleotide and the position of the mismatch. The reduced melting temperature is measured by performing a melting curve analysis. This method may, of course, also be applied by using hybridization probes matching the mutant and having a mismatch with the wild type.

More than one SNP can be simultaneously genotyped combining the use of the two different fluorescent labels with the design of probes with different melting temperatures. Nevertheless, it is difficult to perform more than four-plex PCR *(13)*. The main advantage of this system is the high sensitivity *(13)*.

2.1.1.2. TAQMAN ASSAY (APPLIED BIOSYSTEMS)

The TaqMan assay is based in the 5' nuclease activity of Taq polymerase that displaces and cleaves the oligonucleotide probes hybridized to the target DNA, generating a fluorescent signal *(14,15)*. Two TaqMan probes that differ at the polymorphic site are required; one probe is complementary to the wild-type allele and the other to the variant allele. These probes have different fluorescent dyes attached to the 5' end and a quencher attached to the 3' end *(16)*. When the probes are intact, the quencher interacts with the fluorophore by FRET, quenching their fluorescence. During the PCR annealing step, the TaqMan probes hybridize to the target DNA. In the extension step, the 5' fluorescent dye is cleaved by the 5' nuclease activity of the Taq polymerase, leading to an increase in fluorescence of the reporter dye (**Fig. 2B**). Mismatch probes are displaced without fragmentation. The genotype of a sample is determined by measuring the signal intensity of the two different dyes.

A three-plex has been described *(17)* using six different reporter dyes. However, the detection was performed in a luminescence spectrometer after PCR because the real-time PCR instrument normally used in this assay is not able to measure more than four dyes.

Another detection method that can be used in TaqMan assays is fluorescence polarization (FP) *(18)*. When a fluorophore is excited by plane-polarized light, its emissions remains polarized if the molecule is still and the angle between the exciting plane and the emitting plane is a function of the mass of the molecule when other parameters are kept constant. In principle, any genotyping method in which the product of the allelic discrimination reaction is substantially larger or smaller than the starting fluorescent molecule can use FP as a detection method. Because the TaqMan probe is labeled with a fluorescent dye and the starting probe has a much higher molecular weight than the cleavage products, the FP changes drastically in a positive reaction.

2.1.1.3. MOLECULAR BEACONS

Molecular beacons are oligonucleotides probes that have two complementary sequences flanking the complementary sequence to the target DNA, with a fluorophore in the 5' end and a quencher in the 3' end (**Fig. 2C**). The probe adopts a hairpin-loop conformation when not hybridized to the target, and the fluorophore is quenched by the quencher and, therefore, no fluorescence is emitted. When the molecular beacon is bound to a perfectly complementary target, the fluorophore and the quencher are separated and fluorescence appears *(19)*. For SNP typing, two molecular beacons are used, one specific for the wild-type allele and the other specific for the mutant allele. Each of them is labeled with different fluorophores allowing allelic discrimination in one PCR *(20)*.

Different targets can be detected in the same reaction. This is accomplished using different molecular beacons for each target and attaching a different color fluorophore to each *(21)*. The number of different fluorophores that can be used in the same reaction is limited by the detection capability of available instruments. Instruments that can be used to perform PCR while simultaneously monitoring fluorescence in real-time use a monochromatic light source, such as a laser or light-emitting diodes. By using wavelength-shifting molecular beacons, this problem is solved. These probes emit fluorescent light in a distinct range of colors even though they are excited by the same monochromatic light source *(22)*. This approach increases the multiplex capability for SNP typing.

The principal advantage of homogenous hybridization methods is that no post-PCR process is necessary because PCR and detection are performed in the same reaction. This allows for high-throughput genotyping of a few SNPs in many samples, but the method has the serious drawback of limited multiplexing capability.

2.1.2. Array Hybridization and Fluorescence Detection

In this approach, short oligonucleotides are attached to a solid support, to create a microarray, and are hybridized with fluorescent-labeled PCR products containing the SNP sequence. This is more suitable to analyze many SNPs in parallel. However, the efficiency of the hybridization and the stability of hybrids depend not only on the polymorphic site but also on the SNP flanking sequence *(23)*. Therefore it is very difficult to design optimum conditions to simultaneously analyze a large number of SNPs. This difficulty is overcome in the GeneChip system (Affymetrix) using tens of ASO probes for each SNP. The probes include all possible sequences at the polymorphic site and some nucleotides that flank the SNP: a technique referred to as tiling strategy *(24,25)*. The GeneChip is produced with parallel light-directed chemistry to synthesize specific oligonucleotide probes covalently bound at defined locations on a chip *(26,27)*. This method is designed for genotyping a large number of SNPs at a scale that far exceeds current forensic requirements.

2.2. Primer Extension

Primer extension is based on the ability of DNA polymerase to incorporate specific deoxyribonucleotides that are complementary to the sequence of the template DNA. There are several variations of the primer extension reaction; however, they can be divided into two main types of reaction. First, there is the minisequencing reaction or single nucleotide primer extension, where the polymorphic base is determined by the addition of the ddNTP complementary to the base interrogated by a DNA polymerase. Second, there is the allele-specific extension, where the DNA polymerase amplifies only if the primers have a perfect match with the template (**Fig. 1**). One other alternative approach for DNA sequencing is pyrosequencing, which is also based on the DNA polymerase reaction *(28,29)*.

2.2.1. Minisequencing

In the minisequencing reaction (**Fig. 1**), a primer that anneals to its target DNA immediately adjacent to the SNP is extended by a DNA polymerase with a single nucleotide that is complementary to the polymorphic site *(30–32)*. This method is based on the high accuracy of nucleotide incorporation by DNA polymerases.

The detection of SNPs in the human genome, and also in other large genomes, requires the previous PCR amplification of the region that flanks the variable site. This is a requirement in most of the technologies used for genotyping SNPs. Before the minisequencing reaction, it is necessary to remove the excess PCR reagents, such as PCR primers and dNTPs, from the previous PCR amplification to obtain the specific product from the primer extension.

There are different technologies for analyzing the primer extension products. The use of labeled nucleotide or unlabeled nucleotide, ddNTP combined with dNTP or only ddNTP, in the minisequencing reaction depends on the method selected for detecting the products.

The capability of multiplexing depends also on the technology used. The most common technologies used for analyzing minisequencing products are SNaPshot (Applied Biosystems), matrix-assisted laser desorption ionization time-of-flight mass spectrometry (MALDI-TOF MS) , and microarrays.

2.2.1.1. SNaPSHOT (APPLIED BIOSYSTEMS)

The SNaPshot multiplex single-base extension reaction uses fluorescent ddNTPs. An unlabeled primer is positioned with the 3' end at the base immediately upstream to the SNP site and is extended with a single ddNTP that is labeled with a fluorescent dye. Each ddNTP is assigned one fluorescent dye. Multiplex reactions can be accomplished by spatial separation of the minisequencing products using "tails" at the 5' end of the SNaPshot primers with varying lengths of nonhuman sequence. The products are then separated electrophoretically in an automated capillary DNA sequencer. It is possible to perform a 10-plex according to the manufacturer's protocol, but larger multiplexes have been developed *(33,34)*.

2.2.1.2. MALDI-TOF MS

MALDI-TOF MS measures the molecular weight of the products formed in a minisequencing reaction. Therefore, it is the most direct method of detection compared with the other assay formats that infer the identity of the products by monitoring the fluorescence emitted by labeled molecules. The mass of the base added to the extended primer is determined by the incremental mass of ddNMP residues added *(35)*. The smallest mass difference is between ddA and ddT: 9 Daltons. The resolution of MALDI-TOF MS is very high; therefore, it is possible to distinguish which ddNTP has been incorporated in the primer extension.

Minisequencing products are deposited onto a matrix on the surface of a plate or a chip. The matrix and the DNA product are hit with a pulse from a laser beam in a process known as desorption. Energy from the laser beam is transferred to the matrix and it is vaporized, resulting in a small amount of the DNA product being expelled into a flight tube. The DNA product is subsequently accelerated towards a detector as it becomes charged when an electrical field pulse is applied to the flight tube. The time between application of the electrical field pulse and collision of the DNA product with the detector is referred to as the time of flight. This is a very precise measure of the molecular weight of the DNA products because molecular mass correlates directly with time of flight: lighter molecules flying faster and hitting the detector quicker than heavier molecules. Specific software converts this time of flight into an exact mass.

There are several approaches for typing SNPs with MALDI-TOF. The PROBE assay (MassEXTEND, Sequenom) combines the use of ddNTP with dNTPs in the extension reaction to increase mass differences between the alleles of a SNP. *(36)*. In the PinPoint assay (Applied Biosystems), only ddNTPs are used *(35)*. Despite the fact that the smallest mass difference of 9 Daltons can be detected, it is difficult to distinguish between A/T, A/A, and T/T genotypes *(37)*.

One limitation of MALDI-TOF analysis is the purity of the sample required by the assay. This problem is solved in the GOOD assay *(38)*, which increases the sensitivity using modification primers. Although this requires more reaction steps, all the reagents can be added to a single tube.

If the minisequencing products have nonoverlapping mass, the assay can be multiplexing *(39)*. This can be achieved adding a nonhuman tail sequence at the 5' end of the primer, as in the SNaPshot reaction. A 12-plex has been described by Ross et al. *(40)* and even a 20-plex by Kim et al *(41)*.

2.2.1.3. Microarrays

The microarray format also is suitable for genotyping SNPs with minisequencing, which can be performed on the chip surface or in solution. In the first case, minisequencing primers are attached to a chip (**Fig. 3**). This reaction is also known as arrayed primer extension *(42,43)*. The primers are

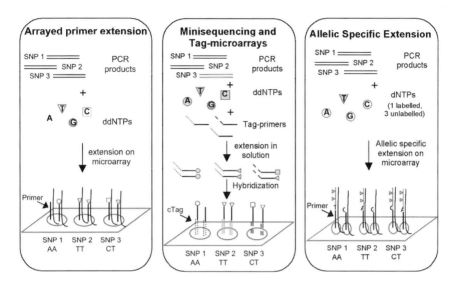

Fig. 3. SNP typing technologies with microarrays.

extended by a DNA polymerase with labeled ddNTPs and the microarray is scanned to measure fluorescence. In the second case, the SNPs are genotyping by a single base extension using minisequencing primers with a unique sequence tag at the 5' end *(44,45)*. Each SNP has a distinct identifying tag. The product of the multiplex minisequencing reaction performed in solution is hybridized to the reverse complementary sequences of the tags arrayed onto the chip (**Fig. 3**).

In Pastinen et al. *(46)*, an "array of arrays" format for slides was described. This allows the analysis of up to 80 different samples per slide by creating different hybridization chambers with silicon rubber grids.

2.2.1.4. FP

As previously described, FP can be used for detecting any allelic discrimination product where the initial molecules have different sizes. In the case of minisequencing, the primer is extended by the dye-terminator that is specific for the allele present on the template, increasing approximately 10-fold the molecular weight of the fluorophore *(47)*.

2.2.2. Pyrosequencing

Pyrosequencing is a sequencing-by-synthesis method. This technology uses an enzyme cascade system, consisting of four enzymes and specific substrates, to produce light whenever a nucleotide is complementary to the template DNA strand *(28,29)*. This light signal is detected, the base registered, and the next nucleotide added. If the added nucleotide is not complementary to the next base in the template, no light will be generated. The detection is based on the pyrophosphate released during the DNA polymerase reaction. The reaction mixture consists of single-stranded DNA with an annealed primer, DNA polymerase, ATP sulfurylase, luciferase, and apyrase. The four nucleotides are added to the mixture in a defined order (i.e., CGAT). If the added nucleotide forms a base pair, the DNA polymerase incorporates the nucleotide and pyrophosphate will consequently be released. The released pyrophosphate will be converted to ATP by ATP sulfurylase. Luciferase then uses the ATP to generate detectable light. The light intensity is proportional to the number of incorporated nucleotides. The excess of each nucleotide will be degraded by apyrase. If the added nucleotide does not form an incorporated base pair with DNA template no light will be produced.

Pyrosequencing provides rapid real-time determination of 20–30 base pairs of target DNA. With this technology, the SNP alleles are determined, including adjacent base positions as a built in control.

The limiting factors of pyrosequencing are the template preparation required and the degree of multiplexing. Before analysis, PCR products need to be converted to single stranded template onto which a sequencing primer is annealed. This is achieved using biotinylated PCR products. In addition, as with real time PCR, the method has the problem of limited multiplex capability.

2.2.3. Allele-Specific Extension

Allele-specific extension relies on the difference in extension efficiency of DNA polymerase between primers with matched and mismatched 3' ends. DNA polymerase extends a primer only when the 3' end is perfectly complementary to the DNA template (**Fig. 1**). Two primers are required, one for each allele of a SNP. By detecting which primer forms the product, the genotype of a sample can be determined. The product of this reaction can be detected on a microarray using fluorescently labeled nucleotides (*48*).

Another variant of this reaction is the use of allelic-specific primers: where the matching primer allows the amplification of a specific allele in a sample. In this case, the reaction is called allele-specific PCR. The detection of the appropriate PCR products allows the genotyping of the sample (*49,50*). The use of tag-primers allows the specific identification of each PCR product, in some cases based on melting curve analysis (*51*) and in other cases on the detection of fluorescent tags (*52*).

2.3. ASO Ligation

DNA ligase is highly specific in repairing nicks (a missing phosphodiester bond) in the DNA. Landergren et al., (*53*) described the oligonucleotide ligation assay (OLA) as a method for SNP typing based on the ability of ligase to

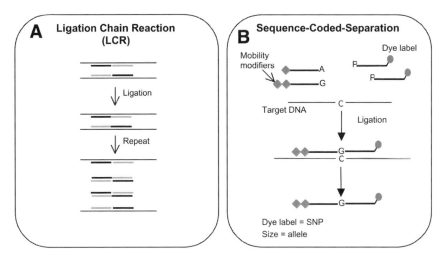

Fig. 4. Representation of ligase chain reaction (**A**) and sequence-coded separation of OLA reactions (**B**).

covalently join two oligonucleotides when they hybridize next to one another on a DNA template. The OLA assay requires that three probes are designed, one common and two allele specific. The common probe anneals to the target DNA immediately downstream of the SNP. One allelic probe has at the 3' end the nucleotide complementary to one allele, with the other allelic probe complementary to the alternative allele. These two allelic probes compete to anneal to the DNA target adjacent to the common probe. This generates a double stranded region containing a nick at the allele site. Only the allelic probe perfectly matched to the target will be ligated to the common probe by the DNA ligase (**Fig. 1**). The use of thermostable DNA ligase allows repeated thermal cycles, resulting in a linear increase in ligation products. If both strands of genomic DNA are used as targets for oligonucleotide hybridization, the increasing of ligation products can be exponential. This reaction is called ligase chain reaction *(54)*. Two sets of oligonucleotides, complementary to each target strand, are used. The ligation products from the first ligation reaction can then be the targets for the next round of ligation (**Fig 4**). Different assay formats have been developed for detecting the ligated product. The use of biotin on the common probe and a reporter group on the allelic specific probe allows for product capture and detection *(53)*. Other assays have replaced the biotin with mobility modifiers and the allelic specific probes have been labeled with different fluorescent dyes, enabling the ligation products to be discriminated by size and color *(55)*. The use of mobility modifiers and fluorescent dyes allows a multiplexed OLA to be performed where the products of this reaction are resolved electrophoretically under denatured conditions with fluorescent detection

(**Fig. 4**). The mobility modifiers allow the precise regulation of the mobility of each ligation product regardless of oligonucleotide length. This strategy has been termed sequence-coded separation by Grossman et al. *(55)*. In this assay a PCR is performed before the OLA reaction. However, the coupled amplification and oligonucleotide ligation procedure *(56)* combines multiplex amplification and SNP typing in one reaction. This is achieved using PCR primers with high melting temperatures and oligonucleotide ligation probes with lower melting temperatures. All the reagents are added simultaneously to one tube, minimizing the manual work and allowing easy automation. During the first stage of the reaction the PCR primers anneal to the DNA target and amplification occurs at a temperature above the melting temperature of the oligonucleotide ligation probes. In the second stage the temperature is lowered, allowing the probes to hybridize and for ligation to occur. Ligation products are detected using a fluorescence DNA sequencer.

A variation of the coupled amplification and oligonucleotide ligation assay is the dye-labeled oligonucleotide ligation *(57)*. In this case the ligation products are detected by monitoring FRET in real time. Three dye-labeled ligation oligonucleotides are needed for each biallelic marker. The common probe is labeled at 5' end with a donor dye, and the allele-specific probes have an acceptor dye at the 3' end. When ligation occurs, an increase in FRET is detected.

2.4. Invasive Cleavage

The Invader assay (Third Wave Technology) is based on the specificity of recognition, and cleavage, by a Flap endonuclease, of the three-dimensional structure formed when two overlapping oligonucleotides hybridize perfectly to a target DNA *(58,59)*.

The two oligonucleotides required, called "invader oligonucleotide" and "probe," anneal to the target DNA with an overlap of one nucleotide. The invader oligonucleotide is complementary to the sequence on the 3' side of the SNP. The probe is designed with the allelic base at the overlapping fragment and contains two regions, one complementary to one of the alleles of the SNP and the sequence on the 5' side of the polymorphic site and a non complementary 5' arm region (**Fig. 1**). When the allelic base is complementary to the base in the probe, the probe overlaps the 3' end of the invader oligonucleotide, forming the structure that is recognized and cleaved by the Flap endonuclease, releasing the 5' arm probe. If there is a mismatch, the structure formed will not be recognized by the Flap endonuclease and cleavage will not occur. This specificity of substrate structure recognition enables detection of single nucleotide mutations. The 5' arm probe serves as an invader oligonucleotide in a secondary cleavage reaction with a signal probe.

Performing the invasive reaction at elevated temperatures allows for rapid denaturation of the probe after cleavage, enabling the endonuclease to produce multiple cleaved probes per target DNA molecule. Because of this, the signal is amplified and, together with the secondary cleavage reaction, the amplification is exponential. Therefore, the Invader assay is a genotyping method without the requirement of previous PCR amplification *(58,60,61)*, but a large amount of target DNA is needed. In order to increase the sensitivity, this assay can also performed with a PCR step before the invader reaction, known as PCR-Invader assay *(62)*.

Different detection methods can be used, involving different designs of probe. When FRET is the detection method, a reporter dye is placed on the 5' arm and the quencher is placed on the complementary region of the probe *(60,62)*. The cleavage event removes the fluorophore and enhances fluorescence. With FP detection, the probe is labeled with a fluorophore at the 5' end. When the probe is cleaved, the molecular weight of the fluorophore decreases with the corresponding decrease in FP *(63)*. If mass spectrometry is the detection method, probes are designed with different numbers of nucleotides *(64)*.

3. Discussion

SNP genotyping technologies have been developing rapidly in the last few years. As a result, a great variety of different SNP typing protocols have become available for researchers, but there is no single protocol that meets all research needs. The level of throughput required depends on each application. Some applications use few SNP markers but a large sample size, other applications require a large number of SNPs in a few samples and, finally, there are other applications that need large number of both SNPs and samples. For forensic purposes, a medium throughput is required for paternity testing and criminal casework, but a high throughput is necessary to implement criminal DNA databases.

An important limiting step in virtually all these technologies is the PCR amplification. In forensic applications the development of multiplex PCR is essential, not only from the throughput point of view but also as a consequence of the small amount of DNA available to be analyzed in much criminal casework. There are some technologies that analyze SNP markers without a previous PCR, like the Invader assay, but these strategies are not suitable for forensic genetics because of the large amount of DNA required for the analysis. At this point, considerable effort is needed to successfully develop PCR with increased multiplex capability. All the technologies that have limited multiplexing capability should be excluded as candidates for routine forensic analysis; however, they could be useful for estimating the allele frequencies of the SNPs selected SNPs and also for creating large criminal DNA databases.

Another important issue in forensic genetics is the analysis of mixtures. Because of the biallelic nature of the majority of the SNPs, it will be more difficult to detect the presence of a mixture in a sample using these markers. Therefore, the possibility of the quantification of each allele in a sample can help in the determination of the contribution of each component in a mixed profile. Some technologies such as mass spectrometry and pyrosequencing allow the possibility of some quantification. This feature is routinely used for estimating allele frequencies in pooled samples, but could be an advantageous feature useful in forensic genetics. All these aspects need to be taken into account in making the decision about which technology to use, notably the accuracy, sensitivity, flexibility, time-consumption, and cost of the SNP typing technique.

Biotechnology companies have been developing new strategies and have created considerable technical advances for SNP genotyping in the last few years. Rapid technological progress makes it all the more difficult to choose appropriate methods for specific applications, especially as technical advances are published at such regular intervals.

Acknowledgments

This work was supported by grants from Xunta de Galicia ((PGIDT01PX I20806 PR) and Ministerio de Educación y Ciencia (DGCYT.P4.BIO2000-0145-P4-02). B.S. has a fellowship from the Ramón Areces Foundation.

References

1. Sachidanandam, R., Weissman ,D., Schmidt, S. C., Kakol, J. M., Stein, L. D., Marth, G., et al. (2001) A map of human genome sequence variation containing 1.42 million single nucleotide polymorphisms. *Nature* **409,** 928–933.
2. Venter, J. C., Adams, M. D., Myers, E. W., Li, P. W., Mural, R. J., Sutton, G. G., et al. (2001) The sequence of the human genome. *Science* **291,** 1304–1351.
3. Zhao, Z., Fu, Y.X., Hewett-Emmett, D., and Boerwinkle, E. (2003) Investigating single nucleotide polymorphism (SNP) density in the human genome and its implications for molecular evolution. *Gene* **312,** 207–213.
4. The Y Chromosome Consortium. (2002) A nomenclature system for the tree of human Y-chromosomal binary haplogroups. *Genome Res.* **12,** 339–348.
5. Gill, P. (2001) An assessment of the utility of single nucleotide polymorphisms (SNPs) for forensic purposes. *Int. J. Legal Med.* **114,** 204–210.
6. Chakraborty, R., Stivers, D. N., Su, B., Zhong, Y., and Budowle, B. (1999) The utility of short tandem repeat loci beyond human identification: implications for development of new DNA typing systems. *Electrophoresis* **20,** 1682–1696.
7. Gabriel, S. B., Schaffner, S. F., Nguyen, H., Moore, J. M., Roy, J., Blumenstiel, B., et al. (2002) The structure of haplotype blocks in the human genome. *Science* **296,** 2225–2229.

8. Brion, M., Blanco-Verea, A., Lareu, M., Carracedo, A. (in press) 29 Y-chromosome SNP analysis in European populations, in *Progress in Forensic Genetics, 10* (Doutremepuich, C., and Morling, N., eds), Elsevier, Amsterdam.

9. Phillips, C., Lareu, M., Salas, A., Carracedo, A. (in press) Non binary Single Nucleotide Polymorphism markers, in *Progress in Forensic Genetics, 10* (Doutremepuich, C., and Morling, N., eds), Elsevier, Amsterdam.

10. Phillips, C., Lareu, M., Salas, A., Fondevila, M., Berniel, G., Carracedo, A., et al (in press) Population specific single nucleotide polymorphism, in *Progress in Forensic Genetics, 10* (Doutremepuich, C., and Morling, N., eds), Elsevier, Amsterdam.

11. Wallace, R. B., Shaffer, J., Murphy, R. F., Bonner, J., Hirose, T., and Itakura, K. (1979) Hybridization of synthetic oligodeoxyribonucleotides to phi 174 DNA: the effect of single base pair mismatch. *Nucleic Acids Res.* **6,** 3543–3557.

12. Clegg, R. M. (1992) Fluorescence resonance energy transfer and nucleic acids. *Methods Enzymol.* **221,** 353–388.

13. Lareu, M., Puente, J., Sobrino, B., Quintans, B., Brion, M., and Carracedo, A. (2001) The use of the LightCycler for the detection of Y chromosome SNPs. *Forensic Sci. Int.* **118,** 163–168.

14. Holland, P. M., Abramson, R. D., Watson, R., and Gelfand, D. H. (1991) Detection of specific polymerase chain reaction product by utilizing the 5'-3' exonuclease activity of Thermus aquaticus DNA polymerase. *Proc. Natl. Acad. Sci. USA* **88,** 7276–7280.

15. Livak, K. J., Flood, S. J., Marmaro, J., Giusti, W., and Deetz, K. (1995) Oligonucleotides with fluorescent dyes at opposite ends provide a quenched probe system useful for detecting PCR product and nucleic acid hybridization. *PCR Methods Appl.* **4,** 357–362.

16. Livak, K.J. (1999) allelic discrimination using fluorogenic probes and the 5' nuclease assay. *Genet. Anal. Biomol. Engin.* **14,** 143–149.

17. Lee, L. G., Livak, K. J., Mullah, B., Graham, R. J., Vinayak, R. S., and Woudenberg, T. M. (1999) Seven-color, homogeneous detection of six PCR products. *BioTechniques* **27,** 342–349.

18. Latif, S., Bauer-Sardina, I., Ranade, K., Livak, K. J., and Kwok, P. Y. (2001) Fluorescence polarization in homogeneous nucleic acid analysis II: 5'-nuclease assay. *Genome Res.* **11,** 436–440.

19. Tyagi, S., and Kramer, F. R. (1996) Molecular beacons: probes that fluoresce upon hybridization. *Nat. Biotechnol.* **14,** 303–308.

20. Kostrikis, L. G., Tyagi, S., Mhlanga, M. M., Ho, D. D., and Kramer, F. R. (1998) Spectral genotyping of human alleles. *Science* **279,** 1228–1229.

21. Tyagi, S., Bratu, D. P., and Kramer, F. R. (1998) Multicolour molecular beacons for allele discrimination. *Nat. Biotechnol.* **16,** 49–53.

22 Tyagi, S., Marras, S. A. E., and Kramer, F. R. (2000) Wavelength-shifting molecular beacons. *Nat. Biotechnol.* **18,** 1191–1196.

23. Conner, B. J., Reyes, A. A., Morin, C., Itakura, K., Teplitz, R. L., and Wallace, R. B. (1983) Detection of sickle cell beta S-globin allele by hybridization with synthetic oligonucleotides. *Proc Natl Acad Sci USA* **80,** 278–282.

24. Wang, D. G., Fan, J. B., Siao, C. J., Berno, A., Young, P., Sapolsky, R., et al. (1998) Large-scale identification, mapping, and genotyping of single-nucleotide polymorphisms in the human genome. *Science* **280,** 1077–1082.

25. Mei, R., Galipeau, P. C., Prass, C., Berno, A., Ghandour, G., Patil, N., et al. (2000) Genome-wide detection of allelic imbalance using human SNPs and high-density DNA arrays. *Genome Res.* **10,** 1126–1137.

26. Fodor, S. P., Read, J. L., Pirrung, M. C., Stryer, L., Lu, A. T., and Solas, D. (1991) Light-directed, spatially addressable parallel chemical synthesis. *Science* **251,** 767–773.

27. Pease, A. C., Solas, D., Sullivan, E. J., Cronin, M. T., Holmes, C. P., and Fodor, S. P. (1994) Light-generated oligonucleotide arrays for rapid DNA sequence analysis. *Proc Natl Acad Sci USA* **91,** 5022–5026.

28. Ronaghi, M., Karamohamed, S., Pettersson, B., Uhlen, M., and Nyren, P. (1996) Real-time DNA sequencing using detection of pyrophosphate release. *Anal. Biochem.* **242,** 84–89.

29. Ronaghi, M., Uhlen, M., and Nyrén, P., (1998) A sequencing method based on real-time pyrophosphate. *Science* **281,** 363–365.

30. Syvanen, A. C., Aalto-Setala, K., Harju, L., Kontula, K., and Soderlund, H. (1990) A primer-guided nucleotide incorporation assay in the genotyping of apolipoprotein E. *Genomics* **8,** 684–692.

31. Sokolov, B. P. (1990) Primer extension technique for the detection of single nucleotide in genomic DNA. *Nucleic Acids Res.* **18,** 3671.

32. Kuppuswamy, M. N., Hoffmann, J. W., Kasper, C. K., Spitzer, S. G., Groce, S. L., and Bajaj, S. P. (1991) Single nucleotide primer extension to detect genetic diseases: experimental application to hemophilia B (factor IX) and cystic fibrosis genes. *Proc. Natl. Acad. Sci. USA* **88,** 1143–1147.

33. Sanchez, J., Børsting, C., Hallenberg, C., Buchard, A., Hernandez, A., and Morling, N. (2003) Multiplex PCR and minisequencing of SNPs—a model with 35 Y chromosome SNPs. *Forensic Sci. Int.* **137,** 74–84.

34. Quintans, B., Alvarez-Iglesias, V., Salas, A., Phillips, C., Lareu, M., and Carracedo, A. (2004) Typing of mitochondrial coding region SNPs of forensic and anthropological interest using SNaPshot minisequencing. *Forensic Sci. Int.* **140,** 251.

35. Haff, L. A., and Smirnov, I. P. (1997) Single-nucleotide polymorphism identification assays using a thermostable DNA polymerase and delayed extraction MALDI-TOF mass spectrometry. *Genome Res.* **7,** 378–388.

36. Braun, A., Little, D. P., and Koster, H. (1997) Detecting CFTR gene mutations by using primer oligo base extension and mass spectrometry. *Clin. Chem.* **43,** 1151–1158.

37. Fei, Z., Ono, T., and Smith, L. M. (1998) MALDI-TOF mass spectrometric typing of single nucleotide polymorphisms with mass-tagged ddNTPs. *Nucleic Acids Res.* **26,** 2827–2828.

38. Sauer, S., Lechner, D., Berlin, K., Lehrach, H., Escary, J. L., Fox, N., et al. (2000) A novel procedure for efficient genotyping of single nucleotide polymorphisms. *Nucleic Acids Res.* **28,** E13.

39. Haff, L. A., and Smirnov, I. P. (1997) Multiplex genotyping of PCR products with MassTag-labeled primers. *Nucleic Acids Res.* **25,** 3749–3750.

40. Ross, P., Hall, L., Smirnov, I., and Haff, L. (1998) High level multiplex genotyping by MALDI-TOF mass spectrometry. *Nat. Biotechnol.* **16,** 1347–1351.

41. Kim, S., Shi, S., Bonome, T., Ulz, M. E., Edwards, J. R., Fodstad, H., et al. (2003) Multiplex genotyping of the human bcta2-adrenergic receptor gene using solid-phase capturable dideoxynucleotides and mass spectrometry. *Anal. Biochem.* **316,** 251–258.

42. Shumaker, J. M., Metspalu, A., and Caskey, C. T. (1996) Mutation detection by solid phase primer extension. *Hum Mutat.* **7,** 346–354.

43. Pastinen, T., Kurg, A., Metspalu, A., Peltonen, L., and Syvanen, A. C. (1997) Minisequencing: a specific tool for DNA analysis and diagnostics on oligonucleotide arrays. *Genome Res.* **7,** 606–614.

44. Fan, J. B., Chen, X., Halushka, M. K., Berno, A., Huang, X., Ryder, T., et al. (2000) Parallel genotyping of human SNPs using generic high-density oligonucleotide tag arrays. *Genome Res.* **10,** 853–860.

45. Hirschhorn, J. N., Sklar, P., Lindblad-Toh, K., Lim, Y. M., Ruiz-Gutierrez, M., Bolk, S., et al. (2000) SBE-TAGS: an array-based method for efficient single-nucleotide polymorphism genotyping. *Proc. Natl. Acad. Sci. USA* **97,** 12,164–12,169.

46. Pastinen, T., Raitio, M., Lindroos, K., Tainola, P., Peltonen, L., and Syvänen, A. C. (2000) A system for specific, high-throughput genotyping by allele-specific primer extension on micoarrays. *Genome Res.* **10,** 1031–1042.

47. Chen, X., Levine, L., and Kwok, P. Y. (1999) Fluorescence polarization in homogeneous nucleic acid analysis. *Genome Res.* **9,** 492–498.

48. Pastinen, T., Raitio, M., Lindroos, K., Tainola, P., Peltonen, L., and Syvanen, A. C. (2000) A system for specific, high-throughput genotyping by allele-specific primer extension on microarrays. *Genome Res.* **10,** 1031–1042.

49. Newton, C. R., Graham, A., Heptinstall, L. E., Powell, S. J., Summers, C., Kalsheker, N., et al. (1989) Analysis of any point mutation in DNA. The amplification refractory mutation system (ARMS). *Nucleic Acids Res.* **17,** 2503–2516.

50. Okayama, H., Curiel, D. T., Brantly, M. L., Holmes, M. D., and Crystal, R. G. (1989) Rapid, nonradioactive detection of mutations in the human genome by allele-specific amplification. *J. Lab. Clin. Med.* **114,** 105–113.

51. Germer, S., and Higuchi, R. (1999) Single-tube genotyping without oligonucleotide probes. *Genome Res.* **9,** 72–78.

52. Myakishev, M. V., Khripin, Y., Hu, S., and Hamer, D. H. (2001) High-throughput SNP genotyping by allele-specific PCR with universal energy-transfer-labeled primers. *Genome Res.* **11,** 163–169.

53. Landergren, U., Kaiser, R., Sanders, J., and Hood, L. (1988) A ligase-mediated gene detection technique. *Science* **241,** 1077–1080.

54. Barany, F. (1991) The ligase chain reaction in a PCR world. *PCR Methods Appl.* **1,** 5–16.

55. Grossman, P. D., Bloch, W., Brinson, E., Chang, C. C., Eggerding, F. A., Fung, S., et al. (1994) High-density multiplex detection of nucleic acid sequences: oli-

gonucleotide ligation assay and sequence-coded separation. *Nucleic Acids Res.* **22,** 4527–4534.

56. Eggerding, F. A. (1995) A one-step Coupled Amplification and Oligonucleotide Ligation procedure for multiplex genetic typing. *PCR Methods Appl.* **4,** 337–345.

57. Chen, X., Livak, K. J., and Kwok, P. Y. (1998) A homogeneous, ligase-mediated DNA diagnostic test. *Genome Res.* **8,** 549–556.

58. Lyamichev, V., Mast, A. L., Hall, J. G., Prudent, J. R., Kaiser, M. W., Takova, T., et al. (1999) Polymorphism identification and quantitative detection of genomic DNA by invasive cleavage of oligonucleotide probes. *Nat. Biotechnol.* **17,** 292–296.

59. Kaiser, M. W., Lyamicheva, N., Ma, W., Miller, C., Neri, B., Fors, L., et al. (1999) A comparison of eubacterial and archaeal structure-specific 5'-exonucleases. *J. Biol. Chem.* **274,** 21387–21394.

60. Ryan, D., Nuccie, B., and Arvan, D. (1999) Non-PCR-dependent detection of the factor V Leiden mutation from genomic DNA using a homogeneous Invader microtiter plate assay. *Mol. Diagn.* **4,** 135–144.

61. Hall, J. G., Eis, P. S., Law, S. M., Reynaldo, L. P., Prudent, J. R., Marshall, D. J., et al. (2000) Sensitive detection of DNA polymorphisms by the serial invasive signal amplification reaction. *Proc. Natl. Acad. Sci. USA* **97,** 8272–8277.

62. Mein, C. A., Barratt, B. J., Dunn, M. G., Siegmund, T., Smith, A. N., Esposito, L., et al. (2000) Evaluation of single nucleotide polymorphism typing with Invader on PCR amplicons and its automation. *Genome Res.* **10,** 330–343.

63. Hsu, T. M., Law, S. M., Duan, S., Neri, B. P., and Kwok, P. Y. (2001) Genotyping single-nucleotide polymorphisms by the invader assay with dual-color fluorescence polarization detection. *Clin. Chem.* **47,** 1373–1377.

64. Griffin, T. J., Hall, J. G., Prudent, J. R., and Smith, L. M. (1999) Direct genetic analysis by matrix-assisted laser desorption/ionization mass spectrometry. *Proc. Natl. Acad. Sci. USA* **96,** 6301–6306.

9

Genotyping SNPs With the LightCycler

María Victoria Lareu and Clara Ruiz-Ponte

Summary

Here, a single nucleotide polymorphism typing methodology is described based on polymerase chain reaction monitoring, in real time, of fluorescently labeled amplified products using the LightCycler. The main advantages of the system are the time required for the analysis (about 20 min), combined with the robustness, accuracy, and the sensitivity of the method.

Key Words: SNPs; LightCycler; forensic science; DNA analysis; PCR on-line; real-time PCR.

1. Introduction

The study of single nucleotide polymorphism (SNPs) is becoming an increasingly important part of forensic genetics analysis. SNP loci are widespread and are adaptable to analysis from small amplicons, presenting the possibility of typing degraded deoxyribonucleic acid (DNA). One drawback of SNPs is the reduced discrimination resulting from having only two alleles compared with the much higher variability shown by short tandem repeats (STRs). This problem can be addressed by using high-throughput technologies that are less time consuming and give one the opportunity to automatically analyze large multiplexes. In comparison, the classical methods for typing SNPs are time-consuming and involve the use of restriction enzymes followed by polyacrylamide gel electrophoresis and silver staining (1). Improved methods for SNP analysis have been proposed, such as the use of DNA microarrays (including electronically activated microchips), matrix-assisted laser desorption ionization time-of-flight (MALDI-TOF) mass spectrometry, pyrosequencing, or Taq Man SNP assay (2). Other methods proposed for SNP analysis, such as heteroduplex

From: *Methods in Molecular Biology, vol. 297: Forensic DNA Typing Protocols*
Edited by: A. Carracedo © Humana Press Inc., Totowa, NJ

analysis by denaturating high performance liquid chromatography, are not robust enough for forensic analysis because of the difficulties in producing consistent and reproducible heteroduplex patterns *(3,4)*. However, denaturating high performance liquid chromatography *(5)* methods using denaturing gradients are robust and should be explored.

Among the new methodologies for SNP analysis worth consideration, one is on-line fluorescent polymerase chain reaction (PCR) monitoring in real time *(6,7)*. Several fluorescent formats and systems are available for correlating the fluorescent signals to the amount of PCR product amplified. The LightCycler (Roche Molecular Biochemicals, Mannheim, Germany) is an ultrarapid thermal cycler that allows one to monitor amplified PCR product in real time. The combination of using air for heating and fine capillaries to hold up to 20 µL of sample is essential in reducing the time for a single PCR cycle to less than 30 s. Therefore, a complete PCR run of 30 cycles can be typically performed in 20 min.

Real-time PCR allows quantification of target DNA using fluorescent hybridization probes or double-stranded dyes, such as SYBR Green I. The use of fluorescent hybridization probes with the LightCycler instrument offers the additional advantage of genotyping by melting curve analysis. Genotyping using hybridization probes is based on the principle of fluorescence resonance energy transfer (FRET; **Fig. 1**). FRET occurs when the donor fluorophore is excited photometrically and transfers its energy to the acceptor fluorophore. Then, the acceptor fluorophore emits fluorescence at a longer wavelength and is consequently detected by the instrument. This phenomenon only occurs when the two probes hybridize to the target together and in close proximity. The probes are designed to hybridize between the amplification primers. Fluorescein is the donor fluorophore and is usually the label attached to the 3' end of the probe whereas the 5' end of the adjacent probe is labeled with an acceptor fluorophore (either LCRed640 or LCRed705). The probe that spans the altered sequence is called the mutation probe. This probe can be complementary to the mutation or to the wild-type allele. If a mismatch occurs between the probe and the target DNA, the melting temperature (Tm) will decrease and detected differences in Tm thus allow the identification of alternative alleles at a SNP site.

There are different formats and strategies for PCR monitoring using the LightCycler. We have successfully used the LightCycler for Y chromosome SNP analysis for forensic applications *(8)* and autosomal SNP typing *(9)*. The strategy described will illustrate the methods used for SNP genotyping using fluorescent hybridization probes and melting curve analysis.

We successfully developed singleplexes of four different SNPs (M9, sY81, SRY-1532, and SRY-2627) in addition to two duplexes (M9 with sY81 plus SRY-1532 with SRY-2627). The simultaneous amplification and analysis of

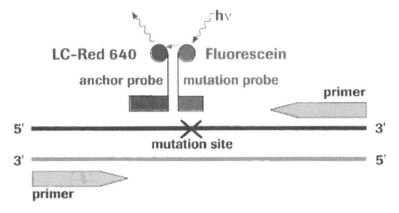

Fig. 1. FRET principle and hybridization probe design.

the four SNPs is also possible. It appears difficult to implement more than a four with the current LightCycler methodology. The genotyping accuracy was checked by testing a number of samples with this technology and conventional restriction enzyme analysis. In all cases, the results showed complete concordance, providing 100% accuracy *(8)*. As an example of autosomal SNP typing, we describe the strategy used to genotype a SNP: PMP22 located in 17p11.2 region.

2. Materials

2.1. Equipment

1. LightCycler Instrument (Roche Diagnostics, Mannheim, Germany).
2. LightCycler software version 3.3 (Roche Diagnostics).

2.2. Reagents

1. Amplification oligonucleotides (TIB MOLBIOL, Berlin, Germany).
2. Fluorescent hybridization probes (TIB MOLBIOL, Berlin, Germany). n.b. probes are light sensitive; store in dark at –20°C.
3. LightCycler-DNA Master Hybridization Probes (Roche Diagnostics).
4. Wizard Genomic DNA Purification Kit (Promega, Madison, WI).

3. Methods

3.1. Y Chromosome SNPs

3.1.1. Primers and Hybridization Probes Design

The primers used for sY81 and M9 amplifications were as previously described by Seielstad et al. *(10)* and Underhill et al. *(5)*, respectively. For SRY-1532 amplification the forward primer previously described by Santos et al. *(11)* was used with an alternative reverse primer SRY-1532, developed to avoid dimer forma-tion with the anchor probe. For the SRY-2627 SNP, the SRY gene sequence (Gene Bank database accession no. L08063) was used for the selection of primers.

To calculate the melting point and test for possible primer-primer interac-tions, the program designed by Williamstone Enterprises was used (http:// www.williamstone.com/primers/calculator). To test for possible repetitive sequences, primers were aligned with the GenBank nucleotide database at the National Center for Biotechnology Information (NCBI) using the Basic Local Alignment Search Tool (BLAST) program. The unlabeled oligonucle-otides used as amplification primers are listed in **Table 1**.

The fluorogenic sequence specific hybridization probes (*see* **Table 2**) were designed according to guidelines recommended by Roche Molecular Biochemicals (Technical Note LC 6/99; *see* **Note 1**). The upstream probe was labeled with fluorescein as donor fluorophore at the 3' end; the other probe was labeled at the 5' end with either LightCycler-Red 640 (sY81 and M9) or LightCycler-Red 705 (SRY-1532 and SRY-2627).

Genotyping with two hybridization probes is possible using the probe with the lowest stability ("sensor probe") positioned directly over the mutation to be detected and a longer "anchor probe" that recognizes an adjacent sequence. It is well known that a hybridization probe spanning one mismatch can still hybridize to the target sequence but will dissociate at a lower melting tempera-ture than a probe with a perfect match; therefore, polymorphic alleles can be distinguished by the Tm of the sensor probe. Unlabeled primers and fluorescently labeled hybridization probes were synthesized by TIB MOLBIOL (Berlin, Germany).

3.1.2. Rapid Cycle PCR and Melting Curve Analysis

PCR and melting curve analysis were performed in a 32-sample rapid fluo-rescent thermal cycler with three-color fluorescence monitoring capability (LightCycler). Each SNP was amplified at a 20 µL final volume using the fol-lowing:

1. 10 ng of genomic human DNA.
2. 0.25 µmol/L each primer,
3. 0.1 µmol/L anchor and sensor probe.
4. 2 µL of 10X LightCycler-DNA Master Hybridization Probes (Roche Molecular Biochemicals) containing Taq DNA polymerase, Taq PCR buffer, a dNTP mix-ture, and 10 mmol/L $MgCl_2$. The final Mg^{2+} concentration in the reaction mix-ture was adjusted to 3 mmol/L.

Samples were loaded into composite glass disposable capillaries, capped, briefly centrifuged, and placed in the LightCycler sample carousel.

Table 1
Primer Sequences Used for Y-SNP Amplifications

SNP	Size (bp)	Forward primer	Reverse primer
sY81	209	5' AGGCACTGGTCAGAATGAAG3'	5'AATGGAAAATACAGCTCCCC3'
M9	341	5'GCAGCATATAAAACTTTCAGG3'	5'AAAACCTAACTTTGCTCAAGC3'
SRY-1532	165	5'TCCTTAGCAACCATTAATCTGG3'	5'ATAGCAAAAAATGACACAAGGCA3'
SRY-2627	376	5'GAACTCCTTTACTGGGGTGATG3'	5'ATACGTGATGGTGACTGAACAG3'

Table 2
Sequence-Specific Hybridization Probes

SNP	GBD no.	Hybridization probes[a]
sY81	S76940	AAAATGTAGGTTTTATTATTATATTTCATTGT-X (Anchor)
		LCRed 640-AACAAAAGTCC**G**TGAGAT-P (Sensor)
M9	G42825	CAGAACTGCAAAGAAACGGCCTAA-X (Anchor)
		LCRed 640-TGGTTGAAT**G**CTCTTTATTTTTCTT-P (Sensor)
SRY-1532	L08063	ATCATTCAGTATCTGGCCTCTTGTATCT-X (Anchor)
		LCRed 705-CTTTTTCACACA**G**TGTAACATTTTCAA-P (Sensor)
SRY-2627	L08063	CCACAGGGTGC**T**CCACAGGGT-X (Sensor)
		LCRed 705-AAGCCCCATGCCCTACAGGGTGAAG-P (Anchor)

[a]Nucleotide bases in bold type are involved in genotyping at each SNP.
X indicates fluorescein.
P indicates a 3' phosphate.

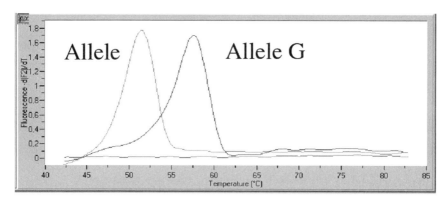

Fig. 2. SNP sY81 amplification and melting curve analysis of the two alleles of the system (allele A and allele G).

Figure 2 shows the graph of the sY81 amplification and the melting curve analysis of the two alleles of the system. In every case, each allele in each SNP was clearly distinguished.

For multiplex (quadruple) amplification, identical reagent concentrations were used, the only difference being the primer concentrations used: 1) 0.2 µ*M* each sY81 primer, 2) 0.6 µ*M* each M9 primer, 3) 0.5 µ*M* each SRY-1532 primer, and 4) and 0.2 µ*M* each SRY-2627 primer.

Table 3
Experimental Conditions for the Four Y-SNPs

Program	Cycles	Segment 1[a]	Segment 2[a]		Segment 3[a]
Denaturation	1	95°C for 30 s			
			SY81	60°C for 10 s	72°C for 8 s
			M9	59°C for 10 s	72°C for 13 s
			SRY-1532	60°C for 10 s	72°C for 7 s
Amplification	40	95°C for 0 s	SRY-2627	60°C for 10 s	72°C for 15 s
			SRY-1532/2627	61°C for 10 s	72°C for 15 s
			SY81/M9	59°C for 10 s	72°C for 13 s
			Quadruplex	60°C for 10 s	72°C for 15 s
Melting	1	95°C for 0 s		40°C for 60 s	85°C for 0 s
Cooling	1	40°C for 0 s			

[a]The temperature transition rate was 20°C/s, except in the segment 3 of the melting program, where it was 0.2°C/s.

Table 4
Melting Temperatures of the Four Y-SNPs Analyzed

	Average melting temperatures			
SNP	Allele 0	Allele 1	Mismatch	Label
SY81	51.35°C	57.48°C	G–T	LCRed-640
M9	57.85°C	61.78°C	G–C	LCRed-640
SRY-1532	59.26°C	64.02°C	G–T	LCRed-705
SRY-2627	65.68°C	68.57°C	T–G	LCRed-705

The LightCycler protocol for sequence-specific detection and analysis of DNA with hybridization probes contains four cycling programs: initial denaturation of template DNA, amplification of target DNA, melting curve analysis (for identification of mutated sequences), and cooling of the instrument. All programs used, except for the amplification program, were identical in all assays (including multiplexes). The protocol is shown in **Table 3**.

The melting temperatures of the four SNPs analyzed are shown in **Table 4** (*see* **Note 2**). The SNPs labeled with the same fluorophore have different Tm values so without overlap. They can be accurately distinguished and typed.

An advantage of genotyping Y chromosome SNPs with the LightCycler is that these loci are much more sensitive when used in the detection of male

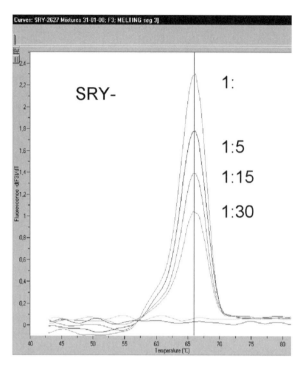

Fig. 3. SRY-2627 analyzed in male–female mixtures at different proportions.

DNA in male–female mixtures compared with Y chromosome STRs (**Fig. 3**; *see* **Note 3**).

3.2. Autosomal SNPs: Genotyping SNP: PMP22 Located in 17p11.2 Region

3.2.1. Hybridization Probe Design

Primers and probes were designed by TIB MOLBIOL, with sequences and Tm listed in **Table 5**.

3.2.2. Rapid Cycle PCR

Amplification was performed using the LightCycler DNA Master Hybridization Probes reagent (Roche Molecular Biochemicals) in a 20-μL final volume reaction containing: 0.4 μmol/L of each primer, 0.1 μmol/L of each probe, 2 μL of DNA sample (MgCl$_2$ final concentration was 4 mM).

After a pulse centrifugation in a microcentrifuge to fill the cuvets, the sealed capillaries were placed into the LC rotor. The reaction mixture was denatured at

Table 5
Oligonucleotides (GenBank Accession No. AC005703)

	Sequence (5'-3')	Position	Length	GC (%)	Tm (°C)
	Primers				
F	CCATGGCCAGCTCTCCTAAC	186862–186881	20	60	66.16
R	CATTCCGCAGACTTTGATGC	187099–187080	20	50	63.58
	Probes				
Anchor	TTCCAAATTCTTGCTGGTAAGTTG TGGAT-F	187027–187055	29	37.9	68.52
Sensor	LCRed640-TAAAGTCCATGTGGAAGCG GGGT	187058–187080	23	52.2	69.70

Tm, melting temperature.

95°C for 2 min followed by 31 cycles of (95°C for 0 s, ramp rate, 20°C/s), annealing (55°C for 10 s, ramp rate, 20°C/s), and extension (72°C for 5 s, ramp rate, 20°C/s).

3.2.3. Melting Curve Analysis and Genotyping

After amplification, melting curves were determined by a denaturation step at 95°C for 2 min followed by holding the reaction at 55°C for 10 s and then heating slowly to 80°C with a linear rate of 0.2°C/s. Fluorescence was monitored continually during the melting stage. As the temperature increased, the detection probe dissociated first from the allele with the mismatch and at later point in time, from the perfectly matched allele.

Melting curves were obtained by plotting fluorescence (F) vs temperature (T) and were seen as loss of fluorescent signal as the probes melted from the PCR product (**Fig. 4a**). The LightCycler software calculated the rate of change of fluorescence (–dF/dT) vs T. These derivative melting curves discriminate different alleles by differences in Tm (**Fig. 4b**). The SNP analyzed was a substitution of a C-T. The difference in Tm between the two alleles is 7°C (*see* **Note 4**).

4. Notes

1. For the design of specific hybridization probes, sequence was selected to delay displacement of the probe by the polymerase and to allow for maximum hybridization time, both hybridization probes for each SNP were placed as far away as possible from the extension primers and with the Tm set 5–10°C higher than the Tm of the primers. To avoid extension by the Taq polymerase, the 3' end of the downstream probe was phosphorylated. Only when the two probes are hybrid-

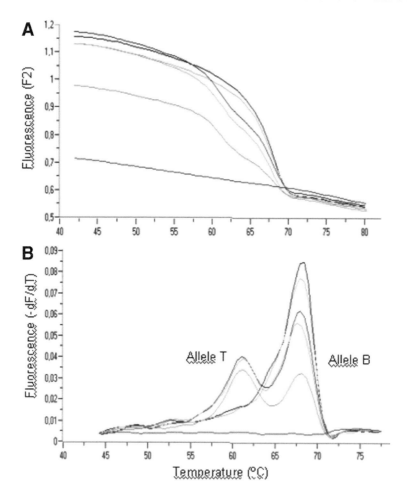

Fig. 4. Hybridization melting curves of five samples. (A) Melting curves, probes dissociating from the target DNA results in decreasing fluorescence. (B) Derivative melting curves. The negative derivative of the melting curves versus temperature in a melting "peak."

ized and in close proximity, does FRET occur. To achieve optimal energy transfer, the spacing between each of the probes was chosen not to exceed more than one to four bases because a greater distance would lead to a loss of the fluorescence signal.

2. Genotyping using fluorescent hybridization probes offers the possibility of multiplex reactions with amplified products distinguished either by Tm, color, or both. Multiplex by color uses different acceptor fluorophores (LCRed640 and LCRed705) that are detected in different fluorescent channels on the LightCycler. A color compensation file is required to correct fluorescent at each temperature

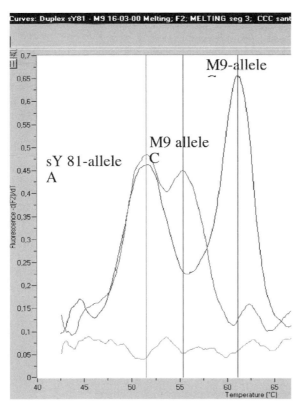

Fig. 5. Duplex amplification and analysis of M9 and sY81 in two different samples. The sample in blue shows sY81 allele A and M9 allele G. In red sY81 allele A and M9 allele C.

and to correct spectral overlap of dyes between channels. Multiplex by Tm uses the same acceptor fluorophore for the two probes. In this strategy the mutation probes are designed with differences in G-C content or length. Simultaneous analysis of two SNPs can therefore easily be performed as shown in the **Fig. 5**. It is more difficult to design multiplexes for more than two SNPs because it is difficult to avoid the overlapping of melting temperatures of the different alleles. We were able to simultaneously amplify four Y-SNPs in the same reaction with very good results, although some problems did arise. For example, with a sample exhibiting the allele G of the sY81 system (Tm 57–58°C) and the allele C of the M9 system (55–56°C) labeled with the same fluorophore, a single peak is obtained with an intermediate Tm of 56–57°C. Despite this, typing can be made without problems because there is no overlap with the individual Tm of both systems. The same occurs with the allele G of SRY-1532 (63–64°C) and allele C of SRY-

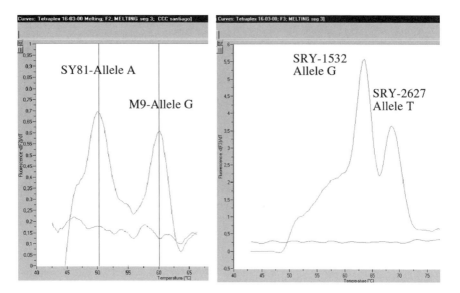

Fig. 6. A sample analyzed with the quadruplex designed with two SNPs (M9 and sY81) labeled with LC-Red 640 (on the left) and two SNPs (SRY-1532 and SRY-2627) labeled with LC-Red 705 (on the right).

2627 (65–66°C), which give a single peak with a Tm of 64–65°C when they occur simultaneously in a sample.

An example of a quadruplex that we have designed is shown in **Fig. 6** with two SNPs (M9 and sY81) labeled with LC-Red 640 and two SNPs (SRY-1532 and SRY-2627) labeled with LC-Red 705.

Multiplexes of more than four SNPs have the additional difficulty that the whole system (including probes and primers) needs to be designed so as to avoid dimer formation. We recommend using singleplex or duplex amplification in forensic casework samples.

3. Mixture samples. 10 mixed male–female DNA samples in different proportions were used in the analysis of different Y-SNPs. It was possible to reliably detect proportions 1 to 300 (male:female) with the SRY-2627 system and up to 1 to 100 with the other SNPs for all the samples analyzed. Occasionally the male component in higher dilutions was detected. In our experience, this sensitivity is much higher compared with STRs, which always exhibited lower sensitivity when the same samples were analyzed and offers new possibilities for the analysis of minimal male DNA in female material, which is of great importance in sexual crimes. More variable results were obtained in real male–female bloodstains, probably because of the individual variation of the amount of DNA in different samples. However, it was always possible to detect male: female mixtures up to 1:50 with the SNPs used.

4. When genotyping by melting curve analysis, it was not always possible to distinguish the two alleles of a heterozygote by the software analysis. One broader curve could be obtained representing the two alleles. This problem is attributable to PCR mixtures and can be resolved by repeating the assay or adjusting the number of degrees selected to calculate the derivative curves. Another solution is to click on the "enable" filter of the LC data analysis software to deactivate the predetermined option of "enable." This provokes melting curves that are not as smooth but are sufficient in discriminating between the two alleles.

Acknowledgments

This work was supported by grants from the Xunta de Galicia (XUGA 20806B97 and PGIDT99PXI20807B). The technical assistance of Meli Rodriguez is highly appreciated.

References

1. Brión, M., Lareu, M. V., Pereira, L., Gonzalez-Neira, A., Salas, A., Prata, M. J., Amorin, A., and Carracedo, A. (2000) Y chromosome lineages in Iberians: Construction of highly informative haplotypes using biallelic markers, STRs and the minisatellite MSY1, in *Progress in Forensic Genetics, Vol. 8* (Sensabaugh, G. F., et al eds.), Elsevier, Amsterdam, pp. 263–265.
2. Carracedo, A., Barros, F., Loidi, L., and Dominguez, F. (1998) Progress in methodology and standards in European molecular genetics laboratories. *Clin. Chim. Acta* **278,** 163–169.
3. Barros, F., Carracedo, A., Lareu, M. V., and Rodríguez-Calvo, M. (1991), Electrophoretic HLADQA1 DNA typing after polymerase chain reaction amplification. *Electrophoresis* **12,** 1041–1045.
4. Barros, F., Lareu, M. V., and Carracedo, A. (1992) Detection of polymorphisms of human DNA after PCR by miniaturized SDS-polyacrylamide gel electrophoresis. *Foren. Sci. Int.* **55,** 27–36.
5. Underhill, P.A., Jin, L., Lin, A.A., Qasim Mehdi, S., Jenkins, T., Vollrath, D., et al. (1997) Detection of numerous Y chromosome biallelic polymorphisms by denaturing high-performance liquid chromatography. *Genome Res.* **7,** 996–1005.
6. Wittwer, C. T., Ririe, K. M., Andrew, R. V., David, D. A., Gundry, R. A., and Balis, U. J. (1997) The LightCycler: a microvolume multi-sample fluorimeter with rapid temperature control. *Biotechniques* **22,** 176–181.
7. Bernard, P. S., Lay, M. J., and Wittwer, C. T. (1998) Integrated amplification and detection of the C677T point mutation in the methylenetetrahydrofolate reductase gene by fluorescence resonance energy transfer and probe melting curves. *Anal. Biochem.* **255,** 101–107.
8. Lareu. M. V., Puente, J., Sobrino, B., Quintans, B., Brión, M., and Carracedo, A. (2001) The use of the LightCycler for the detection of Y chromosome SNPs. *Foren. Sci. Int.* **118,** 163–168

9. Ruiz-Ponte C., Loidi L., Vega A., Carracedo A., and Barros F. (2000) Rapid real-time fluorescent PCR gene dosage test for the diagnosis of DNA duplications and deletions. *Clin. Chem.* **46,** 1574–1582

10. Seielstad, M. T., Hebert, J. M., Lin, A. A., Underhill, P. A., Ibrahim, M., Vollrath, D., et al. (1994) Construction of human Y-chromosomal haplotypes using a new polymorphic A to G transition. *Hum. Mol. Genet.* **12,** 2159–2161.

11. Santos, F. R., Pandya, A., Tyler-Smith, C., Pena, S., Schanfield, M., Leonard, W. R et al. (1999) The Central Siberian origin for native American Y chromosomes. *Am. J. Hum. Genet.* **64,** 619–628.

10

Universal Tag Arrays in Forensic SNP Analysis

Marie Allen and Anna-Maria Divne

Summary

Microarray-based single nucleotide polymorphism (SNP) genotyping enables simultaneous and rapid detection of a large number of markers and is thus an attractive method for forensic individual acid identification. This assay relies on a one-color detection system and minisequencing in solution before hybridization to universal tag arrays. The minisequencing reaction is based on incorporation of a fluorescent dideoxynucleotide to a primer containing a tag-sequence flanking the position to be interrogated. This one-color system detects C and T polymorphisms in separate reactions on multiple polymerase chain reaction targets with the fluorophore TAMRA coupled to the respective dideoxynucleotide. After incorporation, tagged primer sequences are hybridized through their complementary sequence on the array, and positive signals are detected by a confocal laser-scanner.

Key Words: Microarrays; universal tag-arrays; minisequencing; forensic; SNP.

1. Introduction

The field of microarray-based deoxyribonucleic acid (DNA) analysis has expanded greatly during recent years and provides a powerful tool for the rapid and cost-effective detection of a large number of polymorphisms. This chapter describes the protocols for a microarray-based single nucleotide polymorphism (SNP) detection system, which is under development for analysis of forensic material. Markers for 21 polymorphisms in the mitochondrial genome and 12 nuclear SNPs were designed for simultaneous or separate analysis of forensic samples. This system is based on a limited number of markers, and a fully developed system will require approx 40–50 nuclear SNP markers to achieve a discrimination power similar to what is obtained using nuclear STR-markers *(1)*. The combination of nuclear and mitochondrial markers allow different

From: *Methods in Molecular Biology, vol. 297: Forensic DNA Typing Protocols*
Edited by: A. Carracedo © Humana Press Inc., Totowa, NJ

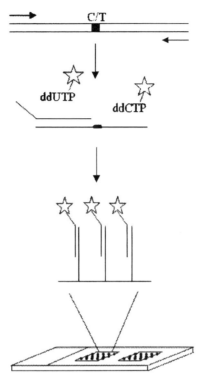

Fig. 1. The region of interest is amplified and used as template in the minisequencing reaction. Fluorescently labeled ddNTPs are incorporated at the SNP site in the 3' end of the minisequencing primer. The primers are then hybridized through their complementary zip addresses to the zip codes on the array

types of materials to be analyzed on the same platform. A sample with larger DNA amounts enables detection of the nuclear markers, whereas smaller amounts can be analyzed using the mitochondrial part of the chip. As forensic samples often contain highly degraded DNA, the polymerase chain reaction (PCR) design of very small amplicons (74–130 base pairs) increase the sensitivity.

Figures 1 and **2** illustrate the outline of a one-color microarray-based SNP detection system and its experimental procedure. The region of interest is first amplified by PCR and the SNP is detected by minisequencing in solution before hybridization onto universal tag arrays. The minisequencing primer is designed to contain two different sequences, one that is complementary to the region located 20 base pairs upstream of the SNP and one tag-sequence (zip address) that is complementary to the oligonucleotide (zip code) printed on the chip. In the minisequencing reaction, primers are extended with fluorescent dideoxynucleotides at the polymorphic site, and the solution is thereafter placed

EXPERIMENTAL PROCEDURE

1. Printing, blocking and washing of slides.

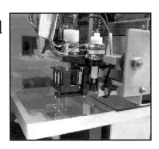

2. PCR and minisequencing

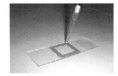

3. Hybridization and washing

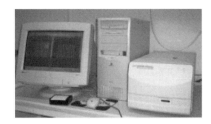

4. Scanning and quantification

Fig. 2. Overview of the experimental procedure. Oligonucleotides are printed on slides using a 417 arrayer (Affymetrix) with a capacity of 42 slides. After washing and blocking of the slide surface, slides are ready for hybridization experiments. After PCR and minisequencing the solution is placed in a hybridization chamber on the slide. Hybridization is carried out for 2 h and the slides are thereafter washed. The slides are scanned in the laser scanner ScanArray 5000 and the results are read and quantified by the software provided with the instrument.

in a reaction chamber on the microarray. The zip address sequences are hybridized to their complementary zip code on the array, and positive signals are detected by a confocal laser-scanner. The arrays are produced with an in-house robotic arrayer using slides with aldehyde chemistry.

2. Materials

2.1. Oligonucleotides

The 39-mer zip code oligonucleotides contain 15 T residues as a spacer coupled to an aminolinker C7 at the 3' end.

2.2. PCR Primer Design

PCR reverse primers carry phosphorothioate in the first five bases in the 5'-end.

2.3. Array Preparation and Blocking Procedure

1. NaHCO$_3$, pH 9.0.
2. Phosphate-buffered saline (PBS).
3. 99.5% Ethanol.
4. Sodium dodecyl sulfate (SDS).
5. NaBH$_4$ (fire hazard, creates toxic gas in contact with water; Sigma; St Louis, MO).
6. Silylated Slides, aldehyde groups (ArrayIt/TeleChem, Sunnyvale, CA).
7. GMS 417 Arrayer (Affymetrix, Santa Clara, CA).

2.4. PCR Amplification and Purification

1. AmpliTaq™ Gold Polymerase 5 U/µL (Applied Biosystems, Foster City, CA).
2. 1X PCR Taq Gold buffer (Applied Biosystems).
3. dNTPs.
4. MgCl$_2$.
5. QIAquick™ PCR Purification Kit (MERCK Eurolab, Germany).
6. T7 Gene Exonuclease 50 U/µL (USB Corporation, Cleveland, OH).
7. T7 Gene Exonuclease 6 Reaction Buffer (USB Corporation).

2.5. Multiplex Minisequencing

1. Thermo Sequenase™NA polymerase 32 U/µL (unstable in diluted aliquots) (Amersham Bioscience, Piscataway, NJ).
2. Thermo Sequenase Reaction Buffer.
3. ddATP, ddGTP.
4. Fluorescently labeled ddCTP-TAMRA and ddUTP-TAMRA (light-sensitive; NEN Life Science, Boston, MA).

2.6 Hybridization of Minisequencing Products to Zip Code Arrays

1. 15 × 15 or 9 × 9-mm Frame Seal Incubation Chambers (MJ Research, Watertown, MA, USA)
2. Saline sodium citrate (SSC).
3. *N*-lauroyl sarcosine (Sigma).
4. SDS.
5. Scan Array 5000 with autoloader function (Packard BioScience, Wellesley, MA).

3. Methods

3.1. Chip Design

A total of 33 mitochondrial and nuclear SNP markers with allele frequencies close to 0.5, among European populations, were chosen to design a forensic chip. Frequencies and locations of 10 autosomal nuclear markers were obtained from the HGbase database of human SNPs (http://hgybase.cgb.ki.se) with the exception of markers 2629 and XY, which corresponds to SNP PD-1.5 *(2)* and a SNP for sex determination *(3)*, respectively, **Table 1**.

3.2. Oligonucleotides

To enable covalent binding to the aldehyde groups on the microscopic slide, an aminolinker C7 is attached in the 3' end. To further improve hybridization, the spotted zip code contains a spacer of 15 T residues after the aminolinker at the 3' end. The 39-mer oligonucleotide also comprises a 24-mer zip code complementary to a corresponding zip address in the minisequencing primer. The design of the zip codes and their complementary zip addresses were followed as described by Gerry et al. 1999 *(5)*. In short, the zip code sequences consist of six tetramers, each of which differs from all others by at least two bases and all were designed to have similar Tm- values. Each minisequencing primer covers 20 bases upstream of the SNP and is tagged with a zip address in the 5' end (*see* **Notes 1** and **2**).

3.3. PCR Primer Design

PCR primer pairs covering SNP containing regions were designed to amplify fragments of lengths between 74 and 130 base pairs using the Primer Express 3.1 package software (Applied Biosystems). Reverse primers carry phosphothioate in the last six bases in the 3' end to protect the strand from degradation during exonuclease treatment.

3.4. Array Preparation and Blocking Procedure

1. Prepare spot solutions with a final concentration of 60 μM zip code oligonucleotide; 200 mM NaHCO$_3$, pH 9.0; and 0.07 % SDS in a 96-microtiter plate. Print two sets of 4 × 6 oligonucleotide arrays with two vertical replicates on Silylated Slides (**Fig. 3**) with reactive aldehyde groups using a 417 Arrayer. To obtain the dense spot pattern shown in **Fig. 3** using a four-pin-head arrayer, two consecutive rounds of printing is performed using the same preprogrammed pattern.
2. Before hybridization, remove uncoupled oligonucleotides and block unbound aldehyde residues by sequential washing in 0.2% SDS for 2 min, ddH$_2$O for 2 min, 0.5 g of NaBH$_4$ resuspended in 150 mL of 1X PBS and 50 mL of 99.5% ethanol for 5 min, 0.2% SDS for 2 min, followed by ddH$_2$O twice for 2 min.
3. Dry the slides by fan or put the slides in a slide box that fits a plate centrifuge and spin the slides at 82g for about 1 min. Incubate printed arrays for 12 h at room temperature and store at 4°C until use. Arrays are spotted with 3 μM of the control oligonucleotide sequence 5'-aminolinkC6-Poly (dT)$_{35}$-GACT-TAMRA-3' at the upper left corner and the lower right corner of the array. The TAMRA control is used as a control of successful binding to the support (*see* **Notes 3–5**).

Table 1
Location and Frequencies of the SNPs Detected by the Forensic Array

SNP name	Frequency in HGVbase (%C/%T)	Location
24	62/38	Xq28
155	45/55	20p11.21
2397	47/53	8p22
2629	52.5/47.5[a]	2q37.3
3288	45/55	11q23.1
3412	25/75	6p24-p23
5175	77/23	20q13.13
8075	67/33	11q23
8093	68/32	2p24-23
8101	65/35	16q13.2
8102	59/41	16q13.2
XY	50/50[b]	Xp21.3, Yp11.3
mt146		HVII
mt150		—
mt152		—
mt195		—
mt295		—
mt4216		Coding region
mt7028		—
mt10463		—
mt12705		—
mt14766		—
mt16126		HVI
mt16186		—
mt16189		—
mt16192		—
mt16223		—
mt16224		—
mt16256		—
mt16270		—
mt16294		—
mt16311		—
mt16519		Non coding region

The mt-polymorphisms detected are represented by their number according to the revised Cambridge reference sequence *(4)*

[a]Frequency obtained from previous work in our laboratory *(2)*.
[b]SNP obtained from Reynolds et al. *(3)*.

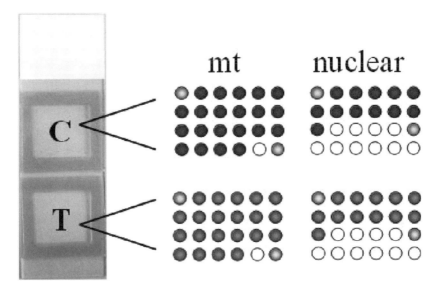

Fig. 3. Array pattern. Triplicates of the zip codes for the mitochondrial DNA and nuclear DNA markers are printed in two sets of 4 × 6-arrays. The two sets are divided into two separate areas on the slide to allow separate C and T reactions. Light grey spots denote reference spots of a TAMRA-labeled control oligonucleotide. Empty spots are printed with water or reagent blanks. The grey frames on the slide shows the thin adhesive hybridization chamber (size 15 × 15 mm)

3.5. PCR Amplification and Purification

1. Perform PCR amplifications of mitochondrial and nuclear DNA in 50-µL single or multiplex reactions.
2. Treat amplified products with 0.27 units/µL T7 gene exonuclease 6 in 1X T7 gene exonuclease 6 reaction buffer at 37°C for 15 min followed by inactivation of the enzyme at 80°C for 15 min. If dsDNA is used, go directly to step 3.
3. Pool single or double-stranded PCR products two and two and purify them by using the QIAquick™ PCR purification kit. Pool the purified PCR fragments into one mitochondrial and/or one nuclear reaction and resuspend the residual pellets in elution buffer or DI water to yield 2.25 times concentrated products. PCR amplifications of DNA from case material are performed as above with the following exceptions: the reactions are performed in 25-µL duplex reactions containing 0.25 µ*M* of the primers and 1 ng of DNA (*see* **Note 6**).

3.6. Multiplex Minisequencing

Perform two separate C and T minisequencing reactions in 30- or 15-µL volumes containing 5 µL of pooled, concentrated single-stranded PCR products, 0.25 µ*M* each of ddATP and ddGTP, 0.25 µ*M* of either ddCTP or ddTTP, and 1.6 μM of the fluorescently labeled ddCTP-TAMRA or ddUTP-TAMRA (NEN Life Science), 0.5 μM of each zip address, 1X Thermo Sequenase reaction buffer, and 0.32 U/μL Thermo Sequenase enzyme. The cycling procedure is performed by preheating at 95°C for 1 min followed by 10 cycles at 94°C for 15 s, 50°C for 30 s, 68°C for 1 min, 10 cycles at 94°C for 15 s, 45°C for 30 s, 68°C for 1 min, and 10 cycles at 94°C for 15 s, 40°C for 30 s, 68°C for 1 min in a 9700 thermal cycler (Applied Biosystems; *see* **Notes 7–9**).

3.7. Hybridization of Minisequencing Products to Zip Code Arrays

1. Preincubate the arrays in 4X SSC for 10 min and dry the slides by fan or centrifugation. Place two separate reaction chambers (15 × 15 or 9 × 9-mm Frame Seal Incubation Chambers) on the slides and hybridize the mitochondrial and nuclear minisequencing reactions on separate arrays or pooled together on the same array. For separate reactions, 10 µL of the C or T-minisequencing reaction are diluted with 40 µL or 20 µL of SSC (depending on the size of the incubation chamber) to yield a final concentration of 4X SSC. For pooled reactions, 9 µL of the nuclear and 15 µL of the mitochondrial reaction are added in a total volume of 30 µL.
2. Pipet the solution on the slide and carefully place the adhesive, plastic cover lid on top of the hybridization chamber. Start at one side of the frame and press it to cover the whole chamber. Press hard on the side of the frame to assure strong adhesion to the slide.
3. Put the slides in a rotating slide holder or in tubes that fit a rotisserie in a hybridization oven. Place cellstoff paper in the ends of the glass tubes for fixation and so that the slides don't break during rotation. Conduct hybridization at 50°C for 1–2 h (*see* **Notes 10** and **11**).
4. Remove the hybridization chambers. Wash slides in 6X SSC/0.05% *N*-lauroyl Sarcosine 2 × 5 min at room temperature and in 0.2X SSC/0.1%SDS for 3 × 15 min at 50°C on a shaker. Dry slides by fan or by using a plate centrifuge. Slides are thereafter ready for scanning.

3.8. Image Analysis

1. Positive signals on the arrays are detected using the confocal laser scanner Scan Array 5000 with autoloader function (Packard Biochip). Scan the slides using the ScanArray® version 2.11 software and start at default settings of PMT and laser (80, 80 respectively) and adjust if necessary.
2. Quantify the results by importing the scan images into the QuantArray® software one by one. The first image will be given a red color and the next a green color. If this order is used consequently, red spots will always denote the incorporation of a certain ddNTP in a one- or two-color system. Spots are analyzed using an adaptive quantitation method with a p value of 0.0001, and signal intensities are read using total intensities. As controls for background signals, four to six spots of reagent blanks and nonprinted positions outside the array are quantified and compared to the other spots on the array. The lowest acceptable level for identifica-

tion of a true positive signal is set to two times the background signal (*see* **Notes 12–14**).
3. The text file generated by the quantifying software is further imported into MS Excel for calculations of mean values of the triplicate spots and background-subtracted signals. A summary of the scanning and quantification procedure is shown in **Fig. 4**, and an example of the results from mtDNA and nDNA genotyping is shown in **Fig. 5**.

4. Notes

1. Microarray analysis of SNPs can be achieved by different strategies, either by direct extension or ligation of a hybridized PCR product or probe sequence on the chip *(6–10)* or an indirect detection by hybridization of ligated or extended target sequences to probes on the array *(5,11–13)*.
2. Clustered polymorphisms within a few base pairs, which are common in the hypervariable region of the mitochondrial genome, can affect the incorporation efficiency of the dideoxynucleotide by destabilizing the priming event and result in a reduction or complete loss of signal *(7)*. To reduce expected loss of signal from mismatches, the minisequencing primer may be designed with degenerate positions where mismatches are expected *(14)*.
3. To obtain homogenous spots and improve the spot quality, a detergent like SDS can be used, which decreases the surface tension. Be careful not to add too much as it can lead to spreading of the solution. Different surface chemistries require optimization of the spot solution.
4. To increase sensitivity, the binding to the solid support is an important factor. One strategy is to evaluate the binding capacity for adjustment of the amount of spotted oligonucleotide. Concentrations of 20–120 µM (in increments of 20 µM) showed the largest increase in signal intensity at 60 µM; only a minor increase was observed above this concentration. Comparisons of 20, 40, and 60 µM oligonucleotides showed approximately a 1.5- to 2-fold increase in signal intensity for each increment. A choice of a solid support with a porous gel layer on top can theoretically bind a larger proportion of the spotted oligonucleotides and thereby decrease the need for a compensating higher oligonucleotide concentration.
5. Carryover between microtiter plate wells during spotting may be observed depending on the technology used for spotting or the sensitivity of the solid support. Spotting a suitable serial dilution of a control oligonucleotide followed by three to four water blanks can be used to evaluate carryover. Design the experiment so that spotting of only water blanks using the same pin follows every round of completed spotting of a certain oligonucleotide concentration.
6. If an analysis of both mitochondrial DNA and nuclear DNA is performed, keep the mitochondrial and nuclear reactions separately throughout the amplification and purification steps. However, in the following minisequencing reaction, the PCR products may be pooled into one reaction.
7. A cycling procedure is preferable to minimize self-complementary binding between minisequencing primers.

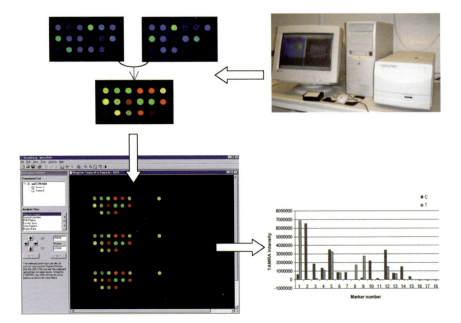

Fig. 4. Scanning and quantification procedure. The two areas on the slide are scanned separately and imported into the quantitation software QuantArray®. The scan images are given different colors and are thereafter superimposed into one picture. Signals from spots that are located on the same place in the overlaid image will appear as yellow spots. The pictures show results from a nuclear array where the reference spots of the mitochondrial DNA array (not used in this hybridization experiment) are seen to the right of the nuclear DNA array. The data are saved as a text file that is imported into an Excel worksheet for further calculations of mean values of the triplicate spots. The results can be displayed graphically in a bar diagram or in other desired forms. The bars show background subtracted signal intensities from 15 SNPs starting at spot number 3 (row no 1, column no. 3 in each array) in the quantitation image. In this experiment, the first spots in the upper left represent two different control oligonucleotides, which are not included in the bar diagram. Bars number 16–18 are quantified spots outside the array that are compared to the detected signal.

8. To decrease cost and work load, we used a system that only detects C and T polymorphims in two separate reactions. This may be achieved by using differently labeled ddCTP and ddUTP in one reaction that is hybridized on one array on the slide, or as in this system where the same fluorophore is coupled to ddNTPs and thereafter hybridized in two separate chambers on one slide. Both strategies have been evaluated, and the one-color system was chosen as the results were easier to interpret. A limitation with this system is that the minisequencing primer cannot be designed for detection on the other DNA strand, which reduces the

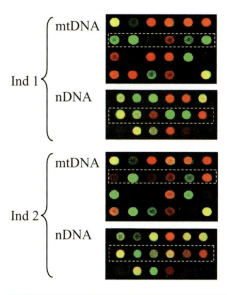

Row and column		R2C1	R2C2	R2C3	R2C4	R2C5	R2C6
Ind 1	mtDNA	T	T	T	C	T	C
	nDNA	CT	CT	CC	TT	TT	CC
Ind 2	mtDNA	C	T	C	C	T	C
	nDNA	CT	**TT**	CT	CT	CC	CC

Fig. 5. Mitochondrial DNA variants and nuclear DNA genotypes from two different individuals. The table shows the typing results fom the spots within the dashed area on each array. The bold letters indicate differences in the selected area between the individuals. Pictures of the nuclear arrays do not represent the current array design and only one reference spot in the upper left corner was included in this particular experiment. The lack of a few signals on the mitochondrial DNA part is caused by a destabilizing mismatch in the primerbinding site (*see* **Note 2**).

number of informative SNPs, especially in the mitochondrial genome. A four-color system can also be used to detect all possible variants.

9. Initial testing of on-chip extension (where the hybridization of the PCR-product and extension of printed minisequencing primers takes place in the same reaction on the chip) and hybridization to zip code arrays using a small subset of mtDNA markers, showed that performing the minisequencing separately in solution produced an increased number of successful experiments and higher signal intensities.

10. The standard parameters to obtain specific hybridization such as temperature and stringency of wash solutions have to be considered but also the volume and movement of the liquid in the hybridization chamber.

11. To test potential crosshybridizations between different zip addresses and zip codes, each zip address may be run in separate minisequencing reactions followed by separate hybridization reactions on the array.
12. In the QuantArray software, three different quantitation methods can be used. The adaptive method is suitable if the spots are nonhomogenous in size or shape. The signal intensity can be presented as total, mean, or median intensity as desired.
13. Quantify spots outside the array and spots that only contain water to get an estimate of the background signal. Avoid scanning at maximum PMT and laser, unless the spots are very weak, as it may produce saturated spots and increase the background signal and the risk of photo bleaching. Inclusion of a control oligonucleotide on the array as a control for adhesion to the surface and as reference during quantitation is recommended.
14. If different fluorophores are used that have overlapping emission spectra, the signals in the two channels have to be normalized.

Acknowledgment

This work was supported by grants from the Beijer Foundation and the Swedish Research Council for Medical Sciences (MFR grants K2002-31P-12577-05C and K2002-31X-13095-04B).

References

1. Gill, P. (2001) An assessment of the utility of single nucleotide polymorphisms (SNPs) for forensic purposes. *Int. J. Legal Med.* **114,** 204–210.
2. Prokunina, L., Castillejo-Lopez, C., Oberg, F., Gunnarsson, I., Berg, L., Magnusson, V., et al. (2002) A regulatory polymorphism in PDCD1 is associated with susceptibility to systemic lupus erythematosus in humans. *Nat. Genet.* **32,** 666–669.
3. Reynolds, R., & Varlaro, J. (1996) Gender determination of forensic samples using PCR amplification of ZFX/ZFY gene sequences. *J. Forensic Sci.* **41,** 279–286.
4. Andrews, R. M., Kubacka, I., Chinnery, P. F., Lightowlers, R. N., Turnbull, D. M., and Howell, N. (1999) Reanalysis and revision of the Cambridge reference sequence for human mitochondrial DNA. *Nat. Genet.* **23,** 147.
5. Gerry, N. P., Witowski, N. E., Day, J., Hammer, R. P., Barany, G., and Barany, F. (1999) Universal DNA microarray method for multiplex detection of low abundance point mutations. *J. Mol. Biol.* **292,** 251–262.
6. Syvanen, A. C. (1999) From gels to chips: "minisequencing" primer extension for analysis of point mutations and single nucleotide polymorphisms. *Hum Mutat.* **13,** 1–10.
7. Dubiley, S., Kirillov, E., and Mirzabekov, A. (1999). Polymorphism analysis and gene detection by minisequencing on an array of gel-immobilized primers. *Nucleic Acids Res.* **27,** e19.
8. Fortina, P., Delgrosso, K., Sakazume, T., Santacroce, R., Moutereau, S., Su, H. J.,

Graves, D., McKenzie, S., and Surrey, S. (2000). Simple two-color array-based approach for mutation detection. *Eur. J. Hum. Genet.* **8**, 884–94.

9. Pastinen, T., Raitio, M., Lindroos, K., Tainola, P., Peltonen, L., and Syvanen, A. C. (2000). A system for specific, high-throughput genotyping by allele-specific primer extension on microarrays. *Genome Res.* **10**, 1031–1042.

10. Landegren, U. (1993). Ligation-based DNA diagnostics. *Bioessays* **15**, 761–5.

11. Guo, Z., Guilfoyle, R. A., Thiel, A. J., Wang, R., and Smith, L. M. (1994). Direct fluorescence analysis of genetic polymorphisms by hybridization with oligonucleotide arrays on glass supports. *Nucleic Acids Res.* **22**, 5456–5465.

12. Hirschhorn, J. N., Sklar, P., Lindblad-Toh, K., Lim, Y. M., Ruiz-Gutierrez, M., Bolk, S., et al. (2000). SBE-TAGS: an array-based method for efficient single-nucleotide polymorphism genotyping. *Proc. Natl. Acad. Sci. USA* **97**, 12,164–12,169.

13. Fan, J. B., Chen, X., Halushka, M. K., Berno, A., Huang, X., Ryder, T., et al. (2000). Parallel genotyping of human SNPs using generic high-density oligonucleotide tag arrays. *Genome Res.* **10**, 853–860.

14. Knoth, K., Roberds, S., Poteet, C., and Tamkun, M. (1988). Highly degenerate, inosine-containing primers specifically amplify rare cDNA using the polymerase chain reaction. *Nucleic Acids Res.* **16**, 10,932.

11

SNP Typing on the NanoChip Electronic Microarray

Claus Børsting, Juan J. Sanchez, and Niels Morling

Summary

We describe a single nucleotide polymorphism (SNP) typing protocol developed for the NanoChip electronic microarray. The NanoChip array consists of 100 electrodes covered by a thin hydrogel layer containing streptavidin. An electric currency can be applied to one, several, or all electrodes at the same time according to a loading protocol generated by the user. Biotinylated deoxyribonucleic acid (DNA) is directed to the pad(s) via the electronic field(s) and bound to streptavidin in the hydrogel layer. Subsequently, fluorescently labeled reporter oligos and a stabilizer oligo are hybridized to the bound DNA. Base stacking between the short reporter and the longer stabilizer oligo stabilizes the binding of a matching reporter, whereas the binding of a reporter carrying a mismatch in the SNP position will be relatively weak. Thermal stringency is applied to the NanoChip array according to a reader protocol generated by the user and the fluorescent label on the matching reporter is detected.

Key Words: NanoChip microarray; nanogen molecular biology workstation; electronic addressing of DNA; hybridization; base stacking effect; SNP typing.

1. Introduction

In recent years, the number of different methods for determination of single nucleotide polymorphisms (SNPs) has increased dramatically *(1,2)*. Hybridization of a labeled target specific probe to endonuclease-digested genomic deoxyribonucleic acid (DNA) was the first technique to be widely used that did not require actual sequencing of the target DNA. However, this method can be applied only to SNPs in endonuclease-recognition sites (restriction fragment length polymorphisms), and in order to use hybridization techniques for SNP detection, a more general approach was needed.

From: *Methods in Molecular Biology, vol. 297: Forensic DNA Typing Protocols*
Edited by: A. Carracedo © Humana Press Inc., Totowa, NJ

The difference in hybridization energy between a perfect match and a single nucleotide mismatch is very small, and it may be very difficult to find the conditions where discrimination is possible. However, the difference can be increased by exploitation of the so-called base stacking effect: Two short oligos placed right next to each other bind stronger to a DNA target than either of the oligos alone because of noncovalent interactions between the two oligos *(3,4)*. The SNP typing protocol developed for the NanoChip electronic microarray *(5,6)* makes use of this phenomenon (**Fig. 1**). The NanoChip array consists of 100 electrodes with a diameter of 80 μm in a 10 × 10 format covered with a thin hydrogel layer containing streptavidin. Biotin-labeled polymerase chain reaction (PCR) products are electronically directed to the pads and bound to streptavidin, allowing a fast and efficient way to concentrate the target DNA. Two fluorescently labeled reporter oligos, one for each SNP allele, and one stabilizer oligo are hybridized to the target DNA on the pads. The reporter oligos are short (8–16 bp), whereas the stabilizer oligo is relatively long (25–30 bp). The SNP is positioned at the 3' end of the reporter, and the 5' end of the stabilizer oligo hybridizes to the neighboring base. Thus, the binding of the matching reporter is stabilized by the stabilizer oligo, whereas the reporter carrying a mismatch in the 3' end binds weakly to the target and can be removed by applying thermal stringency. Finally, the fluorescent label on the matching reporter is excited by laser light and detected by a CCD camera.

Here, we describe the NanoChip SNP typing protocol in detail, and we discuss alternatives to the standard protocol. In addition, we describe how to analyze small multiplexes, and we comment on some of the problems involved. The NanoChip electronic microarray can be used for other applications than SNP typing, but these techniques are outside the scope of this chapter, and they are described elsewhere *(7–12)*.

2. Materials

1. High-performance liquid chromatography purified oligonucleotides.
2. Purified genomic DNA.
3. Taq polymerase, polymerase buffer, 25 mM MgCl$_2$, dNTPs.
4. Thermal cycler.
5. MultiScreen® PCR plates (Millipore, Copenhagen, Denmark).
6. MultiScreen® separation system (Millipore).
7. MinElute™ PCR purification kit (Qiagen, Albertslund, Denmark).
8. Nanogen® Molecular Biology Workstation (Nanogen, Helmond, Netherlands).
9. NanoChip® H2 cartridge (Nanogen, Helmond, Netherlands), stored at 4°C.
10. n*LAB*™ 1.12.16L software (Nanogen, San Diego, CA).
11. 96-well Nunc™ plates (Merck Eurolab, Albertslund, Denmark).

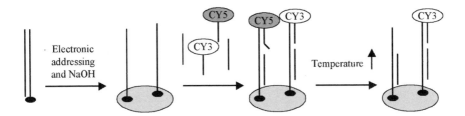

Fig. 1. Diagram of the NanoChip SNP typing protocol.

12. Twin conductivity meter B-173 (Horiba Europe GmbH, Salzbach, Germany).
13. 1.41 mS/cm calibration solution (Horiba Europe GmbH).
14. 50 m*M* histidine (Nanogen), stored at 4°C. Usually, the 50 m*M* histidine solution is stable for 1–2 wk at 4°C.
15. 100 m*M* histidine (Nanogen), stored at –20°C.
16. High salt buffer: 500 m*M* NaCl, 50 m*M* NaH$_2$PO$_4$, pH 7.0.
17. Low salt buffer: 50 m*M* NaH$_2$PO$_4$, pH 7.0
18. 0.1 *N* NaOH.

3. Methods

The methods described below outline 1) the initial planning by the computer leading to the design of the PCR product, and to the design of the reporter and stabilizer oligos, 2) the PCR purification protocols, 3) the loading and reading of the NanoChip microarray, and 4) the multiplexing protocol.

3.1. Work in Silica

The initial work in front of the computer is pivotal for the outcome of the experiment. Spending a few extra hours searching the various SNP and genomic databases (*see* **Note 1**), as well as analyzing the primer and oligo design carefully (*see* **Note 2**) may easily save days or weeks later on.

3.1.1. Design of PCR product

1. Search the genomic databases for the sequence surrounding the SNP (*see* **Note 1**).
2. Search the databases for homologous and repetitive sequences (*see* **Note 1**).
3. Search the SNP databases for additional SNPs in the target sequence (*see* **Note 1**).
4. Use primer software to find the most promising position for the primers (*see* **Notes 2** and **3**). Look for similar sequences in any homologous sequence found above and select unique primer binding sites.
5. Use the primer sequences to search the genomic databases for homologous sequences. If strong homology is found, search for different primer binding sites.

Table 1
Base Stacking Energies Calculated
by the Nearest Neighbor Algorithm

			5' end of stabilizer		
	ΔG	A	C	G	T
3'end of reporter	A	−5.37	−10.5	−6.78	−6.57
	C	−6.57	−8.26	−9.69	−6.78
	G	−9.81	−14.6	−8.26	−10.5
	T	−3.82	−9.81	−6.57	−5.37

From ref. *13*.

3.1.2. Design of Reporter and Stabilizer Oligos

1. Calculate the theoretical melting temperature (Tm) of the reporter in 50 m*M* Na$^+$ (the concentration in the stringent wash buffer) using the nearest neighbor algorithm (*see* **Note 2**). Tm should be between 31 and 42°C, thus, depending on the G/C content, the reporter will be between 8 and 16 nt. long.
2. Calculate the free energy of any primer dimer formation and hairpin structures in the reporter (*see* **Note 2**).
3. Determine the free energy of the base stacking effect (*see* **Table 1** and **Note 4**).
4. Select the best reporter design (*see* **Note 5** and **6**).
5. When the reporters have been selected, calculate the Tm and the free energy of any primer dimer formation and hairpin structure in the stabilizer (*see* **Note 7**). The Tm of the stabilizer should be approx 60°C.
6. Order the PCR primers (*see* **Note 8**), the fluorescently labeled reporters, and the stabilizer oligo (*see* **Note 9**).

3.2. Purification of PCR Products

   Below, we describe two efficient methods for purification of PCR products, but other methods may be equally efficient. The Millipore protocol is based on a 96-well plate system with high throughput, whereas the Qiagen protocol is based on single spin columns that are useful for purification of a small number of samples (*see* **Note 10**).

3.2.1. Millipore Purification Protocol

1. Place the MultiScreen® PCR plate on the Millipore manifold.
2. Add 50–250 µL sample per well.
3. Start the pump and set the pressure at 8–10 inch Hg.
4. When the fluid is sucked through, stop the pump and add 100 µL ddH$_2$O.
5. Start the pump and set the pressure at 8–10 inch Hg.
6. When the water is sucked through, stop the pump and add 60 µL ddH$_2$O or 60 µL 50 m*M* histidine to each well.

7. Place the MultiScreen PCR plate on a shaking table for 5 min.
8. Recover the dissolved DNA from the wells.

3.2.2. Qiagen Purification Protocol

1. Add 5X volume of PB buffer to the PCR reaction and mix.
2. Place the MinElute™ spin column in the 2-mL collection tube and add the sample.
3. Spin for 1 min at 10,000g and discard the flow-through.
4. Add 750 µL PE buffer.
5. Spin for 1 min at 10,000g, discard the flow-through, and spin again.
6. Place the spin column in a clean Eppendorf tube.
7. Add 30 µL ddH$_2$O and leave the column for 1 min.
8. Spin for 1 min at 10,000g.

3.3. Nanogen Molecular Biology Workstation

The Nanogen Molecular Biology Workstation consists of a loader and a reader. In the loader, DNA samples, oligos, and controls are moved from a 96-well plate and electronically addressed to the NanoChip array. The reader contains a temperature controller and a robotic system that will perform the stringent washes (*see* **Note 11**). In addition, the reader contains two lasers (excitation at 635 nm and 532 nm) and a detector (emission at 660–720 nm and 550–600 nm) for the collection of the fluorescent signal. The loader and the reader are equipped with barcode scanners that register the barcode on the NanoChip array and ensure the identity of the NanoChip array throughout the experiment from loading of the array to analysis of the collected data.

3.3.1. Loading Protocol

1. Test the conductivity of the 50 mM histidine solution using a conductivity meter. The conductivity should be less than 100 µS/cm.
2. Place the bottle with 50 mM histidine in the left-hand drawer on the loader. Make sure that the trash bottle is in place.
3. Place the bottles with low and high salt buffer in the reader. Make sure that the trash bottle is in place.
4. Turn on the Nanogen Molecular Biology Workstation (the reader first). The instrument will prime all fluid lines automatically when turned on.
5. Make 60 µL 50 mM histidine solutions (*see* **Note 12**) of your samples, oligos, and controls in a 96-well plate (*see* **Note 13**). Three controls are needed: 1) a 50 mM histidine solution is used for background subtraction, 2) a heterozygote control is used for normalization of the fluorescent signals (*see* **Note 14**), and 3) two homozygous controls (one for each allele) are used as positive controls.
6. Logon to the Nanogen Molecular Biology Workstation and go to "Loader protocols."
7. Click on "New," select the desired plate format (96 or 384 wells), and create a Target/Amplicon submap (*see* **Note 15**). An image of the 96-well plate and the NanoChip array is displayed.

8. Click on a well and name the sample in the well. The well will be given a distinct color.
9. Click on the pad(s) where the sample should be addressed. The pads will be given the same color as the well. Right-click on a pad to set the amplitude and the duration of the electronic addressing (default is 2000 V and 120 s).
10. When all samples in the 96-well plate have been defined and all submaps created, save the file.
11. Click on "Loader run." A panel with start, stop, pause, and eject buttons is displayed.
12. Place the 96-well plate and the NanoChip array(s) in the front drawer of the loader.
13. Press the start button in the panel. The loader will perform a conductivity test of every pad on the NanoChip array(s). If the conductivity test fails, the loader protocol will pause.
14. When the loader protocol is completed, remove the NanoChip array and the 96-well plate.
15. Replace the 50 mM histidine bottle in the left-hand drawer with a water bottle and shutdown the loader. The loader will automatically prime the fluid lines before it can be turned off.

3.3.2. Hybridization of Reporters and Stabilizer Oligo

1. Add 150 µL 0.1 N NaOH to the NanoChip array and leave the array for 3 min on the table to denature the PCR products (this step can be performed as part of the loader protocol).
2. Wash the NanoChip array three times with 150 µL high salt buffer and leave the last wash in the NanoChip array for 3–5 min to ensure that the permeation layer is saturated with high salt buffer.
3. Mix 1 µM of each reporter and 250 nM stabilizer in 150 µL high salt buffer.
4. Add the mix to the NanoChip array and leave the array on the table for 5 min.
5. Wash the NanoChip array three times with 150 µL high salt buffer and leave the last wash in the NanoChip array.

3.3.3. Reader Protocol

1. Logon to the Nanogen Molecular Biology Workstation, go to "Reader protocol" and click on "New." A window with the reader protocol will be displayed. The first "General" stage of the protocol is automatically listed. Information about the experiment can be entered here.
2. Create the desired stages of the protocol (*see* **Notes 16** and **17**).
3. Save the file.
4. Click on "Reader run." A panel with start, stop, pause and eject buttons is displayed.
5. Insert the NanoChip array into the Reader.
6. Select the initial temperature to 24°C and instruct the Reader to fill the NanoChip array with low salt buffer. A live picture of the NanoChip array will be displayed.

7. Mark the corner pads on the array and click on the "Set pads" button.
8. Press the start button in the panel.
9. When the reader protocol is completed, eject the NanoChip array.
10. Replace the bottles with low and high salt buffer with water bottles and shutdown the reader. The reader will automatically prime the fluid lines before it can be turned off.

3.3.4. Data Analysis

1. Logon to the Nanogen Molecular Biology Workstation and go to "Cartridges."
2. Click on the desired NanoChip array and click on the n*LAB*™ button. A window containing all the experiments (*see* **Note 18**) performed with the selected NanoChip array is displayed.
3. Click on "NanoChip® Config." A summary of all the submaps from the loader protocol(s) will be displayed.
4. Click on "Edit" and create a capture layer (*see* **Note 19**) that covers all samples and controls. The histidine control should be defined separately within the layer.
5. Remove any samples from the target layer that will not need to be analyzed and save the configuration.
6. Click on "Analysis tools" and select the desired scan(s) for analysis.
7. Click on "Analyze selected data" and select the histidine control for background subtraction.
8. Select the heterozygote control for normalization of the fluorescent signal (*see* **Note 20**).
9. Set the minimum signal-to-noise ratio for an accepted call (default is 5:1).
10. Set the minimum normalized signal-to-signal ratio for a homozygotic SNP call (default is 5:1).
11. Set the maximum normalized signal-to-signal ratio for a heterozygotic SNP call (default is 2:1).
12. Select the desired scan(s) for analysis and click on "Generate summary." A bar diagram and a table with the analyzed data is displayed (*see* **Note 21**).

3.4. Analysis of Multiplex PCRs

If different amplicons are addressed to the same pad on the NanoChip array *(14,15)* or several interesting SNPs are located on the same amplicon *(16)*, more than one SNP needs to be analyzed in the same pad. This is done by sequential hybridization, analysis, and stripping of the fluorescent reporters and stabilizer oligo (*see* **Subheadings 3.3.2.** and **3.3.3.**). Approximately 10–15 rounds of stripping and hybridization can be performed on the same NanoChip array before the signal strength is affected (*see* **Note 22**).

4. Notes

1. Genome and SNP databases:
   http://www.ncbi.nlm.nih.gov/

http://snp.cshl.org/
http://snpper.chip.org/bio/snpper-enter/ (password required)
http://genome.ornl.gov/
http://genome.ucsc.edu/

2. Oligo design software:
   http://www.molbiol.bbsrc.ac.uk/reviews.html
   http://searchlauncher.bcm.tmc.edu/multi-align/multi-align.html
   http://www-genome.wi.mit.edu/cgi-bin/primer/primer3_www.cgi
   http://biotools.idtdna.com/gateway/
   http://ftp.genome.washington.edu/cgi-bin/RepeatMasker

3. The length of the amplicon is important. Strong fluorescent signals on the NanoChip array have been obtained from as little as 10–30 fmol 50-bp amplicons whereas the hybridization efficiency towards the same SNPs on 200- to 300-bp amplicons was up to 10 times lower *(14)*.

4. Make a list of all possible reporters containing the sequence, the Tm and the free energy of primer dimer formation, hairpin structures, and base stacking effect (for example, *see* **Fig. 2**). Each possible reporter pair (one for each allele) can then be compared and rated against each other. Remember to divide the list in two parts, one for each DNA strand.

5. The best reporter pair (one for each allele) is determined from the following guidelines: 1) the Tm should be between 31°C and 42°C, 2) the theoretical Tm of the two selected reporters must not differ by more than 2°C, 3) avoid the lowest base stacking energies (T:A, A:A and T:T) if possible, 4) the base stacking energies should be similar if possible, and if this is not possible, the reporter with the highest Tm should have the lowest base stacking energy, 5) avoid strong hairpin structures ($\Delta G < -7$ kcal/mol) and palindromic sequences longer than four nucleotides.

6. A reporter pair can work even though the reporter pair does not fulfill all the guidelines mentioned in **Note 5**. Similarly, a reporter pair is not guarantied to work even though the reporter pair fulfills all the guidelines. Often, it is necessary to design new reporters because it is impossible to normalize the fluorescent signal (*see* **Subheading 3.3.4.** and **Note 20**). Recently, a universal reporter system was described *(16)*, where the fluorescent reporter binds to the tail of another oligo consisting of a 3' target specific sequence and a 5' universal sequence. In this way, only one pair of fluorescent reporters is needed during the assay development phase and different target sequences can be tested at a relatively low cost.

7. If very strong secondary structures ($\Delta G < -10$ kcal/mol) are found in the stabilizer sequence, consider using the other DNA strand. Alternatively, the so-called dot-blot assay could also be used, where the SNP is placed in the middle of the reporter and a stabilizer is not used. This should be the last alternative, because without the base-stacking effect the discrimination between match and mismatch is less.

DNA target sequence

AATTCAAGGGCATTTAGAACA/CCTTTGTCATCTGTTAATATT

Reporter sequence	Length	Tm	Dimer	Hairpin	Basestacking	
GGGCATTTAGAACA	14	40.6	-3.1	+2.1	AC	: -10.5
GGGCATTTAGAACC	14	41.7	-3.1	+1.1	CC	: -8.26
GGCATTTAGAACA	13	35.7	-3.1	+3.3	AC	: -10.5
GGCATTTAGAACC	13	36.9	-3.1	+1.1	CC	: -8.26
GCATTTAGAACA	12	30.0	-3.1	+3.3	AC	: -10.5
GCATTTAGAACC	12	31.4	-3.1	+3.3	CC	: -8.26

Reporter sequence (reverse)	Length	Tm	Dimer	Hairpin	Basestacking	
ACAGATGACAAAGT	14	38.9	-2.0	+1.8	TG	: -6.57
ACAGATGACAAAGG	14	40.1	-2.0	None	GG	: -8.26
CAGATGACAAAGT	13	35.1	-2.0	+3.9	TG	: -6.57
CAGATGACAAAGG	13	36.4	-2.0	None	GG	: -8.26
AGATGACAAAGT	12	30.9	-2.0	+3.9	TG	: -6.57 *
AGATGACAAAGG	12	32.4	-2.0	None	GG	: -8.26 *

Stabilizer sequence	Length	Tm	Dimer	Hairpin
CTTTGTCATCTGTTAATATTCAGAAATGATAAGCC	35	58.6	-7.8	-1.0

Stabilizer sequence (reverse)	Length	Tm	Dimer	Hairpin
GTTCTAAATGCCCTTGAATTGTAAGAA	27	56.0	-5.4	+0.5 *

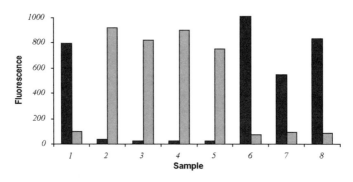

Fig. 2. Analysis of the Y chromosome SNP M173 using the NanoChip SNP typing protocol. Possible reporters in the forward and reverse direction were listed in a table containing the sequence, the length of the reporter, the theoretical Tm in degree centigrade, and the free energy in kcal/mol of the strongest primer dimer, the strongest hairpin and the base stacking effect. A similar table was made for the potential stabilizer oligos. The selected reporters and stabilizer oligo are marked by asterisks. Below the table is shown the normalized results from eight Danish males.

The reverse direction was selected because the forward stabilizer oligo will form a relatively strong primer dimer. Two different reporter pairs (12 and 13 nucleotides long) were tested before the final selection was made because the reporters had unusually high Tm values compared with their theoretical Tm values. In the experiment shown, the NanoChip was analyzed at 42°C.

8. Biotin-labeled oligos are expensive, and the PCR primers may have to be redesigned. Therefore, the PCR should be tested and optimized in the laboratory before the biotin-labeled PCR primer is ordered.
9. Make 8 µL 30 µ*M* aliquots of the reporter oligos and store the aliquots and the stock at –20°C. In this way, we have successfully used oligo stocks that are more than 1 yr old.
10. The recoveries from both the Millipore and the Qiagen protocols are more than 80%. However, PCR products shorter than 100–110 bp are lost in the Millipore protocol. In contrast, we successfully purified 44-bp PCR products with the Qiagen protocol *(14)*.
11. The Nanogen Molecular Biology Workstation can also apply electronic stringency. However, we do not recommend this feature, because electronic stringency is difficult to optimize.
12. It will take approx 8 to 9 h to load the entire NanoChip array. Some of the sample solution will evaporate during this period. If there is too little fluid in the well, the sample solution cannot fill the channels in the NanoChip and there will be no connection between the electrode in the NanoChip array and the electrode in the Loader. Consequently, no DNA will be addressed to the array. Therefore, it is necessary to make 100 µL 50 m*M* histidine solutions if you are going to load the entire array.
13. Make a diagram of the 12 × 8 96-well plate and the 10 × 10 NanoChip microarray, and document where each sample is loaded. This will also facilitate the construction of the loader protocol.
14. The heterozygote control should be a sample with known genotype. The concentration of your heterozygote control and your samples on the NanoChip array must be approximately the same. If this is not the case, you can normalize the signal, but the fluorescent signal from your samples will either be too strong (saturated) or too weak. Therefore, amplify your heterozygote control in the same PCR experiment as your samples and address the heterozygote control in two different concentrations on the NanoChip array. Synthetic oligos can be used as controls if a heterozygote control is not available. However, as mentioned in **Note 3**, the hybridization efficiency depends strongly on the length of your DNA target. Thus, if the PCR product is long and your oligo control is relatively short, you will normalize your signal under one condition and type your samples under another condition.
15. There are four different submaps. Each submap has different default settings. The "capture submap" is used for the electronic addressing of short capture oligos (for capture down protocol, *see* **Note 23**). The "target/amplicon submap" is used for electronic addressing of amplicons. The "passive submap" is used for incubation of the NanoChip array in a solution for any given time. The "target prep submap" is used for electronic denaturation of double-stranded DNA. One loader protocol can contain several different submaps.
16. The first stage should be an initial florescence scan at 24°C. This stage will register the level of fluorescence before any thermal stringency has been applied.

For each temperature you want to test, there are four stages: 1) "Environment" sets the desired temperature, 2) "Fluidics" washes the NanoChip array with 250 μL of wash buffer at 75 μL/s, 3) "Environment" sets the temperature to 24°C, and 4) "Fluorescence" scans the desired pads on the NanoChip array. Once the reader protocol is optimized, it is usually sufficient to analyze two or three different temperatures, but for the initial experiments, analyze six to eight different temperatures near the theoretical Tm of your reporters.

17. In addition to the stages mentioned in **Note 16**, the following stages can be applied to the reader protocol: "Activation" sets the desired amplitude (either electronic stringency or electronic capture); "Conductivity" tests the conductivity of the pads on the NanoChip array; "Image" will take a picture of the NanoChip array; and "Wait" will pause the reader protocol for up to one hour.

18. From this window you have access to detailed information on date and time of every experiment, the electronic addressing of your samples, the conductivity test performed by the loader, temperature measurements during the reader protocol, and results from the florescence scans. The later can be given by either color symbols or numeric values.

19. The analysis tool can only analyze your data if you have created a capture layer, equivalent to a capture submap (*see* **Note 15**). The reason for this peculiarity probably is that the software was developed for the capture down protocol (*see* **Note 23**).

20. If the normalization factor is more than 2, "no designation calls" can occur from the homozygotes carrying the allele with the strongest signal because the background signal from the other channel (the weak one) is multiplied with the normalization factor and, consequently, the signal-to-signal ratio may be less than 5:1. "No calls" from homozygotes carrying the allele with the weakest signal may also occur because the signal-to-noise ratio is less than 5:1 at the temperature where normalization is possible (the temperature window where the fluorescent signal from the heterozygote control is not saturated or too weak, will be very small). A large normalization factor is a sign of poor reporter design, and it usually originates from a large difference in Tm of the two reporters. Therefore, trying a different reporter pair may be warranted.

21. The nLAB™ software contains very few options. If the normalized data is to be presented in any other way than the bar diagram, the data in the table must be transferred to a spreadsheet, and if raw data is to be presented, a "print screen" of the color image of the desired scan must be pasted into another software.

22. If more than one amplicon is addressed to the same pad or the amplicon is long, the risk of cross-hybridization increases. The use of short reporters and the relatively low temperatures at which the reporters bind to their targets complicates the development of large multiplexes. We have experienced several examples of reproducible cross hybridization between a reporter and a different amplicon than the intended target amplicon, even at stringent temperatures (unpublished results). In each case, we redesigned the multiplexes and, instead of one large multiplex, we ended up with several smaller multiplexes. In addition, the presence of differ-

ent amplicons on the same pad decreases the hybridization efficiency *(14)*, most likely because interactions between the amplicons shield the target sequence from the reporters. This can only be avoided by directing the different amplicons to different pads on the NanoChip array (*see* **Note 23**).

23. In the capture down protocol, a 3' biotin-labeled capture oligo is electronically addressed to the NanoChip array. The amplicon is electronically addressed to the same pad and hybridizes to the capture oligo. The fluorescent reporters are hybridized to the amplicon immediately upstream of the capture, resulting in base stacking between the 3' end of the reporter (in case of a perfect match) and the 5' end of the capture. If different captures are addressed to different pads on the NanoChip array, the different amplicons in a multiplex PCR can be bound to different pads and interactions between amplicons can be avoided. We have tried the capture down protocol on 7 different amplicons (in singleplex) using DNA captures. We obtained reproducible results from only one of the amplicons and only if we pooled the DNA from two to four 25-µL PCR reactions and addressed it all to the NanoChip array (unpublished results). We are in the process of testing other capture molecules than DNA, but at the present time, the capture down protocol works for only a small number of assays.

Acknowledgments

We thank Ms. Rikke W. Hansen for technical assistance. The work was supported by grants to Juan J. Sanchez from Ellen and Aage Andersen's Foundation.

References

1. Chen, X., and Sullivan, P. F. (2003) Single nucleotide polymorphism genotyping: biochemistry, protocol, cost and throughput. *Pharmacogenomics J.* **3**, 77–96.
2. Kwok, P. Y. and Chen, X. (2003) Detection of single nucleotide polymorphisms. *Curr. Issues Mol. Biol.* **5**, 43–60.
3. Yershov, G., Barsky, V., Belgovskiy, A., Kirillov, E., Kreindlin, E., Ivanov, I., et al. (1996) DNA analysis and diagnostics on oligonucleotide microchips. *Proc. Natl. Acad. Sci. USA* **93**, 4913–4918.
4. Lane, M. J., Paner, T., Kashin, I., Faldasz, B. D., Li, B., Gallo, F. J., and Benight, A. S. (1997) The thermodynamic advantage of DNA oligonucleotide 'stacking hybridization' reactions: energetics of a DNA nick. *Nucleic Acid Res.* **25**, 611–616.
5. Sosnowski, R. G., Tu, E., Butler, W. F., O'Connell, J. P., and Heller, M. J. (1997) Rapid determination of single base mismatch mutations in DNA hybrids by direct electric field control. *Proc. Natl. Acad. Sci. USA* **94**, 1119–1123.
6. Gilles, P. N., Wu, D. J., Foster, C. B., Dillon, P. J., and Chanock S. J. (1999) Single nucleotide polymorphic discrimination by an electronic dot blot assay on semiconductor microchips. *Nat. Biotechnol.* **17**, 365–370.
7. Huang, Y., Sunghae, J., Duhon, M., Heller, M., Wallace, B., and Xu, X. (2002)

Dielectronic cell separation and gene expression profiling on microelectronic chip arrays. *Anal. Chem.* **74,** 3362–3371.

8. Westin, L., Xu, X., Miller, C., Wang, L., Edman, C. F. and Nerenberg, M. (2000) Anchored multiplex amplification on a microelectronic chip array. *Nat. Biotechnol.* **18,** 199–204.

9. Weidenhammer E. M., Kahl B. F., Wang L., Wang L., Duhon M., Jackson J. A., et al. (2002) Multiplexed, targeted gene expression profiling and genetic analysis on electronic microarrays. *Clin. Chem.* **48,** 1873–1882.

10. Yang J. M., Bell J., Huang Y., Tirado M., Thomas D., Forster A. H., et al. (2002) An integrated, stacked microlaboratory for biological agent detection with DNA and immunoassays. *Biosensors Bioelectronics* **17,** 605–618.

11. Radtkey R., Feng L., Muralhidar M., Duhon M., Canter D., DiPierro D., et al. (2000) Rapid, high fidelity analysis of simple sequence repeats on an electronically active DNA microchip. *Nucleic Acid Res.* **28,** e17.

12. Behrensdorf, H. A., Pignot, M., Windhab, N., and Kappel, A. (2002) Rapid parallel mutation scanning of gene fragments using a microelectronic protein-DNA chip format. *Nucleic Acid Res.* **30,** e64.

13. Saenger W. (1984) Forces stabilizing base associations: hydrogen bonding and basestacking, in *Principles of nucleic acid structure.* Springer-Verlag, New York, pp 116–158.

14. Børsting, C., Sanchez, J. J., and Morling, N. (2004) Multiplex PCR, amplicon size and hybridization efficiency on the NanoChip electronic microarray. *Int. J. Legal Med.* **118,** 75–82 .

15. Thistlethwaite W. A., Moses L. M., Hoffbuhr K. C., Devaney J. M., and Hoffman E. P. (2003) Rapid genotyping of common MeCP2 mutations with an electronic DNA microchip using serial differential hybridization. *J. Mol. Diag.* **5,** 121–126.

16. Santacroce R., Ratti A., Caroli F., Foglieni B., Ferraris A., Cremonesi L., et al. (2002) Analysis of clinically relevant single-nucleotide polymorphisms by use of microelectronic array technology. *Clin. Chem.* **48,** 2124–2130.

17. Cooper K. L. F., and Goering R. V. (2003) Development of a universal probe for electronic microarray and its application in characterization of the *Staphylococcus aureus pol*C gene. *J. Mol. Diag.* **5,** 28–33.

12

Genotyping SNPs Using a UV-Photocleavable Oligonucleotide in MALDI-TOF MS

Peter M. Vallone, Kristina Fahr, and Markus Kostrzewa

Summary

Matrix-assisted laser desorption time-of-flight mass spectrometry coupled with allele-specific primer extension is a proven method for typing single nucleotide polymorphisms (SNPs). A novel modification upon this methodology is the incorporation of a photocleavable linker within the extension primer. After completion of the primer extension reaction, photocleavage of the extension products results in two deoxyribonucleic acid (DNA) fragments of lower mass. Typically, the smaller cleavage product, which contains the genotyping information, is in the range of 1000–3000 Daltons. The decrease in primer mass allows for higher sensitivity in mass spectrometric measurement and increases the potential for higher levels of multiplexing. The disturbing mass spectrometric analysis peaks caused by salt adducts and doubly charged ions are diminished when analyzing lower-mass DNA fragments. Here, we illustrate the methodology for using photocleavable modified extension primers for detection of SNPs located on the Y chromosome.

Genomic templates were prepared from anonymous male donors. Five regions of the Y chromosome containing the SNP markers M9, M42, M45, M89, and M96 were amplified by polymerase chain reaction, treated with shrimp alkaline phosphatase, and subjected to primer extension reactions using primers containing a photocleavable building block at specific sites. After elongation, the extension primers were desalted and subjected to ultraviolet irradiation to cleave the products at the photocleavable site. Subsequently, the small fragments derived from the 3' ends of the molecules containing the genotype information were analyzed by matrix-assisted laser desorption ionization time-of-flight using a 3-hydroxypicolinic acid matrix.

Key Words: MALDI-TOF MS; primer extension; multiplex; SNP; PCR; genotype; Y chromosome.

From: *Methods in Molecular Biology, vol. 297: Forensic DNA Typing Protocols*
Edited by: A. Carracedo © Humana Press Inc., Totowa, NJ

1. Introduction

Genotyping single nucleotide polymorphisms (SNPs) by matrix-assisted laser desorption ionization time-of-flight (MALDI-TOF MS) is a well-established method *(1–4)*. For cost-efficiency reasons, multiplexing at high levels is necessary for the high-throughout analyses that are necessary for unbiased genetic profiling. One approach for increasing the information content of data acquisition is to use smaller analytes, and so make use of a larger spectrum size *(5–8)*. Classical primer extension reactions are limited by the necessity of using analytes with a large-enough molecular weight to form a stable duplex previous to elongation (at least 15–18 bases; approx 5000–8000 Daltons). By using an extension primer of a typical length (18–30 nucleotides) with an internal photocleavable building block, the resulting extension product can be shortened before mass spectrometric analysis at the discretion of the experimenter *(5)*. The ability to control the mass of the fragment analyzed by MALDI-TOF MS allows for greater freedom in the design of extension primers that must anneal under identical experimental conditions. Uniform hybridization of extension primers is critical for the success of multiple primer extension events occurring in the same reaction. With respect to the position of the photocleavable linker within the extension primer, the fragments analyzed by MALDI-TOF MS after ultraviolet (UV) cleavage are in the range of 1000–3000 Daltons. The relatively small mass window (maximum 2000 Daltons) in which the cleaved fragments are analyzed allows for greater uniformity in analyte ionization and sensitivity.

Genetic markers located on the nonrecombining region of the Y chromosome are useful from a standpoint of evolutionary studies *(9)*. These same sites have potential use as genetic markers for human identification, for example, in forensics. In an ongoing project probing the forensic utility of Y chromosome SNPs for human identity purposes, we illustrate the usage of photocleavable extension primers in allele-specific primer extension reactions in combination with MALDI-TOF MS for typing five Y SNPs discovered by denaturing high-performance liquid chromatography *(10; see* **Note 1**).

2. Materials

1. Oligonucleotide synthesis and purity: Oligonucleotides used for polymerase chain reaction (PCR) were purchased from Qiagen Operon (Alameda, CA). Oligonucleotides were delivered lyophilized and desalted. Stock solutions of 100 μM were prepared by adding in the appropriate volumes of deionized water. The integrity of each oligonucleotide was confirmed by mass spectrometry *(11)*. The PCR primer sequences can be found in **Table 1**.
   Bruker Daltonik (Leipzig, Germany) kindly provided extension primers containing the photocleavable linker. The photocleavable linker (PC-*O*-nitrophenyl-CE-

Table 1
PCR Primers

Locus	Sequence 5' to 3'	Amplicon length
M9F	GCAGCATATAAAACTTTCAGG	340
M9R	AAAACCTAACTTTGCTCAAGC	
M42F	AGCTATTGTATTCACCAGTTG	134
M42R	TTTTAGCAAGTTAAGTCACCAGC	
M45F	GCTGGCAAGACACTTCTGAG	206
M45R	GTGACAGTGGCACCAAAGGTC	
M89F	AGAAGCAGATTGATGTCCCACT	530
M89R	TCCAGTTAGGAGATCCCCTCA	
M96F	GTTGCCCTCTCACAGAGCAC	440
M96R	AAGGTCACTGGAAGGATTGC	

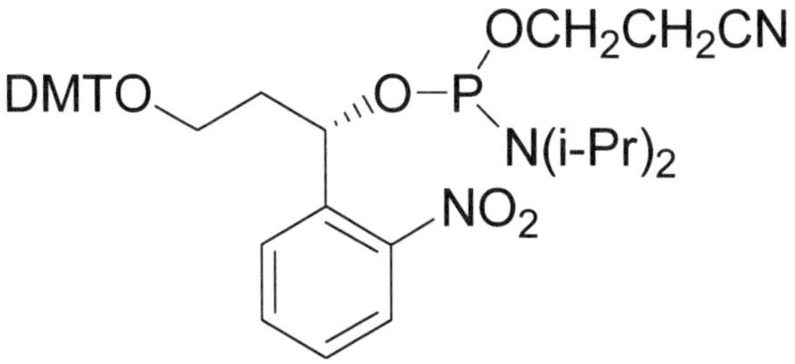

Fig. 1. Photocleavable phosphoramdite linker.

phosphoramidite [*o*-nitrophenyl-1-*O*-(2-cyanoethyl-*N*,*N*-diisopropylphosphora-midyl)-3-*O*-(4,4'-dimethoxy-triphenylmethyl)-1,3-propandiol], which can be obtained commercially from Bruker Daltonik (Germany), can be used to synthesize the primers (ref. *12*; *see* **Fig. 1**). The extension primers containing the photocleavable linker were stored in the dark at 4°C. The sequences of the extension primers with the positioning of the photolinker are shown in **Table 2**.

2. PCR reagents: AmpliTaqGold DNA polymerase (Applied Biosystems Foster City, CA), Taq Gold PCR buffer, dNTPs (Promega Corp., Madison, WI), and bovine serum albumin fraction V (Sigma, St. Louis, MO).
3. PCR cleanup: shrimp alkaline phosphatase (SAP; USB Corp., Cleveland, OH) was used to inactivate unincorporated dNTPs.
4. Primer extension reaction reagents: Thermosequenase reaction buffer (Amersham Biosciences, Piscataway, NJ), thermosequenase polymerase (Amersham Biosciences), and ddNTPs (Amersham Biosciences).

Table 2
Extension Primers Containing Photocleavable Linker

Locus	Extension primer sequence	Fragment mass (Daltons)
M9R(C/G)	ACATGTCTAAATTAAAGAAAAATA<u>A</u> A^{OMe}GA^{OMe}G	1362.9
M42R(A/T)	CCAGCTCTCTTTTTCATTAT<u>G</u>TAGT	1268.8
M45F(G/A)	GCAGTGAAAAATTAT<u>AG</u>^{OMe}ATA	1307.8
M89F(C/T)	CTCTTCCTAAGGTTATGTACAAA<u>A</u>ATCT	1228.8
M96F(G/C)	AACTTGGAAAACAGGTCTCTCA<u>T</u>AATA	1261.8

The underlined base designates the position of the photolinker. The photolinker replaces the speci-fied base in the extension primer (this acts similar to an abasic site). AOMe and GOMe are 2'-*O*-methyladenosine and 2'-*O*-methylguanosine, respectively.

5. Thermal cycling: Thermal cycling for PCR and extension assays was conducted using the GeneAmp 9700 (Applied Biosystems) running in 9600-emulation mode (i.e. ramp speeds of 1°C/s).

6. Desalting: The desalting of primer extension reactions was accomplished by using commercially available Genopure oligo™ purification kit, which is based on the specific binding of single-stranded deoxyribonucleic acid (DNA) to the surface of magnetic beads (Bruker Daltonics, Billerica, MA).

7. Photocleavage: Photocleavage of the linker was performed by irradiation with a 254 nm light by a hand-held lamp typically used for gel illumination. (Appligene Oncor, France).

8 MALDI matrix: 3-hydroxypicolinic acid (Bruker Daltonics) and ammonium cit-rate (Sigma) were the components of the MALDI matrix.

9. MALDI plate: A 384-spot AnchorChip™ MALDI sample plate with 600 μ*M* anchor sizes was used (Bruker Daltonik, Bremen, Germany).

10. Mass spectrometry: Mass spectra were collected on a Bruker BIFLEX III time-of-flight mass spectrometer (Bruker Daltonik, Bremen, Germany) equipped with a pulsed nitrogen laser (337.1 nm).

11. Data analysis: Mass spectra were smoothed and enhanced by the application of matrix convolution filters contained in the XMASS 5.0 analysis software pack-age (Bruker Daltonik, Bremen, Germany). Mass spectrometry data were normal-ized to the largest peak in the spectrum as a reference, resulting in relative intensities between 0 and 100%.

3. Methods

3.1. Perform PCR

Approximately 1–2 ng of human template (genomic) DNA was present in amplification reactions. Final PCR reagent concentrations were as fol-lows: 1 unit of AmpliTaqGold DNA polymerase, 1X Taq Gold PCR buffer,

250 μM dNTPs, 2 mM Mg^{2+}, 0.16 mg/mL bovine serum albumin fraction V, and 0.5 μM of each PCR primer.

3.2. PCR Cleanup

After PCR thermal cycling, unincorporated dNTPs were inactivated by adding 2 µL (2 units) of SAP to each PCR. Reactions were mixed briefly by pipetting and incubated at 37°C for 60 min and then 80°C for 20 min (*see* **Note 2**).

3.3. Primer Extension Reaction Conditions

Primer extension reactions were conducted in a total volume of 10 µL. Components; 10 pmol of extension primer, 0.5X thermosequenase reaction buffer, 2 units thermosequenase, 200 μM ddNTPs, 3–5 µL of PCR template. Thermal cycling conditions for extension reactions were as follows: 35 cycles of 94°C for 10 s, 55°C for 60 s, and 72°C for 40 s followed by 72°C for 5 min.

3.4. Desalting

The desalting of primer extension was accomplished by using the protocol contained with the Genopure magnetic bead. A magnetic separation device for 96-well microtiter plates was used to increase throughput. The magnetic beads are coated with a material that allows single stranded DNA to bind with the supplied buffers (*see* **Note 3**).

1. The entire (10 µL) extension reaction is combined with 5 µL of the magnetic bead solution and 50 µL of a binding buffer (supplied with kit) in a 0.2-mL PCR tube.
2. The solution is mixed thoroughly by pipeting and allowed to sit at room temperature for 5 min.
3. The PCR tube is then placed in the magnetic separator for 2 min. During the 2 min, the magnetic beads migrate to the side of the tube in contact with the magnet. The supernatant is then carefully removed with a pipet. It is important not to disturb the beads when removing the supernatant.
4. 100 µL of wash buffer 1 (supplied with kit) is added to the tube. The beads are mixed with the wash buffer. Mixing is accomplished by moving the tube from one side of the magnet to the opposite (approx 20 times). The beads migrate back and forth mixing with wash solution. Beads are collected in the magnet for 30 s, and the supernatant is removed. The bead washing and supernatant removal are repeated two additional times.
5. As 150 µL of wash buffer 2 (supplied with kit) is added to the tube, the beads are mixed with the wash buffer. The bead washing (with wash buffer 2) and supernatant removal is repeated for a total of two washes. The bead pellet (supernatant has been removed) is allowed to dry for 15 min at room temperature.
6. The beads are resuspended in 7 µL of elution buffer (supplied with kit).
7. The beads are collected for a final time in the magnetic separator, and the supernatant is transferred to a clean tube.

3.5. Sample Preparation with 3 HPA Matrix

The stock matrix solution consisted of 0.7 M 3-hydroxypicolinic acid and 0.07 M ammonium citrate in 1:1 water and acetonitrile *(13,14)*. Stock matrix solution was diluted 2.5-fold with water before usage. Samples were spotted onto the MALDI plate using 1 μL of sample and 1 μL of matrix material. The matrix solution was applied to MALDI plate first and allowed to dry before adding the desalted primer extension products. Approximately 15 min were required for completion of the drying process.

3.6. Mass Spectrometry

The following operating voltages were used for signal collection, IS1 = 19.0 kV, IS2 = 15.0 kV, reflector = 20.0 kV, detector 1.7 kV. All spectra were collected in positive ion mode with between 15 and 50 laser shots collected on each sample for signal averaging purposes. Laser power attenuation was adjusted with each sample to obtain optimal sensitivity and resolution. Before data collection, the mass spectrometer was calibrated with 4- and 16-base single-strand DNA oligomers with masses of 1173.8 and 4881.3 Daltons, respectively, where 1 Dalton is equivalent to 1 g/mol.

3.7. Type SNP Based on Measurement of Mass Difference

In mass spectrometric analysis, a signal should be detected from the extension product(s) and potentially from any remaining unextended extension primer. The singleplex spectra for five Y SNP markers are depicted in **Fig. 2**. The SNPs probed are located on the nonrecombining region of the Y chromosome; therefore, all results will be homozygous (i.e., a single extension product). The masses of ddA, ddG, ddC, and ddT are 297, 313, 273, and 288 Daltons, respectively. By subtracting the mass of the extension primer from detected products(s) the identity of the extended base is elucidated.

4. Notes

1. It is assumed that the researcher will have specific SNP sites of interest. Use of the Y chromosome SNP sites was chosen to illustrate the photocleavable extension assays. For discussion of the selection of successful PCR and extension primers, *see* refs. *15* and *16*.
2. PCR cleanup: Digestion (removal) of the PCR primers by Exonuclease I was not required because PCR primer extension products of would be observed out of the mass range of the photocleaved extension primer fragments.
3. Desalting: Desalting primer extension reactions is essential before MALDI analysis. The salts (Mg^{2+} K^+) present in PCR and primer extension reactions will suppress the ionization efficiency of the DNA, thereby decreasing the sensitivity *(17)*. In extreme cases, the presence of salts can completely suppress the analyte

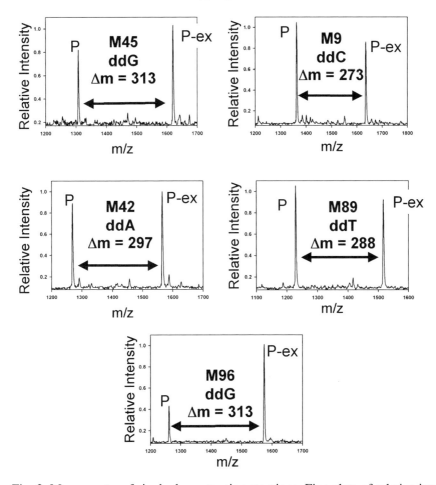

Fig. 2. Mass spectra of singleplex extension reactions. Five plots of relative intensity vs m/z are shown. The five spectra illustrate the data obtained from singleplex mass spectral anaylsis of each of the five Y SNPs. The extended and nonexteneded photocleaved fragments are indicated as P-ex and P, respectively. The mass difference is listed to indicate which ddNTP was incorporated to the primer. The peak heights will vary based on cycling conditions (for extension reaction), extension primer hybridization characteristics and length/sequence of the cleaved fragment.

signal. Desalting also help to remove and low molecular weight stabilizers present in some enzyme solutions. It should also be noted that in **Subheading 3.4, step 2**, the primer extension reaction should not be allowed to bind to the Genopure beads for more than 5 min. Extended incubation may cause low molecular weight stabilizers from the SAP to bind. After release with the desired primer extension products, these stabilizers will obscure genotyping information in the expected

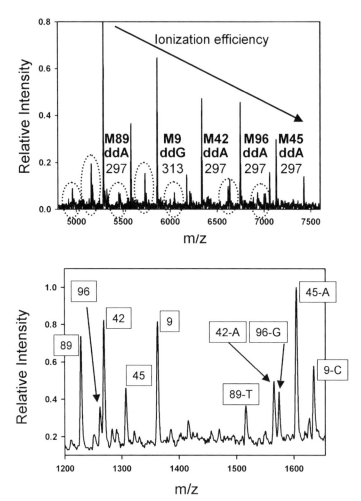

Fig. 3. Comparison of multiplex SNP detection using natural and cleavable exten-sion primers. The top graph of relative intensity vs m/z is typical of a 5 plex using natural or noncleavable extension primers. Salt adducts and depurination artifacts are circled. The peak heights slightly decrease as the analyzed mass range increases (approx 5000–7500 Daltons). It should be noted that the masses of the extension prim-ers must be carefully selected to avoid mass overlap and hybridize at a similar anneal-ing temperature (approx 60°C). Approximately 150 laser shots were required to collect the data shown in the top panel. The bottom graph represents a 5 plex using the photocleavable extension primers. The lower mass range allows for better resolution, more uniform peak heights, and fewer artifacts (depurination and sodium adducts). Approximately 50 laser shots were required to collect the data shown in the bottom panel.

mass range of 1000–3000 Daltons. Alternatively, PCR templates can be "cleaned up" using methods such as the Genopure DS™ purification kit, PurEX DNA™ extraction kit (Edge Biosystems, Gaithersburg, MD), Montage™ PCR (Millipore, Billerica, MA) clean up plates, or similar chromatographic methods for removal or unincorporated primer and dNTPs.

4. Multiplexing: The PCR amplicons can be pooled or generated in multiplex for increased throughput. The extension primer reaction can then also be performed in multiplex. By carefully selecting the length of the analyte masses, all five SNPs can be typed in a single assay. **Figure 3** illustrates the contrast between using non-cleavable and photocleavable extension primers. The five Y SNPs were amplified, extended and analyzed in multiplex.

Acknowledgments

National Institute of Justice (NIJ) funded the work described here through an interagency agreement with the NIST Office of Law Enforcement Standards. Official Disclaimer: Contribution of the U.S. National Institute of Standards and Technology. Certain commercial equipment, instruments, and materials are identified to specify experimental procedures as completely as possible. In no case does such identification imply a recommendation or endorsement by the National Institute of Standards and Technology, nor does it imply that any of the materials, instruments, or equipment identified are necessarily the best available for the purpose.

References

1. Little, D. P., Braun, A., Darnhofer-Demar, B., Frilling, A., Li, Y., McIver, R. T., Jr., et al. (1997) Detection of RET proto-oncogene codon 634 mutations using mass spectrometry. *J. Mol. Med.* **75,** 745–750.
2. Haff, L. A., and Smirnov, I. P. (1997) Single-nucleotide polymorphism identification assays using a thermostable DNA polymerase and delayed extraction MALDI- TOF mass spectrometry. *Genome Res.* **7,** 378–388.
3. Griffin, T. J. and Smith, L. M. (2000) Single-nucleotide polymorphism analysis byMALDI-TOF mass spectrometry. *Trends Biotechnol.* **18,** 77–84.
4. Pusch, W., Wurmbach, J. H., Thiele, H., and Kostrzewa, M. (2002) MALDI-TOF mass spectrometry-based SNP genotyping. *Pharmacogenomics* **3,** 537–548.
5. Sauer, S., Lechner, D., Berlin, K., Lehrach, H., Escary, J. L., Fox, N., and Gut, I. G. (2000) A novel procedure for efficient genotyping of single nucleotide polymorphisms. *Nucleic Acids Res.* **28,** E13.
6. Sauer, S., Lechner, D., Berlin, K., Plancon, C., Heuermann, A., Lehrach, H., et al. (2000) Full flexibility genotyping of single nucleotide polymorphisms by the GOOD assay. *Nucleic Acids Res.* **28,** E100.
7. Sauer, S., Lehrach, H., and Reinhardt, R. (2003) MALDI mass spectrometry analysis of single nucleotide polymorphisms by photocleavage and charge-tagging. *Nucleic Acids Res.* **31,** E63.

8. Sauer, S., and Gut, I. G. (2003) Extension of the GOOD assay for genotyping single nucleotide polymorphisms by matrix-assisted laser desorption/ionization mass spectrometry. *Rapid Commun.Mass Spectrom.* **17,** 1265–1272.
9. Jobling, M. A., and Tyler-Smith, C. (2003) The human Y chromosome: an evolutionary marker comes of age. *Nat. Rev. Genet.* **4,** 598–612.
10. Underhill, P. A., Shen, P., Lin, A. A., Jin, L., Passarino, G., Yang, W. H., et al. (2000) Y chromosome sequence variation and the history of human populations. *Nat. Genet.* **26,** 358–361.
11. Butler, J. M., Devaney, J. M., Marino, M. A., and Vallone, P. M. (2001) Quality control of PCR primers used in multiplex STR amplification reactions. *Forensic Sci. Int.* **119,** 87–96.
12. Ordoukhanian, P., and Taylor, J-S. (1995) Design and synthesis of a versatile photocleavable DNA building block. Application to phototriggered hybridization. *J. Am. Chem. Soc.* **117,** 9570-9571.
13. Wu, K. J., Steding, A., and Becker, C. H. (1993) Matrix-assisted laser desorption time-of-flight mass spectrometry of oligonucleotides using 3-hydroxypicolinic acid as an ultraviolet-sensitive matrix. *Rapid Commun. Mass Spectrom.* **7,** 142–146.
14. Chiu, N. H., Tang, K., Yip, P., Braun, A., Koster, H., and Cantor, C. R. (00) Mass spectrometry of single-stranded restriction fragments captured by an undigested complementary sequence. *Nucleic Acids Res.* **28,** E31.
15. Innis, M. A., Gelfand, D. H., Sninsky, J. J., and White, T.J. (ed.) (1990) *PCR Protocols A Guide to Methods and Application,* Academic Press, San Diego, CA.
16. Kaderali, L., Deshpande, A., Nolan, J. P., and White, P. S. (03) Primer-design for multiplexed genotyping. *Nucleic Acids Res.* **31,** 1796–1802.
17. Shaler, T. A., Wickham, J. N., Sannes, K. A., Wu, K. J., and Becker, C. H. (1996) Effect of impurities on the matrix-assisted laser desorption mass spectra of single-stranded oligodeoxynucleotides. *Anal. Chem.* **68,** 576–579.

13

Mitochondrial D-Loop and Coding Sequence Analysis Using Pyrosequencing

Marie Allen and Hanna Andréasson

Summary

In forensic casework analysis, mitochondrial deoxyribonucleic acid (DNA) often is used when the evidence material contains scarce amounts of DNA. Here, a mitochondrial DNA typing system for D-loop and coding region analysis based on pyrosequencing is described. Pyrosequencing is a real-time, single-tube sequencing-by-synthesis method, in which a cascade of enzymatic reactions yields detectable light. This pyrosequencing system has a higher resolution than the D-loop analysis performed routinely today as it also covers informative positions in the mitochondrial coding region. The system is composed of 16 polymerase chain reaction (PCR) fragments and 24 pyrosequencing reactions with a turn around time for a 96-well plate of less than 3 h after PCR.

Key Words: Forensic science; forensic DNA analysis; forensic evidence material; mitochondrial DNA; D-loop; coding region; polymorphism; sequencing; pyrosequencing; real-time; single-tube; PPi; SSB.

1. Introduction

Because of the high copy number of mitochondrial genomes per cell, mitochondrial deoxyribonucleic acid (DNA) analysis often is used for human identification *(1)* when the forensic evidence contains limited or degraded DNA. Here, we describe a unique, rapid, and easy-to-use typing system for analysis of mitochondrial DNA based on pyrosequencing technology. Pyrosequencing is a novel sequencing-by-synthesis method that is nonelectrophoretic, without need of dyes or specific labels. It is performed in a single-tube format, in which a cascade of enzymatic reactions enables nucleotide incorporation and pyrophosphate (PPi) release to yield detectable light (**Fig. 1**). The nucleotides are

From: *Methods in Molecular Biology, vol. 297: Forensic DNA Typing Protocols*
Edited by: A. Carracedo © Humana Press Inc., Totowa, NJ

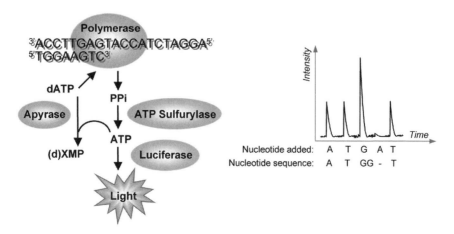

Fig. 1. Left panel, Schematic illustration of the pyrosequencing reaction. Light is produced after enzymatic conversion of PPi, which is released after nucleotide incorporation. The nucleotides are added one at a time in a known order. If a nucleotide is not incorporated, it will be degraded by the enzyme apyrase. Right panel, The light is detected by the pyrosequencing instrument and shown as a peak in a pyrogram, where the peaks represent each nucleotide in the template sequence. When the sequence contains two (or more) identical nucleotides consecutively, they will result in a double peak (or in a proportional higher peak).

added one at a time in a known order, cyclic or directed (directed in respect to the template sequence).

The produced light is detected in real-time using a luminometric detection system and is proportional to incorporated nucleotides and the released PPi (*2–4*). This pyrosequencing system is developed for analysis of the highly polymorphic mitochondrial D-loop as well as short fragments in the mitochondrial coding region (**Fig. 2**).

To achieve a more discriminating analysis than the D-loop sequence analysis alone, the mitochondrial sequencing system has been further developed to include coding sequence polymorphisms. Coding sequence analysis might be especially useful where none or a single difference between different individuals are found, which is common for sequences closely related to the Cambridge reference sequence (*5*). The coding region fragments were chosen based on the diversity determined in 26 Swedish (Nilsson M, Divne A. and Allen M, in preparation) as well as 52 European whole mitochondrial-sequenced individuals (*6*) and cover highly informative polymorphic sites throughout the entire mitochondrial genome. For an optimal discrimination, the complete mitochondrial DNA typing system consists of 16 polymerase chain reaction (PCR)

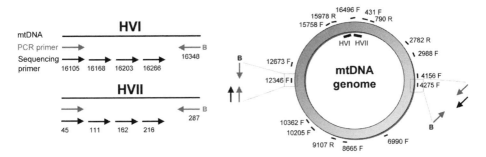

Fig. 2. Left panel, Primer locations for the D-loop fragments. The fragments are named by the 5' nucleotide of the sequencing primer. The reverse PCR primer is biotinylated and the forward PCR primer is used as a sequencing primer together with three internal sequencing primers for each fragment. Right panel, Primer locations for the mitochondrial coding region fragments. The fragments are named by the 5' nucleotide of the sequencing primer. One of the PCR primers is biotinylated and the sequencing is performed using either the non-biotinylated PCR primer or an internal primer. The D-loop location is also shown.

fragments and 24 pyrosequencing reactions: eight D-loop reactions *(7)*, eight haplogroup-indicating reactions, and eight reactions analyzing additional SNPs to enhance the possibility to distinguish between individuals with identical D-loop sequence (**Table 1**). This is a highly flexible system where all fragments can be analyzed at once, or a few coding region fragments can be analyzed as a complement to a previous D-loop analysis

2. Materials

2.1. PCR

1. Human DNA.
2. 10 µM PCR-primers, of which one is biotinylated.
3. 25 mM dNTPs and 25 mM MgCl$_2$.
4. 5 U/µL AmpliTaq Gold® DNA polymerase and 10X GeneAmp® PCR Buffer II (Applied Biosystems, Foster City, CA).
5. Bovine serum albumin (2 mg/mL: Sigma, St. Louis, MO) and 50% glycerol.
6. 96-well PCR plate or single tubes.
7. Strip lids or sealing tape.
8. GeneAmp PCR System 9600 (Applied Biosystems).

2.2. Sample Preparation

1. Streptavidin Sepharose™ HP (Amersham Biosciences).
2. 10 µM Sequencing primer.

Table 1
The Mitochondrial Pyrosequencing System Set Up for Additional Resolution

Haplogroup[a]	Variable position[a]	Sequence primer (5')	Fragment no.	Total[b]
H	7028	6990	1	
J	4216	4156	2	
H1/J1	3010	2988	3	
I	10238	10205	4	
U	12372	12346	5	
K/U2	9055 + 12372	9107 + 12346	6 + 5	
T	15928	15978	7	
T/W	709	790	8	
V	15904	15978	7	8 fragments
H	4336	4275	9	
H	12705	12673	10	
H	15833	15758	11	
H	16519	16496	12	
H	456, 471, 477	431	13	
High freq. (24%)[c]	2706	2782	14	
High freq. (4%)[c], H	8697, 8705	8665	15	
High freq. (44%)[c]	750	790	8	
High freq. (54%)[d]	73	45	D-loop	
High freq. (8%[c], 4%[c])	10398, 10463	10362	16	8 fragments

The first eight fragments are used for haplogroup indication while the additional eight fragments are used to increase the resolution of identical mitochondrial DNA types among different individuals

[a] "/" denotes "or"; "+" denotes "and."
[b] Number of different fragments.
[c] Mitochondrial coding region database by Herrnstadt et al. (*6*).
[d] Mitochondrial D-loop database of 348 Swedish individuals (Nilsson M, and Allen M, in preparation).

3. High-purity water (Milli-Q™ 18.2 $M\,\Omega\times$ cm or equivalent).
4. Binding buffer, pH 7.6: 10 mM Tris-HCl, 2 M NaCl, 1 mM ethylene diamine tetraacetic acid, and 0.1% Tween-20.
5. Denaturation solution: 0.2 M NaOH.
6. Washing buffer. 10 mM Tris-acetate, pH 7.6.
7. Annealing buffer. 20 mM Tris-acetate and 5 mM Mg-acetate, pH 7.6.
8. Eppendorf or Falcon tube.

9. 96-well PCR plate.
10. Strip lids or sealing tape.
11. 96-well MultiScreen® Filter Plate (Millipore Corporation, Billerica, MA).
12. Mixer/shaker for microtiter plates (room temperature).
13. Heating block (80°C).
14. PSQ™96 Sample Prep Thermoplate Low (Pyrosequencing AB, Uppsala, Sweden).
15. Vacuum manifold (220 V/50 Hz; Millipore Corporation).
16. Vacuum source (minimum vacuum 300 mm Hg; Millipore Corporation).
17. Liquid trap flask.

2.3. Pyrosequencing Reaction

1. 220 ng/μL Single-Stranded DNA Binding Protein® (Amersham Pharmacia Biotech AB, Uppsala, Sweden).
2. Enzyme- and Substrate-mixtures, dNTPs (AαS, C, G, and T) (Pyrosequencing AB).
3. PSQ™96 Plate Low (Pyrosequencing AB).
4. PSQ™96 Reagent Cartridge (Pyrosequencing AB).
5. PSQ™96MA System SQA (Pyrosequencing AB).
6. PSQ™96MA SQA software v. 2.02 (Pyrosequencing AB).

2.4. Pyrosequencing Analysis

1. PSQ™96MA SQA software v. 2.02 (Pyrosequencing AB).

3. Methods

The methods described below outlines 1) PCR, 2) sample preparation, 3) pyrosequencing reaction, and 4) pyrosequencing analysis.

3.1. PCR

The mitochondrial D-loop is PCR amplified in two separate reactions (HVI and HVII). Each of the templates is analyzed using four sequencing primers per fragment, including the forward PCR primer. When necessary, the coding region fragments are amplified in 14 separate reactions, followed by analysis in 16 pyrosequencing reactions using either the forward or the reverse PCR primer or an internal sequencing primer. The reactions are incubated for 10 min at 95°C followed by 40 cycles of 30 s at 95°C, 45 s at 60°C (53°C for the coding region primers), and 60 s at 72°C, with a final extension step for 7 min at 72°C in an ABI 9600 instrument (Applied Biosystems).

3.1.1. Control Samples

PCRs for control samples are set up in 70 μL (30 μL for the coding region fragments) containing 1.5 μL of DNA, 200 nM of each primer (**Table 2**), 200 μM of each dNTP, 1.5 mM MgCl$_2$, 2 U AmpliTaq® Gold DNA Polymerase, and 1X GeneAmp® PCR Buffer II.

Table 2
PCR and Sequencing Primers for Pyrosequencing, Named by the 5' Nucleotide

Primer[a]	PCR primer	Sequence primer	T_m (°C)	Sequence (5' to 3')	Dispensation order	SSB required
II 45 F	X	X	55.6	ATGCATTGGTATTTCGTCTG	TCGA	
II 111 F		X	48.2	ACCCTATGTCGCAGTATCT	TCGA	
II 162 F		X	54.4	CGCACCTACGTTCAATATTACA	CTGA	
II 216 F		X	48.3	TTAATGCTTGTAGGACATAATAA	CTGA	
II 287 R-B	X		55.6	TTGTTATGATGTCTGTGTGGAAAG		
C 431 F	X	X	53.6	CACCCCCAACTAACACA	Directed	
C 637 R-B	X		53.1	GTGATGTGAGCCGTCTAA		
C 676 F-B	X		52.3	GCTCTTAGTAAGATTACACATGCA		
C 790 R	X	X	52.8	TAAGCGTTTGAGCTGCA	Directed	
C 2680 F-B	X		51.3	TGACCTGCCCGTGAA		
C 2782 R	X	X	51.8	TAGGACCTGTGGGTTTGTTA	Directed	
C 2988 F	X	X	51.8	CGATGTTGGATCAGGACA	Directed	
C 3216 R-B	X		52.4	GGGTGGGTGTGGGTATAA		
C 4156 F	X	X	52.5	CAACTCATACACCTCCTATGAAA	Directed	
C 4275 F		X	50.2	GATAAAAGAGTTACTTTGATAGAGTAAA	Directed	
C 4367 R-B	X		52.6	TTGGATTCTCAGGGATGG		
C 6990 F	X	X	49.4	CTAGACATCGTACTACACGACA	Directed	X
C 7299 R-B	X		48.8	TTACTGCTGTTAGAGAAATGAA		
C 8665 F	X	X	52	CAATGACTAATCAAACTAACCTCA	Directed	
C 8803 R-B	X		51.1	TAAATGAGTGAGGCAGGAGT		
C 8932 F-B	X		55.1	CCCCTTATCCCCATACTAGTTATTA		
C 9107 R	X	X	54.7	GTGAAGATGATAAGTGTAGAGGGAA	Directed	
C 10205 F	X	X	55.4	CCCTTTCTCCATAAAATTCTTCTTA	Directed	X

C 10362 F	X		55	CTGGCCTATGAGTGACTACAAAA	Directed	X
C 10586 R-B	X		53	CGATAGTATTATTCCTTCTAGGCA		X
C 12346 F	X	X	47.9	CACACTACTATAACCACCCTAA	Directed	X
C 12541 R-B	X	X	49.1	CTCAGTGTCAGTTCGAGATAA		
C 12673 F	X		45.7	AACATTAATCAGTTCTTCAAA	Directed	X
C 12861 R-B	X		46.7	GTTGTATAGGATTGCTTGAA		
C 15588 F	X		51.3	TCCGATCCGTCCCTAA		
C 15758 F		X	51.5	ATCGGAGGACAACCAGTAA	Directed	
C 15978 R-B	X	X	50.6	GGAGTTAAAGACTTTTTCTCTGA		
C 15588 F-B	X	X	51.3	TCCGATCCGTCCCTAA		
C 15978 R	X	X	50.6	GGAGTTAAAGACTTTTTCTCTGA	Directed	X
NC 16496 F	X	X	48.5	GACATCTGGTTCCTACTTCA	Directed	
NC 149 R-B	X	X	47.7	ATGAGGCAGGAATCAAA		
I 16105 F	X	X	55.4	TGCCAGCCACCATGAATA	CTGA	X
I 16168 F		X	50.3	CCAATCCACATCAAAACC	CTGA	X
I 16203 F		X	45.7	AGCAAGTACAGCAATCAA	CTGA	
I 16266 F		X	47.3	CCCACTAGGATACCAACA	CTGA	
I 16348 R-B	X		55.6	GACTGTAATGTGCTATGTACGGTAAA		X

[a] I denotes HVI; II denotes HVII; C denotes coding region; F denotes forward primer; R denotes reverse primer; B denotes biotinylated primer, and NC denotes non-coding.

3.1.2. Evidence Materials

PCR amplification of forensic evidence material is set up in 100 mL (30 μL for the coding region fragments) with 10 μL of DNA, 200 nM of each primer (**Table 2**), 200 μM of each dNTP, 2.4 mM MgCl$_2$, 10 U AmpliTaq® Gold DNA Polymerase, 1.2X GeneAmp® PCR Buffer II, 0.16 mg/mL bovine serum albumin, and 10% glycerol.

3.2. Sample Preparation

The pyrosequencing system is performed on single-stranded PCR products, to which a sequencing primer can be annealed. We have used a method for generating single-stranded DNA that use the binding of biotinylated PCR products to Streptavidin-coated Sepharose beads *(3)*.

3.2.1. Immobilization of PCR Product to Beads

1. Let the solutions reach room temperature (*see* **Note 1**).
2. Shake the Streptavidin Sepharose bottle to obtain a homogenous solution of the beads.
3. Transfer the total required amount of Streptavidin Sepharose beads (4 μL per well) to a tube.
4. To the tube, with Streptavidin beads, add binding buffer to a volume equivalent to the total volume of the PCR product to be used (control samples: 15 μL, evidence: 25 μL per well). Vortex the tube.
5. Mix the PCR product (control samples: 15 μL, evidence: 25 μL per well) with an equal volume (1:1) of the binding buffer-Streptavidin Sepharose bead mix in a 96-well PCR plate. Seal the plate.
6. Incubate at room temperature for 10 min while agitating constantly to keep the beads dispersed, using a mixer/shaker.

3.2.2. Strand Separation

1. Transfer, by pipeting, the immobilized template to a 96-well filter plate (*see* **Note 2**). Place the filter plate on the vacuum manifold and apply vacuum to remove all liquid (**Fig. 3**, **Note 3**).
2. Release the vacuum and add 50 μL of denaturation solution.
3. Incubate for 1 min before applying the vacuum again to remove the denaturation solution.
4. Wash twice with 150 μL of washing buffer; carefully remove all liquid between and after the washing steps (*see* **Note 4**).

3.2.3. Primer Annealing

1. Add 45 μL of annealing buffer per well to the filter plate and resuspend the beads with the immobilized template by pipeting up and down four to five times (one row at the time using a 12-channel pipet).

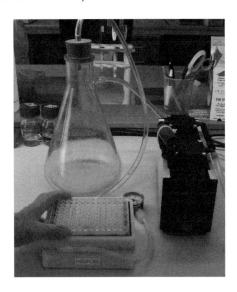

Fig. 3.The vacuum manifold used for the pyrosequencing sample preparation where the templates are strand separated.

2. Transfer 35 μL from the filter plate to a PSQ 96 Plate Low (one row at the time).
3. Add 5 μL of sequencing primer (3 μ*M* in annealing buffer; **Table 2**) to each well (*see* **Note 5**).
4. Heat the plate with the samples at 80°C for 2 min using the PSQ 96 Sample Prep Thermoplate Low. Allow the samples to reach room temperature.
5. When necessary, 2 μL (440 ng) of SSB (**Table 2**) is added to the each primed DNA template before pyrosequencing (*see* **Note 6**).

3.3. Pyrosequencing Reaction

1. Choose method/instrument parameters and enter relevant run/sample information in the sample sheet (PSQ™ 96MA System User Manual; http://www.pyrosequencing.com).
2. Select an appropriate dispensation order for each fragment (**Tables 1** and **3**; **Note 7**).
3. Fill the PSQ 96 reagent cartridge with enzyme, substrate, and separate dNTPs in volumes according to the SQA software (**Fig. 4**).
4. Place the cartridge and PSQ 96 Plate Low with the primed samples to be analyzed in the PSQ 96 instrument.
5. Start the run.
6. After the run, discard the remaining solutions from the cartridge.
7. Rinse the cartridge rigorous by pressing high purity water through the needles, fill the compartments with water and press on the top with a finger. Discard the water and let the cartridge dry on a lint-free tissue.

Table 3
Directed Dispensation Orders

Sequence primer (5')	Dispensation order (5' to 3')
431	TATTCCTCTCACTCCATACTCACTCATCTCATCAATACAACCGCATCTACC AGCACACACACACGCTGCTACCATACCGAACCACAACCAAGACA
790	TTGACTGCGTGGCTGATTGCTGTCATTGATCGGTGATGATTAGAGCTT GGAACTCACTGGAACTGGATTGCTGCATGTGTATCTACTAGAGCTA
2680	GAGCGGACATACACAGCAGACGAGAGACCTATGAGCTTATT ATATGCAACAGTACTACAACCACAGTCTAACTACAC
2988	TCCGTACATGTGCAGCGCTATCAGAAGTCGTTGTCACGATAA GTTCTACGTGAATCTGAGTTCAAGACGGAGTAGCAGTCG
4156	AACTCTACACTGCTCACCTAGCATACTA TATGATCAGATGTCTCATACCATACAT CTCAGCATCCTCAACTAGAAT
4275	TATAGAGCTAACCTATTCTAGACTATGAGA
6990	CGATACTAACGTTGTAGCTCACTTCCACTAATGTCCTATCAATAGGAAGCTG TTATTGGCCATCAATAGGAGGCTTCATTCACTGATTCCTATTCTCAGCTA
8665	AACAATGATCATACATGACACACAATCGCACTAAGGACGACC TGATCGTCTCTATACTAGTATCTATCATTATGCACACTACTC
9107	GTATGTGATATGCTAGGTGCTGCTCATAGTGCATGAGTAGTGCTGCAG TATGTAGCGTAGCGTACGCAGGCTATGTGATGAGTAGCTGATGTTCGA
10205	GTAGCTATACTCTATATTGATCTAGAATGCTCCTTACCTACATGAGCC TACAACACTACTGCCACTATAGTATGTCATCCTCTATATCATCATC
10362	AGATAGACTGAGCGAATTGTATATAGTTACAACGATTGATCGGA CCTCCATATATGATATCATTATTACATGCCTCATTAC
12346	CCTGTACACTCCTATCCATCTTATCGCACTCGTACCTGACACAA CTCATACCATATGTAATCATGTCGCATCACCTTATTATCAGTCTC
12673	TATGCACTACTCATCGTATCCTAATTACATACTATCTAGTTACGC TGACACCAACTATCCACTGTCATCGCTGAGAGGCGTAGAT
15758	GCTACCTTACATCATGACAGTAGCATCGTACTATACT CACACAATCTAATCTATACACCTATCTCTATGACA
15978	TTGTCTGAAGTTCATCTCGTCTACAAGACTGGTGTATAGTT ATACTACAAGACAGGCCATTGAGTTATTGTCATAGG
16496	GGTCAGCATAAGTCACTGACTAATAGCCACACGTCCTTAATA GACATCACGATGATCACAGTCTATCACCTATACACTCACGG

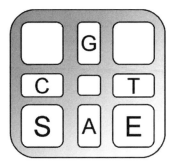

Fig. 4. Enzymes, substrates, and nucleotides are added to the pyrosequencing reaction by the instrument from the PSQ 96 reagent cartridge, where each solution has its specific chamber.

3.4. Pyrosequencing Analysis

1. The sequence data analysis is conducted using the SQA software (PSQ™ 96MA System User Manual; http://www.pyrosequencing.com; **Note 8**). The sequences are visualized in a pyrogram, starting with a substrate peak representing the free PPi in the sample solution from the beginning followed by peaks for each incorporated nucleotide (**Fig. 5**).
2. A few reference peaks can be assigned to assist the software in the analysis of problematic sequences. In addition, the A-peak adjustment integrated in the algorithm of the SQA software can be changed. This might be required because the natural dATP is replaced by dATPαS to prevent interaction with the luciferase reducing the background signal *(3)*.
3. The sequences are aligned to the Cambridge reference sequence *(5)* for comparison and determination of variable positions (**Fig. 6**). The alignments can be illustrated as base-to-base or as best-fit. The sequence is either lined up base by base in the base-by-base alignment whereas the best-fit alignment adjust the alignment to the called master sequence (the Cambridge reference sequence in this case) and gaps are inserted at appropriate positions.
4. Some sequences will require manual editing, due to incorrect base calling by the SQA software when scoring homopolymeric peaks. The problematic regions are easily identified in the alignment and can be corrected, after checking of the pyrograms, by manually removing or adding a nucleotide to the sequence readout (**Figs. 5** and **6**).
5. The pyrosequencing system presented here has been used for mitochondrial analysis of a variety of previously Sanger sequenced and DNA quantified forensic samples. For example, cell material in a sneaker (containing 300 mitochondrial DNA copies per reaction) and a saliva stain from a letter mailed in 1952 (containing 600 mitochondrial DNA copies per reaction) have been pyrosequenced. Moreover, degraded DNA extracted from paraffin embedded tis-

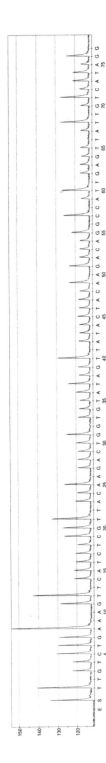

Fig. 5. Pyrogram with the added components (enzyme, substrate, or nucleotides) on the x-axis and light intensity on the y-axis. The height of the peaks is proportional to the number of incorporated nucleotides; however, there is a drop off in peak height over time, which is taken in to account by the software. The substrate peak shows the conversion of free PPi in the sequencing reaction from the start. In this example a directed dispensation order has been used (fragment 15978).

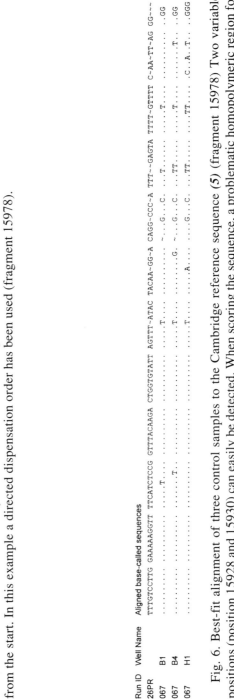

Fig. 6. Best-fit alignment of three control samples to the Cambridge reference sequence (5) (fragment 15978) Two variable positions (position 15928 and 15930) can easily be detected. When scoring the sequence, a problematic homopolymeric region for the SQA algorithm occurs 53–56 nucleotides downstream. However, these errors can easily be edited manually.

sue was successfully analyzed using pyrosequencing (**Fig. 7**). The mitochondrial DNA quantification was performed with a highly sensitive, rapid and reliable real-time 5' exonuclease detection system, using the ABI PRISM® 7700 instrument (Applied Biosystems, Foster City, CA). The system is based on simultaneous amplification of the nuclear retinoblastoma 1 gene (for nuclear quantification) and the mitochondrial tRNA Lys gene (for mitochondrial quantification; ref. *8*).

6. The mitochondrial pyrosequencing system has been used on previously mtDNA analyzed forensic casework materials. In a case in Stockholm, in 1999, a girl and a boy were severely molested by adults who thought that the children were obsessed by demons. In what was thought to be a exorcism ritual, the girl was murdered, and a bible with a small stain was found on the scene of the crime. The mitochondrial DNA analysis showed identical sequences between the stain on the bible and the blood of the 11-yr-old girl (**Fig. 8**).

4. Notes

1. All solutions for sample preparation (binding buffer, denaturation solution, washing buffer, and annealing buffer) are available from Pyrosequencing AB, Uppsala Sweden, separate or together in a PSQ 96 Sample Preparation Kit.

2. There is a PSQ 96 Vacuum Prep Tool available from Pyrosequencing AB to facilitate the production of single-stranded DNA. This hand-held tool with 96 replaceable filter probes is connected to a vacuum source and can be used with or without the use of the PSQ 96 Vacuum Prep Worktable, which has specific holders for all plates and trays used in the strand separation process. A vacuum switch and a manometer are positioned on the front of the table to assist handling and monitoring (**Fig. 9**). These sample preparation tools (PSQ™ Vacuum Prep Workstation; Product Information 014; http://www.pyrosequencing.com) are designed to process up to 96 DNA samples in parallel, from PCR-products to single-stranded sequencing templates, in less than 15 min. Actual hands-on time is less than 1 min, and each set of filter probes can be reused at least 100 times, if simply cleaned (flushing with water) after each use.

3. When using only a few wells of the filter plate, cover the rest of the plate to accelerate the filtration.

4. Excess wash liquid may remain underneath the wells of the filter plate after the wash step. Remove the liquid by gently tapping the filter plate on a piece of lint-free tissue.

5. To save time, dilute the sequencing primer in annealing buffer during the immobilization step and add it to the PSQ 96 Plate Low before the single-stranded template from the filter plate.

6. SSB can alternatively be added to the primed samples in the PSQ 96 Plate Low with the help of the PSQ 96 reagent cartridge (50 µL as a dead volume plus 3.3 µL per well) prior to the actual pyrosequencing run (see PSQ 96 software user manual for details).

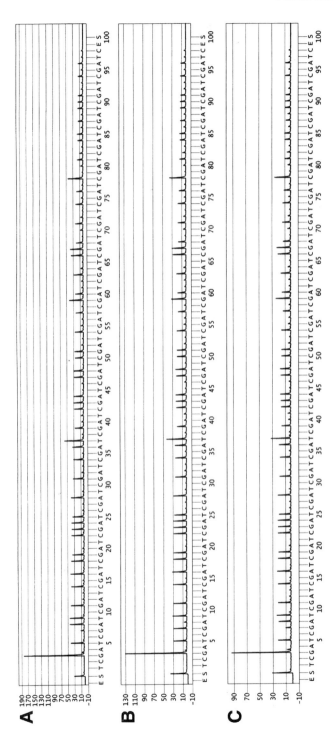

Fig. 7. Pyrosequencing of different evidence materials (fragment 45). A variable position can be seen at nucleotide position 73. Top, DNA sample from a paraffin-embedded tissue. Middle, Cell material from a sneaker. Bottom, Saliva stain from an old letter.

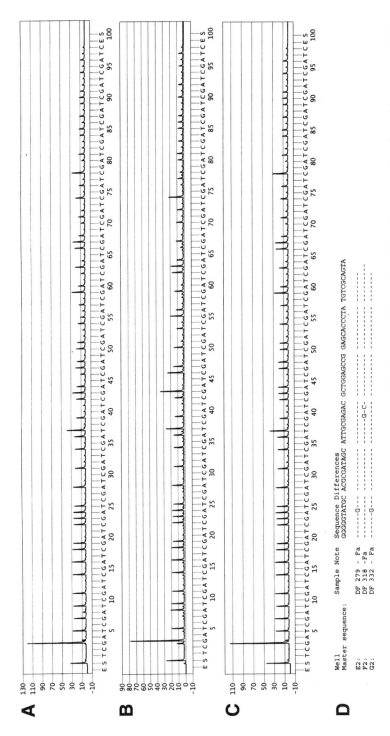

Fig. 8. Pyrosequencing results (fragment 45) in the analysis of casework samples. Top, Pyrogram for the evidence material, a blood stain from a bible. Middle, Reference material from victim 1. Bottom, Reference material from victim 2. Lastly, Base-by-base alignment to the Cambridge reference sequence (*5*) where three variable positions can bee seen, nucleotide 73, 93, and 95. All samples showed identical results in comparison to D-loop Sanger sequencing.

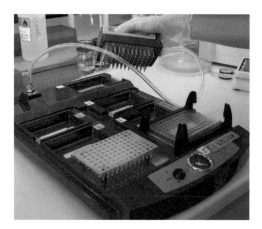

Fig. 9 The PSQ™ Vacuum Prep Workstation that can be used for faster and easier pyrosequencing sample preparation. The Workstation consists of a PSQ 96 Vacuum Prep Tool and a PSQ 96 Vacuum Prep Worktable each to facilitate the sample handling.

7. The dispensation order is entered according to the reference sequence except for positions where differences are expected. When using directed dispensation additional nucleotides are added after homopolymeric regions to limit shifts to occur in the sequence readout.
8. It is possible to work with the SQA software on a client computer connected to the PSQ instrument software via network connection.

Acknowledgments

This work was supported by grants from the Kjell and Märta Beijer Foundation and the Swedish Agency for Innovation System (VINNOVA) P14043-4 A to M.A.

References

1. Allen, M., Engstrom, A. S., Meyers, S., Handt, O., Saldeen, T., von Haeseler, A., et al. (1998) Mitochondrial DNA sequencing of shed hairs and saliva on robbery caps: sensitivity and matching probabilities. *J. Forensic Sci.* **43,** 453–464.
2. Ronaghi, M. (2001) Pyrosequencing sheds light on DNA sequencing. *Genome Res.* **11,** 3–11.
3. Ronaghi, M., Karamohamed, S., Pettersson, B., Uhlen, M., and Nyren, P. (1996) Real-time DNA sequencing using detection of pyrophosphate release. *Anal. Biochem.* **242,** 84–89.
4. Ronaghi, M., Pettersson, B., Uhlen, M., and Nyren, P. (1998) PCR-introduced loop structure as primer in DNA sequencing. *BioTechniques* **25,** 876–788, 880–882, 884.

5. Anderson, S., Bankier, A. T., Barrell, B. G., de Bruijn, M. H., Coulson, A. R., Drouin, J., et al. (1981) Sequence and organization of the human mitochondrial genome. *Nature* **290,** 457–465.

6. Herrnstadt, C., Elson, J. L., Fahy, F., Preston, G., Turnbull, D. M., Anderson, C., et al. (2002) Reduced-median-network analysis of complete mitochondrial DNA coding-region sequences for the major African, Asian, and European haplogroups. *Am. J. Hum Genet.* **70,** 1152–1171.

7. Andreasson, H., Asp, A., Alderborn, A., Gyllensten, U., and Allen, M. (2002) Mitochondrial sequence analysis for forensic identification using pyrosequencing technology. *BioTechniques* **32,** 124–126, **128,** 130–133.

8. Andreasson, H., Gyllensten, U., and Allen, M. (2002) Real-time DNA quantification of nuclear and mitochondrial DNA in forensic analysis. *BioTechniques* **33,** 402–404, 407–411.

14

SNaPshot Typing of Mitochondrial DNA Coding Region Variants

Antonio Salas, Beatriz Quintáns, and Vanesa Álvarez-Iglesias

Summary

We describe a rapid and robust assay to genotype mitochondrial deoxyribonucleic acid (mtDNA) coding region single nucleotide polymorphism (SNPs) using the SNaPshot (Applied Biosystems, Foster City, CA) minisequencing reaction kit. A protocol for mtDNA SNaPshot typing is described in detail, although we emphasize that this method allows great flexibility in the implementation of whatever set of mtDNA SNPs. We discuss the utility of our selection of mtDNA SNPs for molecular anthropologists and forensic geneticists. Firstly, these SNPs allow allocating common mitochondrial West Eurasian haplotypes into their corresponding branches of the mtDNA skeleton, with especial attention to the subdivision of sequences belonging to haplogroup H, the most frequent European haplogroup (40–50%) and the worst phylogenetically characterized in the first and second hypervariable segments (HVS-I/II; by far, the most common segments analyzed by sequencing). Second, the polymorphic positions selected for this multiplex reaction considerably increase the discrimination power of current mitochondrial analysis in the forensic field. The method shows high accuracy and robustness, avoiding both the use of alternative time-consuming classical strategies (i.e., restriction fragment length polymorphism typing) and the requirement of high quantities of DNA template.

Key Words: SNaPshot; SNPs; mtDNA; hypervariable region; human identification.

1. Introduction

The interest in single nucleotide polymorphisms (SNPs) is continuously growing as a result of their numerous applications in medical genetics *(1,2)*, for instance, disease diagnostics and pharmacological response studies, in human and evolutionary genetics (e.g., *3*), and also in the forensics field *(e.g., 4)*.

Mitochondrial deoxyribonucleic acid (mtDNA) molecules have specific features that make them especially useful in forensic casework and human population studies: 1) rapid mutation rate, 2) high copy number per mitochondrion

From: *Methods in Molecular Biology, vol. 297: Forensic DNA Typing Protocols*
Edited by: A. Carracedo © Humana Press Inc., Totowa, NJ

and cell, and 3) it does not recombine and it is maternally inherited as an haplotype block. Analysis of mtDNA polymorphisms has become a useful tool for human population and molecular evolution studies, allowing the inference of patterns of female migrations and peopling of different worldwide populations (e.g., *5,6*). Mutations are recorded in the molecule, and transferred generation to generation mirroring the evolutionary history of the locus. In forensic genetics, polymorphisms of the mtDNA genome are useful for human identification, especially for the analysis of degraded material or samples containing little or no genomic DNA (i.e., skeletal remains and hair shafts; refs, *7–12*). However, the two routinely analyzed mtDNA hypervariable regions (HVS-I and HVS-II) provide limited power of discrimination in a forensic context and, in many cases, provide scarce information in evolutionary studies. Because sequencing of the entire mitochondrial molecule is not practical, the analysis of additional information found in the mtDNA-coding region seems to be a good strategy to short cut this drawback.

Polymerase chain reaction (PCR) amplification followed by restriction fragment analysis (RFLP typing) and manual polyacrylamide gel electrophoresis is a popular technique commonly used for studying point mutations in mtDNA (specially outside the control region). This method has the drawback of being time-consuming, costly, and requiring high amounts of DNA. Note that the later is of particular relevance in the forensic context. During the last few years, new methodologies for high-throughput SNP analysis have been developed. These methods include real-time PCR analysis, microarrays scanning, matrix-assisted laser desorption ionization time-of-flight, pyrosequenc-ing, TaqMan probes, and molecular beacons *(13–15)*. Most of these high-throughput technologies are extremely expensive and therefore cannot be used by a great majority of researchers in standard laboratories. Furthermore, many of them are still in varying phases of development.

Here we show an alternative for SNP typing that is rapid, robust, and relatively cheap. The SNaPshot (Applied Biosystems, Foster City, CA) multiplex reaction is a single-base extension reaction that enables robust multiplex SNP interrogation of PCR-generated templates.

SNaPshot reaction is based on the dideoxy (ddNTP) single-base extension of an unlabeled oligonucleotide at the 3' end of the base immediately adjacent to the SNP (in absence of dNTPs in the reaction). Unlabeled primers (with the 5' end tailed) with varying lengths of noncomplementary oligonucleotide sequences serve as a mobility modifier. In addition, each ddNTP is labeled with different fluorescent dyes. The extended SNaPshot primers used to interrogate different SNPs differ between them by size and color. The resulting products can be separated electrophoretically in a single capillary and analyzed in the presence of a fifth-dye-labeled size standard.

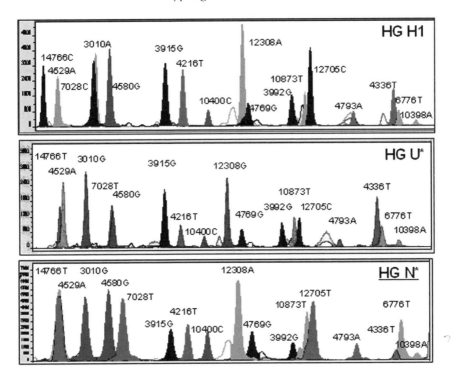

Fig. 1. Electropherograms of 17 SNPs-multiplex assay for three different samples. Polymorphisms refer to the L strand and following the rCRS *(19)*, including those interrogated using minisequencing primers located in H chain (3915, 10400, 4769, 10873, 4793, and 6776).

Here, we describe a method for typing 17 coding region SNPs in two independent multiplex amplifications and one SNaPshot reaction (that is, the two multiplexes amplification products are mixed in a tube and minisequenced in a single reaction). **Figure 1** shows the electropherogram for the 17 coding region mtDNA SNPs. With this technology and using a 16 multicapillary machine, 16 samples can be typed for 17 SNPs in less than 25 min, including capillary filling, sample loading, and separation of the fragments. Thus, 17 SNPs can be analyzed in an approximately maximum number of 920 samples per day.

Note that the method SNaPshot is flexible and performs well with other combinations of SNPs. As we explain below, it is only necessary to optimize SNaPshot reaction conditions depending on the number of SNPs we desire to type, as well as primer amplification, and minisequencing primers. Therefore, SNaPshot has an enormous potential as a substitute technique for SNP typing in more complex platforms, such as matrix-assisted laser desorption/ionization time-of-flight, microarrays technologies, etc. Note, however, that the number of SNPs that can be typed in single SNaPshot reaction is probably limited to a few (probably less than 40).

Therefore, as an example of the potential of the SNaPshot method, we show a protocol to simultaneously genotype 17 mtDNA-selected SNPs for forensic and anthropological applications. The selected markers avoid the use of common time-consuming and expensive strategies when typing individuals of western European ancestry. Special attention has been placed on the subtyping of haplogroup H, which is the most frequent lineage in these populations and the worst characterized when looking at the HVS-I/II segments (the most common mtDNA region analyzed by medical, forensic, and anthropological geneticists).

2. Materials

1. PCR reagents: Human DNA, AmpliTaq Gold® DNA polymerase and 10X GeneAmp® PCR Buffer II (Applied Biosystems), MgCl$_2$, dNTPs, PCR primers (Sigma-Genosys Ltd, Pampisford, Cambs, UK).
2. PCR purification: ExoSap IT (Amershan Biosciences).
3. SNaPshot reaction: Purified PCR products, SNaPshot multiplex kit (Applied Biosystems, Foster City, CA, USA), high-performance liquid chromatography-purified extension primers (Sigma-Genosys Ltd, Pampisford, Cambs, UK).
4. Purification post-extension: Minisequencing product, SAP (Amershan Biosciences).
5. Data analysis: Purified minisequencing product, HiDi™ formamide (Applied Biosystems), GeneScan-120 LIZ size standard (Applied Biosystems), ABI PRISM 3100® Genetic Analyzer (Applied Biosystems), Performance optimum polymer 4 (POP4®), GeneScanTM 3.7 Software (Applied Biosystems).

3. Methods

The SNaPshot multiplex kit (Applied Biosystems) provides all the necessary reagents to perform high-throughput SNP typing in a multicapillary sequencer. Although the manufacture protocol recommends SNP marker sized between 20 and 105 bp, as we will see, bigger amplicon sizes can perfectly be typed. More instructions related to the kit, size standard, software, and matrix standard are provided by the company. Here, we describe a protocol specifically designed for mtDNA typing.

3.1. PCR Multiplex

Two multiplex reactions were designed to type 17 different mtDNA coding region SNPs.

1. Multiplex 1 includes a selection of SNPs defining common European haplogroups (see ref. *16* and references therein).

2. Multiplex 2 exclusively includes polymorphisms defining subhaplogroups inside haplogroup H. The characterization of H sublineages is mainly based on the complete sequences available in Herrnstadt et al. *(17)*.

3.2. Multiplex Primers Design

Primers were designed (except for testing position 12308, which were previously described by Torroni et al. *[18]*), in order to adjust the annealing temperatures and amplicon lengths to the multiplex reactions (**Table 1**).

Primers3 software (http://frodo.wi.mit.edu/cgi-bin/primer3/primer3_www.cgi) was used for primer design. It is recommended to test the primers for possible repetitive sequences. Primer sequences were also screened using the BLAST at the National Center for Biotechnology Information (NCBI) (http://www.ncbi.nlm.nih.gov/blast/blast.cgi).

3.3. Coamplification of PCR Products

Coamplification in the same amplicon can be conducted for those SNPs closely related within the mtDNA molecule. It is important to remember that, for forensic purposes, it is convenient to obtain PCR products of low size to facilitate the analysis of degraded samples or carrying low quantities of DNA. In our set of SNPs, amplicons range from 80 to 224 bp.

3.4. Optimization of PCR Reactives

It is convenient to optimize all PCR reactives to obtain a well-balanced multiplex amplification; special attention should be given to primer concentration, $MgCl_2$, and amount of DNA template. Our multiplex were performed using 10 ng of DNA template in a 25-μL reaction volume comprising 1X Taq Gold Buffer (Applied Biosystems), 200 μM of each dNTP, 2 mM $MgCl_2$, and 0.5 units of AmpliTaq Gold Polymerase (Applied Biosystems). Primers concentrations for Multiplex 1 are between 0.1 μM and 0.4 μM (**Table 1**), and 0.15 μM of each forward and reverse for Multiplex 2.

3.5. Amplification Reaction

We have conducted PCR amplifications in a 9700 Termocycler (Applied Biosystems) according to the following protocol: 1) 95°C preincubation step for 11 min; 2) 32 cycles using the following conditions: denaturation: 94°C for 30 s, annealing at 60°C for 30 s, and extension at 72°C during 1 min; and 3) 15 min of final extension at 72°C. It is convenient to check the multiplex PCR products using polyacrylamide gel electrophoresis (i.e., T9C5), at least while the conditions for the specific multiplex under study are not completely optimized.

Table 1
Coding Region Site (SNP), Primer Sequence (5' to 3'), and Final Concentrations of Each Primer Used for SNPs Amplifications

SNP[a]	Size (bp)	Forward and reverse primers	FC[b] (mM)
PCR-Multiplex 1			
4216	195	CTCTACACAACATATTTTGTCACCAAG GGTTTGAGGGGGAATGCTGGAG	0.30
4529–4580[c]	148	CAACCCGTCATCTACTCTACCAT CTTCTGTGGAACGAGGGTTTATT	0.30
7028	168	CACCGTAGGTGGCCTGACTGGC GTGTAGCCTGAGAATAGGGG	0.15
10398–10400[c]	224	AAATTGCCCTCCTTTTACCCCTA TGTAAATGAGGGGCATTTGG	0.40
10873	123	CATAATTTGAATCAACACAACCACC GTTAGGGGGTCGGAGGAAAAGGTTG	0.10
12308[d]	106	CTGCTAACTCATGCCCCCATG ATTACTTTTATTTGGAGTTGCACCAAGATT	0.40
12705	147	TGTAGCATTGTTCGTTACATGG AGTTGGAATAGGTTGTTAGCGG	0.20
14766	82	TCAACTACAAGAACACCAATGACC GGAGGTCGATGATGAGTGG	0.40
PCR-Multiplex 2			
3010	180	CAATAACTTGACCAACGGAACA CGGTCTGAACTCAGATCACGTA	0.15
3915-3992[c]	158	TAGCAGAGACCAACCGAACC GAAGATTGTAGTGGTGAGGGTGT	0.15
4336	80	GGAGCTTAAACCCCCTTATTTC GATAGGTGGCACGGAGAATTT	0.15
4769-4793[c]	118	CCGGACAATGAACCATAACC TGGGTAACCTCTGGGACTCA	0.15
6776	140	GCTTCCTAGGGTTTATCGTGTG GAGTGTGGCGAGTCAGCTAAA	0.15

[a]SNPs are called by its position in mitochondrial genome according to revised Cambridge Reference Sequence (rCRS; ref. *19*).

[b]FC, final concentration.

[c]Two SNPs are localized in the same amplicon.

[d]Primers reference for this polymorphism: Torroni el al. (*18*). Reverse primer was design by Torroni et al., with a mismatch (underlined) to detect this polymorphism as RFLP.

3.6. SNaPshot Reaction

1. PCR products must be purified to remove primers and unincorporated dNTPs. Post-PCR purification was performed using different protocols varying the concentrations of *Exo*I and SAP (Amershan Biosciences Biotech; data not shown), but better results were obtained using ExoSap IT (Amershan Biosciences Biotech): 2.5 μL of PCR product is incubated with 1 μL of ExoSapIT for 15 min at 37°C followed by 15 min at 80°C for enzyme inactivation.

2. Minisequencing reaction performed in a 9700 Termocycler following recommendations of manufacturer (Applied Biosystems). A total volume of 7 μL should contain 2 μL of kit SNaPshot, 0.2 μM of extension primer for each SNP, and 1 μL of both purified PCR products.

3. The reaction mixture was subjected to 25 single-base extension cycles as follows: denaturation: 96°C for 10 s, annealing at 50°C for 5 s, and extension at 60°C for 30 s. Again, Primers3 software can be used to design extension primers (also called minisequencing primers). Detection of extension products is based on a strategy that combines colors (using different flourocromes to assay A/G and C/T polymorphism) and extension primer sizes (the length of a primer can be modified by the addition of non-homologous tails at the 5' end). Poly (dC) or poly (dGACT) tails are added at the 5' end of the specific part of the primer depending on the polymorphic variant interrogated. The final sizes range between 20 and 57 bp (**Table 2**). All minisequencing primers were purified by high-performance liquid chromatography to remove incomplete primer synthesis products (Sigma-Genosys Ltd, Pampisford, Cambs, UK). After minisequencing reaction, a postextension treatment removes the 5' phosphoryl group of the ddNTPs. The entire volume (7 μL) was treated as follows: 0.7 μL of SAP (Amershan Biosciences) for 60 min at 37°C and 15 min at 80°C for enzyme inactivation.

4. Minisequencing products (1.5 μL) were mixed with 10 μL of HiDi™ formamide and 0.2 μL of GeneScan-120 LIZ size standard (Applied Biosystems) and electrophoresis was performed on an ABI PRISM 3100® Genetic Analyzer (Applied Biosystems).

5. Minisequencing products are then injected electrokinetically for 10 s at 15 kV and electrophoresed for 20 min at 15 kV and 9 μA at 60°C (default module) in a 36-cm length capillary using the performance optimum polymer 4 (POP4®) with the laser set at a constant power of 9.9 mW. SNaPshot patterns can be analyzed using GeneScan™ 3.7 Software (Applied Biosystems).

4. Final Remarks

1. The detected size determined by the automatic sequencer and the real size of some minisequencing products are slightly different. This is caused by differences in electrophoretic mobility, mainly determined by the length, sequence, and the dye use to label the amplicon. To assure the correct differentiation of the extended primer, we estimate that amplicons must differ at least in four nucleotide bases in length.

Table 2
Minisequencing Primer Sequences

SNP	Chain	Base change	Size (bps)	Extension primer[a]	FC (μM)[b]
3010	L	G-A	24	CTCGATGTTGGATCAGGACATCCC	0.10
3915	H	G-A	32	TGACTGACTAAGCCTGAGACTAGTTCGGACTC	0.20
3992	L	C-T	45	TGACTGACTGACTGACTGACTCCCTATTCTTCATAGCCGAATACA	0.30
4216	L	T-C	33	CCCTACCACTCACCTAGCATTACTTATATGA	0.20
4336	L	T-C	55	CTGACTGACTGACTGACTGACTGACTGCTTAAACCCCCTTATTTCTAGGAC	0.20
4529	L	A-T	21	CTTTGCAGGCACACTCATCAC	0.15
4580	L	G-A	28	TTACCTGAGTAGGCCTAGAAATAAACAT	0.10
4769	H	A-G	40	GACTGACTGACTGGGCTATTCCTAGTTTTATTGCTATAGC	0.30
4793	H	A-C	50	GACTGACTGACTGACTGACTGACTCTACTCAGAAGTGAAAGGGGGC	0.40
6776	H	T-C	55	ACTGACTGACTGACTGACTGACTCGTGTGTCTATTCCTACTGTAAATAT	0.30
7028	L	C-T	25	TACACGACACGTACTACGTTGTGTGAGC	0.10
10398	L	A-G	57	GACTGACTGACTGACTGACTGACTGACTATGAGTGACTACAAAAGGATTAGACTGA	0.50
10400	H	C-T	37	CCCCCCCCCGTTTGTTAAACTATATACCAATTC	0.50
10873	H	T-C	45	CCCCCCCCCCCGTTGTTGTTGATTTGGTTAAAAAATAGTAG	0.10
12308	L	A-G	41	CCCCCCCCCCCCCCCCCCCCCCATTGGTCTTAGGCCCCAA	0.40
12705	L	C-T	49	CCCCCCCCCCCCCCCCCAACATTAATCAGTTCTTCAAATATCTACTCAT	0.30
14766	L	C-T	20	AATGACCCAATACGCAAAA	0.30

Second column denotes the chain for primer annealing. Polymorphisms refer to the L strand and follow the standard nomenclature of rCRS (*21*).
[a]The nonspecific primer tail of polyC or polyGACT is underlined.
[b]FC, final concentration.

Table 3
SNP States for the Different Haplogroups Tested Using the SNaPshot Reaction.

rCRS	SNP-HG state																			
	H*	H1	H2	H3	H4	H5	H6	H7	Pre-V	V	HV*	JT	J	U*	K	R*	M*	N*	I	L3*
3010G	G	A	G	G	G	G	G	G	G	G	G	G	G	G	G	G	G	G	G	G
3915G	G	G	G	G	G	G	A	G	G	G	G	G	G	G	G	G	G	G	G	G
3992C	C	C	C	C	T	C	C	C	C	C	C	C	C	C	C	C	C	C	C	C
4216T	T	T	T	T	T	T	T	T	T	T	T	T	C	T	T	T	T	T	T	T
4336T	T	T	T	T	T	C	T	T	T	T	T	T	T	T	T	T	T	T	T	T
4529A	A	A	A	A	A	A	A	A	A	A	A	A	A	A	A	A	A	A	G	A
4580G	G	G	G	G	G	G	G	G	G	A	G	G	G	G	G	G	G	G	G	G
4769A	G	G	A	G	G	G	G	G	G	G	G	G	G	G	G	G	G	G	G	G
4793A	A	A	A	A	A	A	A	C	A	A	A	A	A	A	A	A	A	A	A	A
6776T	T	T	T	C	T	T	T	T	T	T	T	T	T	T	T	T	T	T	T	T
7028C	C	C	C	C	C	C	C	C	T	T	T	T	T	T	T	T	T	T	T	T
10398A	A	A	A	A	A	A	A	A	A	A	A	A	A	A	A	A	G	A	G	G
10400C	C	C	C	C	C	C	C	C	C	C	C	C	C	C	C	C	T	C	C	C
10873T	T	T	T	T	T	T	T	T	T	T	T	T	T	T	T	T	C	T	T	C
12308A	A	A	A	A	A	A	A	A	A	A	A	A	A	G	G	A	A	A	A	A
12705C	C	C	C	C	C	C	C	C	C	C	C	C	C	C	C	C	T	T	T	T
14766C	C	C	C	C	C	C	C	C	C	C	T	T	T	T	T	T	T	T	T	T

The first column indicates the variants corresponding to the rCRS (*19*). Nucleotide differences with respect to the rCRS are indicated (underlined) in the next columns according to each mtDNA haplogroup. In those cases where HVS-I segment is phylogenetically informative (*16*), we have found a complete correlation with the coding region mtDNA SNP variants (data not shown).

2. As seen in the electropherograms, some fragments display a stronger fluorescent signal than others (even after color compensation with corresponding matrix) as a result of the nature of the minisequencing chemistry; therefore, the same SNP can be detected by the automatic sequencer as a higher or lower peak depending on the inserted ddNTPs. In general, guanines labeled with dR100 bring a higher signal than the others ddNTPs. However, this fact does not alter the readability of the electropherogram.

3. All the samples SNaPshot typed in this experiment were previously sequenced for the mtDNA HVS-I region. There was good phylogenetic agreement *(16)* between HVS-I segments and the coding region SNPs typed (**Table 3**).

   The forensic utility of the SNPs selected are clearly manifested when looking at the most frequent European lineage (H; 40–50%). Haplogroup H represents 45% of our samples (a similar value is found in other European populations or of European ancestry). The use of the SNaPshot reaction allows to subtype this haplogroup in 6 different sublineages with the following frequencies: 1) H* (23%); 2) H1 (variant 3010A; 39%); 3) H2 (variant 4769A; 7%); 4) H3 (variant 6776C; 18%); 5) H4 (variant 3992T; 6%); 6) H5 (variant 4336C; 6%); and 7) H6 (variant 3915A; 1%). We did not find any representative of H7 (4793G). The maximum increment in haplotype diversity corresponds to the most common HVS-I sequence in Europe, the rCRS in HVS-I *(19)*. There are a total of 44 identical rCRS HVS-I sequences in our (northwest Spain) sample, 18% of them are H*, 41% H1, 5% H2, 20% H3, 14% H4, and 2% HV* (all of them 7028C; haplotype diversity increase from 0 to 0.737 in this specific set of samples). Other HVS-I haplotypes also gain in discrimination power when using this set of coding region SNPs. For instance, there are four sequences characterized by the only transition at position 16380, two of them harbor 7028T-12308G (U*), one of them is 6776C-7028C (H3), and the other is 7028T-14766T (R*).

4. Mitochondrial coding region SNPs are especially useful for human population genetics. The use of multiplexes appears as the best methodology for typing small amounts of SNPs. The need of low quantity of DNA template is valuable in many anthropological studies. Here, polymorphic sites were selected to assess major haplogroups and subhaplogruops of the mtDNA European phylogeny, with special focus on those with ambiguous HVS-I motifs *(16)*, including the most common haplogroup in Europe (H; 40–50% of the European mtDNA sequences). H-sequences have not diagnostic positions in HVS-I and II segments and are by far the most common regions analyzed in the clinical, forensic, and human population genetic literature. A subclassification of these lineages is therefore necessary to disentangle population relationships in Europe.

Acknowledgments

This work was supported by grants from the Ministerio de Educación y Ciencia (DGCYT-P4. BIO2000-0145-P4-02), Ministerio de Sanidad (FIS 01/0024), and the Xunta de Galicia (PGIDT-01-PXI-20806-PR and PGIDIT02 PXIC20804PN). AS has a research contract with the University of Santiago de Compostela.

References

1. Evans, W. E., and Relling, M. V. (1999) Pharmacogenomics: translating functional genomics into rational therapeutics. *Science* **286**, 487–491.
2. Gwee, P. C., Tang, K., Chua, J. M. Z., Lee, E. J. D., Chong, S. S., and Lee, C. G. L. (2003) Simultaneous genotyping of seven single-nucleotide polymorphisms in the MDR1 gene by single-tube multiplex minisequencing. *Clin. Chem.* **49**, 672–676
3. Jobling, M., and Tyler-Smith, C. (2000) The human Y chromosome: an evolutionary marker comes of age. *TIG* **16**, 356–362
4. Jobling, M., Pandya, A., and Tyler-Smith, C. (1997) The Y chromosome in forensic analysis and paternity testing. *Int. J. Legal Med.* **110**, 118–124.
5. Salas, A., Richards, M., De la Fe, T., Lareu, M. V., Sobrino, B., Sánchez-Diz, P., Macaulay, V., and Carracedo, A. (2002) The making of the African mtDNA landscape. *Am. J. Hum. Genet.* **71**, 1082–1111.
6. Underhill, P., Passarino, G., Lin, A. A., Shen, P., Mirazon Lahr, M., Foley, R. A., et al. (2001) The phylogeography of Y chromosome binary haplotypes and the origins of modern human populations. *Ann. Hum. Genet.* **65**, 43–62.
7. Wilson, M. R., DiZinno, J. A., Polanskey, D., Replogle, J., and Budowle, B. (1995) Validation of mitochondrial DNA sequencing for forensic casework analysis. *Int. J. Legal Med.* **108**, 68–74.
8. Tully, G., Bär, W., Brinkmann, B., Carracedo, A., Gill, P., Morling, N., et al. (2001) Considerations by the European DNA profiling (EDNAP) group on the working practices, nomenclature and interpretation of mitochondrial DNA profiles. *Forensic Sci. Int.* **124**, 83–91.
9. Salas, A., Lareu, M. V., and Carracedo, A. (2001) Heteroplasmy in mtDNA and the weight of evidence in forensic mtDNA analysis: a case report. *Int. J. Legal Med.* **114**, 186–190.
10. Salas, A., Rasmussen, E. M., Lareu, M. V., Morling, N., Carracedo, A. (2001) Fluorescent SSCP of overlapping fragments (FSSCP-OF): a highly sensitive method for the screening of mitochondrial DNA variation. *Forensic Sci. Int.* **124**, 97–103.
11. Alonso, A., Martin, P., Albarran, C., Garcia, P., Primorac, D., Garcia, O., et al. (2003) Specific quantification of human genomes from low copy number DNA samples in forensic and ancient DNA studies. *Croat. Med. J.* **44**, 273–280.
12. Prieto, L., Montesino, M., Salas, A., Alonso, A., Albarran, C., Alvarez S, et al. (2003) The 2000–2001 GEP-ISFG Collaborative Exercise on mtDNA: assessing the cause of unsuccessful mtDNA PCR amplification of hair shaft samples. *Forensic Sci. Int.* **134**, 46–53.
13. Syvänen, A. C. (2001)Accessing genetic variation: genotyping single nucleotide polymorphisms. *Nat. Rev. Gent.* **2**, 930–942.
14. Carracedo, A., Barros, F., Loidi, L., and Domínguez, F. (1998) Progress in methodology and standards in European molecular genetics laboratories. *Clin. Chim. Acta* **278**, 163–169.
15. Lareu, M. V., Puente, J., Sobrino, B., Quintáns, B., Brión, M., and Carracedo, A. (2001) The use of the LightCycler for the detection of Y chromosome SNPs. *Forensic Sci. Int.* **118**, 163–168.

16. Richards, M., Macaulay, V., Hickey, E., Vega, E., Sykes, B., Guida, V., et al. (2000) Tracing European founder lineages in the Near Eastern mtDNA pool. *Am. J. Hum Genet.* **67,** 1251–1276.
17. Herrnstadt, C., Elson JL, Fahy E, Preston G, Turnbull DM, Anderson C, et al. (2002) Reduced-median-network analysis of complete mitochondrial DNA coding-region sequences for the major African, Asian, and European haplogroups. *Am. J. Hum Genet.* **70,** 1152–1171.
18. Torroni, A., Huoponen, K., Francalacci, P., Petrozzi, M., Morelli, L., Scozzari, R., et al. (1996) Classification of European mtDNAs from an analysis of three European populations. *Genetics* **144,**, 1835–1850
19. Andrews, R. M., Kubacka, I., Chinnery, P. F., Lightowlers, R. N., Turnbull, D. M., and Howell, N. (1999) Reanalysis and revision of the Cambridge reference sequence for human mitochondrial DNA. *Nat. Genet.* **23,** 147.

15

Typing of Y Chromosome SNPs With Multiplex PCR Methods

Juan J. Sanchez, Claus Børsting, and Niels Morling

Summary

We describe a method for the simultaneous typing of Y-chromosome single nucleotide polymorphism (SNP) markers by means of multiplex polymerase chain reaction (PCR) strategies that allow the detection of 35 Y chromosome SNPs on 25 amplicons from 100 to 200 pg of chromosomal deoxyribonucleic acid (DNA). Multiplex PCR amplification of the DNA was performed with slight modifications of standard PCR conditions. Single-base extension (SBE) was performed using the SNaPshot kit containing fluorescently labeled ddNTPs. The extended primers were detected on an ABI 3100 sequencer. The most important factors for the creation of larger SNP typing PCR multiplexes include careful selection of primers for the primary amplification and the SBE reaction, use of DNA primers with homogenous composition, and balancing the primer concentrations for both the amplification and the SBE reactions.

Key Words: Y chromosome; single nucleotide polymorphism; multiplex PCR; single-base extension; genotyping.

1. Introduction

Typing for single nucleotide polymorphism (SNP) markers in forensic genetics is of interest in certain situations, for example, when only partly degraded deoxyribonucleic acid (DNA) is available for typing. Typing of Y chromosome markers (short tandem repeats [STRs] and SNPs) may be of special interest in cases with mixed stains with a large proportion of female DNA and a small proportion of male DNA. To obtain a weight of the evidence from SNP typing that is comparable to that of STR typing with, for example, 10 autosomal STRs, 50–100 autosomal SNPs must be typed (1). A reliable, complete

From: *Methods in Molecular Biology, vol. 297: Forensic DNA Typing Protocols*
Edited by: A. Carracedo © Humana Press Inc., Totowa, NJ

STR profile can be obtained from as few as 100–200 pg of intact DNA. If SNP typing is going to be used in forensic cases with limited amounts of DNA, it is important that all SNPs can be typed from 100 to 1000 pg of DNA. One way to obtain this amount is to amplify a number of DNA regions in multiplex polymerase chain reaction (PCR). Other methods exist, including an initial random amplification of DNA and other DNA-amplification methods *(2)*. The subsequent SNP typing may be performed with assays that are already available, such as primer extension, hybridization, and melting point analysis.

To study the possibilities of typing large number of SNPs for forensic casework, we decided to analyze the Y chromosome SNPs because Y chromosome SNPs have only one allele and the results are simple to interpret. We chose to amplify the chromosomal DNA by PCR because we had most experience with this technology, although other methods are available. We chose the single-base extension (SBE) method with subsequent detection of fluorescently labeled primers on an ABI 3100 sequencer because this technology was well established for SNP typing in small multiplexes.

Here, we describe the methods for the development of a SNP typing package containing 35 SNPs on 25 amplified DNA fragments on the Y chromosome. We have successfully used this strategy to build other large SNP multiplexes, so we anticipate that the strategy can be used by others. A few considerations concerning the strategy and specific comments for the development of multiplex PCR Y chromosome SNP typing packages and practical experiences are offered.

2. Materials

2.1. PCR for Target Amplification

1. DNA purification: QIAamp DNA Blood Mini Kit (Qiagen, Hagen, Germany) or FTA paper (Whatman International, Cambridge, UK).
2. Assay for DNA quantification: SYBR Green I using a LightCycler instrument (Roche Diagnostics GmbH, Germany) or Hoechst 33258 (Molecular Probes Inc., Eugene, OR) using a Hoefer DyNA Quant 200 instrument (Molecular Vision) and calf thymus DNA standard (Sigma-Aldrich, St. Louis, MO).
3. High-performance liquid chromatography-purified PCR primers (TAG A/S, Copenhagen, Denmark).
4. Tris/ethylenediamine tetraacetic acid (EDTA) buffer solution: 10 mM Tris, 100 mM EDTA, pH 7.5 (Sigma-Aldrich).
5. GeneAmp PCR reagent kit with AmpliTaq Gold DNA polymerase containing 10X PCR buffer and 25 mM $MgCl_2$ from Applied Biosystems (AB), Foster City, CA.
6. PCR nucleotide mix, 25 mM (Amersham Biosciences, Uppsala, Sweden; Invitrogen, Groningen, The Netherlands).
7. PCR instrument GeneAmp 9600 thermal cycler (PerkinElmer, Wellesley, MA; *(see* **Note 1**).

2.2. Electrophoresis

2.2.1. Using Polyacrylamide Gels

1. 40% acrylamide/bisacrylamide 29:1 solution (Bio-Rad Laboratories, Hercules, CA).
2. TBE: 89 mM Tris-base, 89 mM boric acid, 2 mM EDTA, pH 8.3 (Sigma-Aldrich).
3. TEMED (Tetramethylethylenediamine; Bio-Rad).
4. 10-bp ladder (Invitrogen, Groningen, The Netherlands).
5. Ethidium bromide (Sigma-Aldrich).

2.2.2. Terminal Transferase Nucleotide Labeling

1. R6G-ddATP (PerkinElmer Life Science).
2. Terminal Transferase (20 units/µL) and 5X TdT reaction buffer (Roche Diagnostics GmbH, Germany).

2.3. Single-Base Extension Assay

2.3.1. Purification of the PCR Template Amplification Product

1. MinElute PCR purification spin column (Qiagen, Hagen, Germany).
2. *Escherichia coli* exonuclease I (*Exo*I), shrimp alkaline phosphatase (SAP) and ExoSAP-IT (USB Corporation, Cleveland, OH).

2.3.2. Reaction and Electrophoresis

1. ABI Prism SNaPshot Multiplex kit (AB).
2. HiDi formamide (Invitrogene).
3. Gel or capillary electrophoresis platform for detection of fluorescently labeled oligonucleotides.

2.4. Databases with Genetic Information

2.4.1. DNA Sequences and SNPs

The following web sites offer free information about DNA sequences, SNPs, chromosome position, surrounding sequence, association with genes, etc.

http://www.ncbi.nlm.nih.gov/SNP/ (NCBI and NHGRI dbSNP)
http://snp.cshl.org/ (SNP Consortium)
http://hgbase.interactiva.de or http://hgvbase.cgb.ki.se/ (intragenic SNPs)
http://snp.ims.u-tokyo.ac.jp/ (Japanese SNP database)
http://www.ensembl.org/ (EMBL-EBI and Sanger Institute)
http://www-genome.wi.mit.edu/snp/human (Whitehead Institute/MIT Centre for Genome Research)
http://ihg.gsf.de/ihg/databases.html (Genetic information servers and databases).
http://lpg.nci.nih.gov/GAI (Cancer Genome Anatomy Project).

2.4.2. PCR Primer Design

The following web sites offer free assistance for the design of DNA primers. Other sites exist.

> http://www.molbiol.bbsrc.ac.uk/reviews.html (reviews of primer design programs)
>
> http://ftp.genome.washington.edu/cgi-bin/RepeatMasker (screen for interspaced repeats and low complexity DNA sequences)
>
> http://www-genome.wi.mit.edu/cgi-bin/primer/primer3_www.cgi (primer design program with easy to use interface and good help pages)
>
> http://biotools.idtdna.com/gateway/ (primer and probe design tool, secondary structure prediction and comprehensive oligo analysis)
>
> http://www.zaik.uni-koeln.de/AFS/Projects/Bioinformatics/sbeprimer.html (primer design program for multiplex SBE-based genotyping).

2.4.3. DNA Sequence Alignment

The following web sites can all be used for alignment. We use them primarily to check for ambiguous or homologous sequences.

> http://searchlauncher.bcm.tmc.edu/multi-align/multi-align.html
>
> http://genome.ucsc.edu/cgi-bin/hgGateway?org=human
>
> http://www.ncbi.nlm.nih.gov/blast/
>
> http://www.sanger.ac.uk/HGP/blast_server.shtml
>
> http://genes.mit.edu/GENSCAN.html
>
> http://genome.ornl.gov/
>
> http://www.ncbi.nlm.nih.gov/genome/sts/epcr.cgi
>
> http://www.ddbj.nig.ac.jp/E-mail/homology.html
>
> http://www.ebi.ac.uk/services/.

3. Methods

The process of designing a Y chromosome multiplex PCR package for SNP typing includes the establishment of 1) multiplex PCR amplification of a number of DNA fragments, the concentrations of which are balanced, and 2) a multiplex SBE reaction that gives balanced amounts of SBE products that can be detected unequivocally so that clear SNP types can be recorded.

In the first amplification phase, it is important to choose a strategy that allows a combination of 1) flexibility in choosing primers, 2) highly specific reactions, and 3) uniform amplification of PCR products. Once the PCR conditions have been selected and a multiplex PCR package has been developed, the addition of further amplicons can only be performed if the new primers can work under the conditions chosen. If two or more packages have been developed, interchanges of amplicons between the packages can be performed only if the amplicons can be amplified under similar conditions. We decided to use PCR conditions primarily defined by a theoretical melting temperature of 60 ± 5°C at a salt concentration of 180 m*M* and a purine:pyrimidine ratio close to 1:1. It is important to be able to detect all the amplicons in order to analyse the products for homogeneity and estimate the yield of the PCR amplification so that, at the end, a balanced PCR multiplex consisting of homogeneous amplicons can be obtained. We chose to detect the individual amplicons by their electrophoretic mobility in gels and, therefore, the sizes of the amplicons differ by at least four base pairs. For forensic purposes, one should consider the size range of the amplicons. Ideally, the amplicon sizes should be as small as possible in order to be able to analyse heavily degraded DNA. We ended up with amplicon sizes in the range of 79 to 180 bp.

In our experience, the greatest problems in creating a multiplex PCR is to ensure that the primers do not interact, that the primers are specific, that each primer batch consists of homogeneous molecules, and that the concentrations of the primers are balanced in such a way that the multiplex reaction gives equal amounts of each amplicon.

In the multiplex SBE reaction, it is important to be able to obtain an equal number of extended primers for each SNP, and it is also important that the primers can be separated under the chosen electrophoretic conditions to obtain clear SNP typing results. SBE is performed as a thermal cycling reaction with one annealing step and one denaturation step. The annealing temperature is 50–60°C and consequently, the SBE primers must have a minimal length of 17–18 nt. The synthesis of oligonucleotides longer than 80–90 nt is presently very costly, and the quality of the primers vary considerably between vendors when the size of the primers are longer than 60–70 nt. In general, it is possible to separate extended SBE primers on an ABI 3100 sequencer, if the primers differ by 4 nt, although there may be difficulties in separating some primers that are shorter than 30–35 nt because the electrophoretic mobility of short primers depend strongly on the nucleotide composition. In a four colour fluorescence system like the SNaPshot kit, two different biallelic SNPs can be detected within the same 4-nt window. Thus, with a range from 18 to 100 nt and 4-nt windows, approx 40 SNPs may be detected in a single experiment.

The establishment of detection primers of various lengths necessitates that the primers contain a 5' tail with nucleotides that do not influence the hybridisation process. This can be done by adding polymers of A, G, T, or C or by adding random nucleotide sequences that do not bind to human DNA. If two or more packages have been developed, interchanges of amplicons and SBE primers between the packages can be performed only if both the amplicons and the SBE primers are compatible.

In the sections below, special emphasis is put on information about the tools that can be used for obtaining the DNA sequences, polymorphisms, detailed information about annealing, etc., design rules for the primers multiplexes, the reaction components and the cycling conditions of the multiplex PCR reaction, and SBE assays capable of detecting multiple SNPs in a single reaction.

3.1. DNA Preparation

Rather clean DNA is needed for multiplex PCR amplification. We use QIAamp, Chelex, and phenol/chloroform-prepared DNA or cells spotted on FTA paper.

3.2. Obtaining the DNA Sequences

The sequences surrounding the selected SNPs are collected from genome databases (e.g., dbSNP or SNP Consortium, *see* **Subheading 2.4.1.**). It is essential for successful multiplex PCR that the DNA sequences are correct. Furthermore, it is important to check for other SNPs in the flanking region (e.g., using the BLAST option, *see* **Subheading 2.4.3.**), where the amplification primers are expected to bind and to check for homologous and repetitive regions, which are especially abundant on the Y chromosome *(3)*.

3.3. Primer Design Strategy for Multiplex PCR Amplification

The major problem in designing large multiplexes is to obtain a balanced amplification of a number of DNA fragments in the same tube under the same conditions. By applying the same design rules to each primer in the multiplex (*see* **Subheading 3.3.1.**), the likelihood of obtaining a balanced amount of PCR products in the multiplex is increased. Similar reaction conditions to some extent also require similar amplicon sizes. However, the amplicons in the multiplex must differ by size so that the amount of each amplicon can be assessed in order to balance the multiplex PCR (*see* **Subheading 3.3.3.**).

Computer programs are used for predicting the best PCR primers for a target sequence (*see* **Subheading 2.4.2.**). The programs will predict which regions are free of secondary structures, and the software will suggest primer location based on conditions given by the user.

3.3.1. Initial Primer Evaluation

1. Use the software (*see* **Subheading 2.4.2.**) to find the best primer sites. We work with a theoretical melting temperature of the primers of 60C ± 5°C at a salt concentration of 180 mM. Primers between 18 and 35 nt will usually work (*see* **Note 2**). The purine: pyrimidine ratio should be close to 1:1. If the template sequence prevents this, the primers can be extended or shortened to compensate for the difference in G + C content. Primers should have one to two G/Cs at the 3' end if possible. However, the last 7 nt. in the 3' end of the primer must not contain more than four G/Cs (*see* **Note 3**).

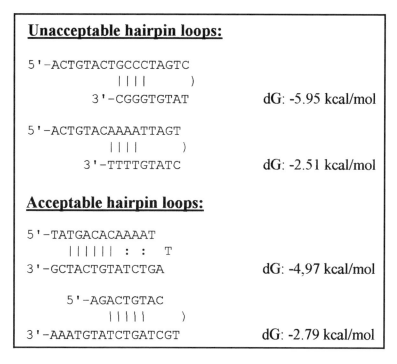

Fig. 1. Examples of acceptable and unacceptable hairpin loops in primers.

2. Calculate the free energy of possible hairpins and primer-dimers (*see* **Note 4**). Primer-dimer formation in the 3' end must be avoided. If primer-dimer formation is suspected in the 3' end, it should be no longer than four nucleotides or dG < −3.0 kcal/mol. Similarly, hairpin loops where the 3' end is part of the hairpin stem must be avoided. In general, hairpin loops with dG < −5.0 kcal/mol should be avoided (*see* **Fig. 1**).
3. Check the primer sequences to avoid similarities with repetitive sequences or with other loci in the genome, for example, by a BLAST search.
4. Test each primer in the multiplex for primer-primer interactions using the same criteria as above.
5. Test each primer for homology to other amplicons in the multiplex.

3.3.2. Quality of DNA Primers

One of the single most import factors for a successful outcome of multiplex PCR is the quality of the DNA primers. The primers should be purified by high-performance liquid chromatography, and the length should be homogeneous (*see* **Note 5**). The quality of the oligonucleotides can be checked directly by mass spectrometry or by extending the primers with fluorescently labelled nucleotides using the terminal transferase method (*see* **Subheading 3.3.3.1**) and analyzing the extended primers on an ABI 3100. **Figure 2** shows an example of a reasonably homogenous oligonucleotide preparation and a preparation with a broad distribution of DNA oligonucleotides of various lengths that will destroy any multiplex PCR reaction.

3.3.3. Test of the Primers in Singleplex PCR and Construction of the Multiplex

1. Test the selected primer pair in singleplex PCR, e.g., with 10 ng template DNA in a 25-µL reaction volume containing 1X PCR buffer, 1.5 mM MgCl$_2$, 200 µM of each dNTP, 0.4 µM of each primer, and 0.6 units of AmpliTaq Gold DNA polymerase (*see* **Subheadings 3.4.** and **3.5.** for thermocycling conditions).
2. Analyze the PCR products by polyacrylamide gel electrophoresis or on ABI 3100 after labeling of the PCR product with the terminal transferase (TdT) method (*see* **Subheading 3.3.3.1.** and **Note 6**) to check whether a single fragment of the correct size is amplified.
3. Combine the primers in sets of 7–12 SNPs and perform the PCR with, for example, 1 ng of DNA in a 50-µL reaction volume containing 1X PCR buffer, 8 mM MgCl$_2$, 400 µM of each dNTP, 0.2 µM of each primer, and 2.5 units of AmpliTaq Gold DNA polymerase (AB; *see* **Subheading 3.4.**).
4. Analyze the PCR products as describe above. Each fragment must be visible and have the correct size.
5. Estimate the amplification efficiency (*see* **Note 7**).
6. Combine the packages of 7–12 amplicons into a final set and adjust the primer concentrations in order to get a balanced set of amplicons (*see* **Subheading 3.4.**).

3.3.3.1. TERMINAL TRANSFERASE PCR PRODUCT LABELING AND DETECTION

1. Make an 8 µM stock of R6G-ddATP (PerkinElmer; cat. no. NEL490).
2. Make the reaction cocktail (for 10 µL of total volume): 2 µL of 5X TdT reaction buffer, 1.25 µL of R6G-ddATP stock (8 µM), 1 µL of terminal transferase (20 Units/µL), and 4.75 µL of ddH$_2$O.
3. Dispense 9 µL per tube and add 1 µL of the PCR product at 0.5–1 ng/µL.
4. Incubate the reaction at 37°C for 1 h.
5. Terminate the reaction by incubation at 75°C for 15 min.
6. Add 1 unit of SAP to remove the 5' phosphoryl groups of the unincorporated fluorescent ddNTPs.
7. Incubate the tube at 37°C for 1 h.
8. Inactivate the SAP by incubation at 75°C for 15 min.
9. Mix 3 µL of the purified product, 16.8 µL of Hi-Di formamide, and 0.2 µL of the GeneScan-120 LIZ™ size standard and spin briefly.
10. Run for 10 s at 3 kV on an ABI 3100 sequencer or similar (use of the internal-line size standard and GeneScan Analysis software (AB) offers a high level of sensitivity and precision in identifying the fragments).

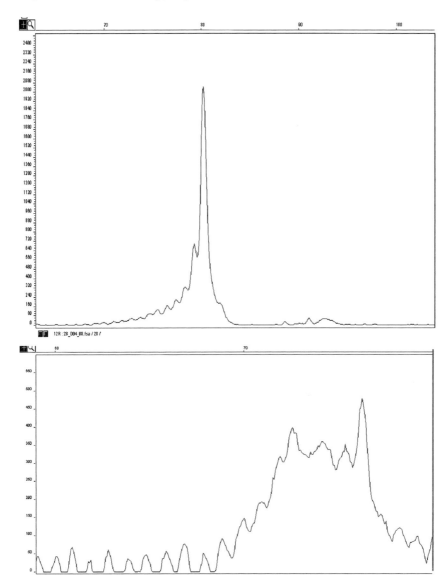

Fig. 2. Examples of oligonucleotide quality. The primers were labeled using the SNaPshot kit (*see* **Note 5**). **A** shows a reasonably homogenous batch of DNA oligonucleotides and **B** shows a poor batch of oligonucleotides.

3.4. Optimization of the SNP Multiplex PCR Template Amplification Reaction

1. We use 2.5 U/50 μL reaction volume of AmpliTaq Gold DNA polymerase (Applied Biosystems), but other polymerases can be used (*see* **Note 8**).
2. Buffer concentration can be altered from 0.8- to 2.0-fold (*see* **Note 9**).
3. Optimize the MgCl$_2$ concentration. We use 8 mM MgCl$_2$ (higher concentrations may inhibit the amplification; *see* **Note 10**).
4. Adjust the amount of dNTPs (proportional to the MgCl$_2$ concentration, 200 μM for each 1.75 mM of MgCl$_2$; *see* **Note 11**).
5. The final concentration of the primers in the multiplex may vary considerably (**Table 1**). In our hands, primer concentrations less than 0.01 μM were insufficient to amplify the fragments in the multiplex, and concentrations greater than 0.5 μM inhibited multiplex PCR probably by increasing primer–primer annealing. The primer mix must be kept on ice at all times in order to avoid artefacts due to hairpin or primer–dimer formation (*see* **Note 12**).
6. Consider the use of dsDNA-destabilizing additives (*see* **Note 13**).

3.5. Optimization of Multiplex Thermocycling Conditions

1. Find the optimal annealing temperatures by titration of the temperatures between, for example, 54°C and 63°C with 3°C intervals (*see* **Note 1**).
2. Find the optimal elongation temperature by titration of the temperatures between 65 and 72°C.

The final conditions of the 35 SNP Y chromosome multiplex were as follows: denaturation at 94°C for 5 min followed by 33 cycles at 95°C, 30 s; 60°C, 30 s; and 65°C, 30 s; followed by a final extension at 65°C for 7 min (*see* **Note 14**).

3.6. Purification of the PCR Template Amplification Product

Unused dNTPs in the PCR amplification multiplex must be removed before the SBE reaction can be performed. We use enzymatic purification by *Escherichia coli* exonuclease I (*Exo*I) and SAP or the ExoSAP-IT kit following this protocol:

1. Six microliters ExoSAP-IT kit (USB Corporation, Cleveland, OH) or 5 units of SAP and 2 units of *Exo*I are added to 15 μL of PCR product and mixed.
2. Incubate at 37°C for 1 h and inactivate the enzyme at 75°C for 15 min.

Other methods may be used (*see* **Note 15**).

3.7. SBE With SNaPshot

3.7.1. Design of SBE Primers

The rules of thumbs for design of amplification primers are also valid for the design of SBE primers. The recommended annealing temperature for the SNaPshot kit is 50°C. However, the SNaPshot kit will, in most cases, work up to 60°C. Thus, specific reactions can be obtained by adjusting the annealing temperature in the range of 50–60°C. Annealing temperatures less than 50°C may cause unspecific reactions.

3.7.2. Primer Tailing Strategy for SBE Assay

Because the reactions are going to be analyzed on the ABI 3100 or a similar unit, the fluorescent colors as well as the size of the extended primers should be considered. Two SNPs with different alleles (e.g., A/G and C/T) can be analysed in a 4-nt size interval. However, for primers shorter than approx 35 nt, the electrophoretic mobility depends strongly on the oligonucleotides composition and, therefore, it is not always possible to predict the exact mobility of the extended primer (**Table 2**). Our strategy for designing tails involves a piece of a "neutral" sequence, for example, a sequence that is not found in the human genome *(4)* and a poly-C tail (**Table 3**). This tail will not in itself influence the hybridization to a significant degree.

3.7.2.1. Test of the Tailed SBE Primers

The length and the homogeneity of each SBE primer as well as the yield of the SBE reaction should be tested (*see* **Subheading 3.3.2.**).

3.7.2.2. Multiplex SBE Primer Mix

The primers are mixed in concentrations corresponding to the signal intensities in the singleplex reactions and titrated. The primer concentration can be adjusted in the range from 0.01 to 0.50 μM to obtain balanced signals from the SBE primers. We use the SNaPshot multiplex kit with the following conditions:

1. 6–10 ng purified PCR product (equivalent to 5–8 fmol of each fragment) in 10 μL.
2. 4–5 μL of SNaPshot reaction mix and 0.01–0.50 μM of each primer.
3. Thermal cycling protocol with a rapid thermal ramp to 96°C for 10 s, 50–60°C for 5 s, and 60°C for 30 s for 25 cycles.
4. Include a positive control (known sample instead of that provided with the kit) and a negative control (sterile water or PCR product from a female).

The amounts of primers must usually be titrated further to obtain balanced reactions. Also, the annealing temperature must be titrated between 50 and 60°C to optimize the reaction. **Table 3** shows the details of the method that allowed simultaneous typing of 35 Y chromosome SNPs.

3.7.2.3. Capillary Electrophoresis and Multicolor Detection on ABI 3100

1. After the SBE reaction, add 1 unit of SAP in order to remove the 5' phosphoryl groups of the unincorporated fluorescent ddNTPs.
2. Incubate at 37°C for 1 h.

Table 1
Y Chromosome SNPs and Primer Sequences for PCR Amplification of 25 Y Chromosome DNA Fragments With 35 SNP loLi

Locus	GenBank or dbSNPs accesion no	Mutation	Forward primer	Reverse primer	µM	Amplicon size (bp)
			PCR primers (5' → 3')			
M2/sY81	Rs3893	A/G	acggaaggagttctaaaattcagg	aaaatacagctcccctttatcct	0.15	128
M9*	Rs3900	C/G	aggaccctgaaatacagaactg	aaatatttcaacatttcacaaaggaa	0.36	186
M17*	Rs3908	4G/3G	cctggtcataacactggaaatc	agctgaccacaaactgatgtaga	0.09	170
M18*	Rs3909	2 bp insertion	cctggtcataacactggaaatc	agctgaccacaaactgatgtaga	0.09	170
M19*	Rs3010	T/A	cctggtcataacactggaaatc	agctgaccacaaactgatgtaga	0.09	170
M32*	AC009977	T/C	tgaccgtcataggctgagaca	ttgaagccccaagagagac	0.07	160
M33*	AC009977	A/C	tgaccgtcataggctgagaca	ttgaagccccaagagagac	0.07	160
M35	Rs1179188	G/C	Agggcatggtcccttctat	tccatgcagactttcggagt	0.42	96
M40/SRY$_{4064}$	AC006040	G/A	tggtctcaatcttcaccctgt	catttcagtaaatgccacacaaga	0.18	119
M45*	Rs2032631	G/A	gagagaggatatcaaaaattggcagt	tgacagtggccaccaaggtc	0.03	138
M46/Tat	AC002531	T/C	tatatggactcgagtgtagacttgtga	ggtgccgtaaaagtgtgaaataatc	0.46	115
M52	AC009977	A/C	Cctcaacttcccagagtgttg	gacgaagcaaacatttcaagagag	0.03	152
M78*	AC010889	C/T	Tgcattactccgtatgttcgac	tggaagcttaccatcttttatga	0.08	132
M81*	Rs2032640	C/T	catctcttaacaaagagagtaaatttgtcc	cattgttacatggcctataatattcagt	0.24	179
M89	Rs2032652	C/T	tggattcagctcttcctaaggttat	ctgctcaggtacacacagagtatca	0.03	135
M96	AC010889	G/C	Tgccctccacagagcactt	ccaccacttgttgctttg	0.27	143
M123	AC010889	G/A	Gttgcccaggaatttgcat	cacagagcaagtgactctcaaag	0.02	88
M139*	AC010137	5G/4G	cccgaaagtttattttattcca	ttctcagacaccaatggtcctatc	0.06	113
M151*	AC010889	G/A	catctcttaacaaagagagtaaatttgtcc	cattgttacatggcctataatattcagt	0.24	179
M153*	AC010137	T/A	cccgaaagtttattttattcca	ttctcagacaccaatggtcctatc	0.06	113
M154*	AC010889	T/C	catctcttaacaaagagagtaaatttgtcc	cattgttacatggcctataatattcagt	0.24	179
M157*	AC010889	A/C	gagagaggatatcaaaaattggcagt	tgacagtggccaccaaggtc	0.03	138
M163*	AC009977	A/C	aggaccctgaaatacagaactg	aaatatttcaacatttcacaaaggaa	0.36	186

Marker	Accession/rs	SNP	Primer 1	Primer 2		
M167/SRY$_{2627}$	AC006040	C/T	Cggaaccactaccagcttca	agttaaggccccacgcagt	0.03	113
M170	Rs2032597	A/C	cagctcttattaagttatgttttcatattctgtg	gtcctcattttacagtgagacacaac	0.07	119
M172	Rs2032604	T/G	Tgagccctccatcagaag	gccaggtacagagaaagtttgg	0.16	179
M173	Rs2032624	A/C	tttcttacaattcaagggcatttag	ctgaaaacaaaacactggcttatca	0.10	81
M175	Rs2032678	-5bp	gatttaaactctgaatcaggcacat	ttctactgatacctttgtttctgttcattc	0.02	79
M212*	Rs2032664	C/A	ccatataaaaacgcagcattcgtt	tggagagaacttgagaaaagtagagaa	0.12	176
M213*	Rs2032665	T/C	ccatataaaaacgcagcattcgtt	tggagagaacttgagaaaagtagagaa	0.12	176
M224*	AC010889	T/C	Tgcattactccgtatgttcgac	tggaagcttaccatctttttatga	0.08	132
SRY$_{10831}$/SRY$_{1532}$	Rs2534636	A/G	tcatccagtccttagcaaccatta	ccacatagggtgaaccttgaaaatg	0.06	150
12f2	AC005820	present/absent	cactgactgatcaaaatgcttacagat	ggatccctccttacacacttatca	0.06	90
92R7	Rs2535813	GA/A	ttaaatccctcctatttgtgctaacc	aatgcatgaacacaaaagacgtaga	0.04	89
P25	Rs150173	C/CA	tggaccatcacctgggtaaagt	ggcagtaaggttgtcacatcacat	0.01	109

*SNP markers on the same DNA fragment: (M9 and M163), (M17, M18 and M19), (M32 and M33), (M45 and M157), (M78 and M224), (M81, M151, and M154), (M139 and M153), and (M212 and M213). All primers were redesigned compared to previously published primers.

Table 2
Differences Between the Observed and the Expected Sizes of the Extended SBE Primers Used in This Study

Expected primer size (nucleotides)	Difference between observed and expected size			
	R6G-ddATP	TAMRA-ddCTP	110-ddGTP	OX-ddUTP
18–30	3.35 ± 1.36	3.25 ± 1.00	2.81 ± 1.26	5.01 ± 0.80
31–60	1.23 ± 0.21	0.87 ± 0.34	0.64 ± 0.45	2.31 ± 0.10
63–100	0.76 ± 0.15	–0.20 ± 0.45	–0.50 ± 0.47	0.97 ± 0.40

3. Inactivate the SAP by incubation at 75°C for 15 min.
4. Mix 1 µL of the purified SBE product, 18.8 µL of Hi-Di formamide, and 0.2 µL of the GeneScan 120 LIZ™ size standard and spin briefly.
5. Run on an ABI Prism 3100 Genetic Analyser with a 36-cm capillary array, POP-4 polymer and 10 s at 3000 V.
6. Analyze using GeneScan Analysis software v. 3.7 (Applied Biosystems). After background subtraction and color separation, peaks can be sorted into bins according to sizes by comparison to the internal size standard. Peaks greater than 400 relative fluorescence units are usually considered positive signals and a SNP type is assigned (*see* **Fig. 3**). Template-related background peaks may be seen in the SNaPshot reaction (*see* **Note 16**).

4. Notes

1. It may be helpful to use a thermocycler with temperature gradient for the optimization of the multiplex PCR.
2. Several attempts have been made to overcome some of the difficulties with conventional multiplex PCR design *(5,6)*. One of the suggested methods is based on the use of primers that are genome specific at their 3' ends and carry common extensions (tails) at their 5' ends (tailed primer strategy). The protocol includes a second step using a higher concentration of tail-specific primers (tags; ref. *6*). All amplicons of the multiplex can then be amplified by just one tag primer. This method, however, does not offer a general solution to large multiplexes. We have compared Y chromosome multiplex systems with tailed primers and conventional primers and found that the tailed primer strategy was less efficient.
3. The primer design guidelines mentioned here are minimal criteria. Primer pairs that fulfil the guidelines, however, may not work in a multiplex reaction because the amplification is too efficient, and, as a consequence, the other fragments in the multiplex are not amplified (*see* **Note 7**). This phenomenon is called PCR bias *(7)*.
4. The alignment score is determined by free energy calculation. The algorithm computes the most stable interaction that the strands can form and returns the free energy change values for the alignment (dG). If dG < 0, the model predicts that

strand pairing may take place, but it does not necessarily mean that a significant interaction will take place in the multiplex reaction.

5. The synthesis process may produce a mix of oligonucleotides of varying lengths. To day, a 99% coupling efficiency is usually obtained. For practical proposes, short oligonucleotides are rather homogeneous, but 50- to 100-mer oligonucleotides tend to be heterogeneous. Therefore, high-quality synthesis and effective check of the product is essential.

6. It is also possible to use the intrinsic Taq DNA polymerase terminal transferase-like activity for analysis of the PCR product(s) by performing a SBE reaction (*see* **Subheading 3.7.2.2.**) without SBE primers. The PCR products are labeled with fluorescent ddATP and can be detected on the ABI 3100. This reaction is more efficient than the TdT method. However, the Taq DNA polymerase terminal transferase-like activity has been shown by others to be sequence dependent *(8,9)*. We performed both assays on several large multiplexes and we never observed any differences in the relative amounts of PCR product(s) detected by the two methods.

7. The amounts of the amplicons in the multiplex must be balanced. This can be obtained by adjusting the primer concentrations. However, if the amount of PCR product differs more than threefold, it may not be possible to balance the multiplex PCR by altering the concentration of the primers, and new primers may have to be designed for one or several of the amplicons. Often, the results from the singleplex PCR will indicate whether the amplification efficiency of the different fragments in the multiplex will be similar. However, the reaction conditions of the multiplex reaction are so different from the singleplex reaction that it is not always possible to predict the results in the multiplex. Therefore, doubtful primer pairs should be tested in the multiplex reaction.

8. Use heat-activated DNA polymerases to reduce primer-dimer formation in the multiplex PCR. Consider the use of a proofreading polymerase.

9. It has been suggested that many primer pairs producing short amplification products (<200 bp) work better at higher KCl concentration in multiplex systems *(10)*. Increasing the concentration of KCl in the PCR buffer 1.6- or 2-fold in our Y SNP reactions did not increase the yield of PCR products significantly and had no effect on the synthesis of fragments >150 bp.

10. The optimal $MgCl_2$ concentration needs to be determined empirically for efficiency of multiplex PCR amplification by testing 2, 4, and 8 mM in the initial experiments.

11. dNTPs are sensitive to repeated freezing and thawing while the storage time is less important *(11)*. We store dNTPs in small aliquots at –20°C for up to 8 mo.

12. We have observed that even with 10 min incubation at 95°C, before the PCR, these constructs are amplified once they have been formed.

13. We do not use dsDNA-destabilizing additives such as bovine serum albumin, dimethyl sulfoxide (DMSO), glycerol, formamide, or betaine. Such additives give variable results in multiplex PCR. For example, betaine makes GC-rich and AT-rich DNA melt at the same temperature *(12)*, possibly by increasing the hydration

Table 3
SBE Primer Sequences Used in the 35 Y Chromosome SNP Package

Locus	Poly (dC)	Neutral sequence (5'→3')	Target-specific sequence (5'→3')	μM	Primer size (nt)
M170	None	None	caacccacactgaaaaaaa	0.02	19
M45	None	caa	ctcagaaggagcttttgc	0.02	22
M139	None	aa	taatctgacttggaaagggg	0.01	22
M2/sY81	None	gacaa	ctttatcctccacagatctca	0.28	26
M46/Tat	None	None	gctctgaaatattaaattaaaacaac	0.25	26
M167/SRY$_{2627}$	None	tgaaagtctgacaa	aagccccacagggtgc	0.35	30
M213	None	tgacaa	tcagaacttaaacatctcgttac	0.02	30
M52	None	tctgacaa	aatatcaagaaaacctatcaaacatcc	0.02	34
P25	None	tcgtgaaagtctgacaa	tgcctgaaacctgcctg	0.04	34
M78	None	gaaagtctgacaa	cttatttgaaatatttggaagggc	0.02	38
92R7	None	gtgaaagtctgacaa	catgaacacaaagacgtagaag	0.01	38
M89	None	cacgtcgtgaaagtctgacaa	aactcaggcaaagtgagagat	0.09	42
M123	None	acgtcgtgaaagtctgacaa	attctaggtattcaggcgatg	0.03	42
M35	None	ggtgccacgtcgtgaaagtctgacaa	tcggagtctgcctgtgtc	0.25	46
M153	None	ggtgccacgtcgtgaaagtctgacaa	gctcaaagggtatgtgaaca	0.02	46
M40/SRY$_{4064}$	None	aaaactaggtgccacgtcgtgaaagtctgacaa	tccaccctgtgatccgct	0.08	50
M154	None	gccacgtcgtgaaagtctgacaa	gttacatggcctataatattcagtaca	0.03	50
M32	None	taggtgccacgtcgtgaaagtctgacaa	agacaagatctgttcagtttatctca	0.50	54
M151	None	aggtgccacgtcgtgaaagtctgacaa	caatctactacatacctacgctatatg	0.02	54
M17	None	actaaactaggtgccacgtcgtgaaagtctgacaa	ccaaaattcacttaaaaaaaccc	0.02	58
M96	None	aactgactaaactaggtgccacgtcgtgaaagtctgacaa	ggaaaacaggtctctcataata	0.15	62
M172	7(dC)	aactgactaaactaggtgccacgtcgtgaaagtctgacaa	caaaccattttgatgctt	0.10	66
M173	3(dC)	aactgactaaactaggtgccacgtcgtgaaagtctgacaa	tacaattcaagggcatttagaac	0.03	66

M19	4(dC)	aactgactaaactaggtgccacgtcgtgaaagtctgacaa	aaactattttgtgaagactgttgta	0.10	70
M224	7(dC)	aactgactaaactaggtgccacgtcgtgaaagtctgacaa	aattgatacacttaacaaagatacttc	0.13	74
SRY_{10831}/SRY_{1532}	10(dC)	aactgactaaactaggtgccacgtcgtgaaagtctgacaa	ttgtatctgactttcacacagt	0.03	74
M18	17(dC)	aactgactaaactaggtgccacgtcgtgaaagtctgacaa	gtttgtggttgctggttgtta	0.05	78
M157	18(dC)	aactgactaaactaggtgccacgtcgtgaaagtctgacaa	caccaaggtcatttgtggt	0.20	78
M81	14(dC)	aactgactaaactaggtgccacgtcgtgaaagtctgacaa	cttggtttgtgagtatactctatgac	0.03	82
M163	25(dC)	aactgactaaactaggtgccacgtcgtgaaagtctgacaa	cacaaaggaatttttttgag	0.51	86
M212	20(dC)	aactgactaaactaggtgccacgtcgtgaaagtctgacaa	gcattcgttaatataaaacacacaaaa	0.20	86
M9	22(dC)	aactgactaaactaggtgccacgtcgtgaaagtctgacaa	catgtctaaattaaagaaaaataaagag	0.40	90
12f2	29(dC)	aactgactaaactaggtgccacgtcgtgaaagtctgacaa	aacatgtaagtctttaatccatctc	0.02	94
M33	29(dC)	aactgactaaactaggtgccacgtcgtgaaagtctgacaa	cagttacaaaagtataatatgtctgagat	0.18	98
M175	46(dC)	aactgactaaactaggtgccacgtcgtgaaagtctgacaa	cacatgcctctcacttctc	0.28	106

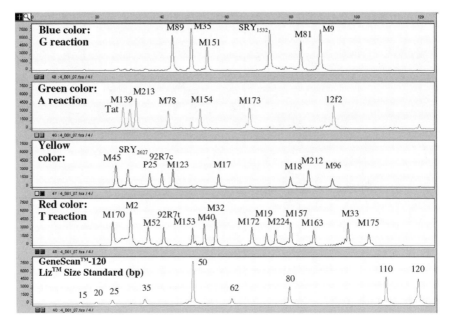

Fig. 3. Electropherogram of peaks corresponding to different primer extension products of the 35 Y chromosome SNP multiplex. The identity of each polymorphism was determined by fragment size and by the incorporated fluorescent ddNTP.

of GC-rich regions *(13)*. Ten percent DMSO decreases the melting temperature of the primers by 5–6°C but DMSO also inhibits Taq DNA polymerase *(14)*. These cosolutes may be useful for some sequences and long PCR products.

14. The touchdown PCR protocol starts with an annealing temperature 5 or 10°C higher than the highest calculated Tm. The annealing temperature is reduced at the rate of 1–3°C in successive PCR cycles until the annealing temperature is the same as the calculated Tm. This increases the specificity of the PCR *(15)* because elongation from unspecific annealing is unlikely during the first cycles. We have not used this strategy because our primers have been designed to work under homogeneous conditions. The technique is especially useful when primers with different melting temperatures must be used together.

15. MinElute PCR purification spin columns (Qiagen, Hagen, Germany) can also be used. In this case, the DNA should be diluted in at least 10 µL of Milli-Q water. The recovery with the Exo I-SAP is usually almost 100% whereas the column purification has a recovery of approx 80%. Spin column and enzymatically purified PCR products give equal satisfactory SBE results. Qiagen purification is preferable if excess of salts is a problem in the detection phase or if a sample needs to be concentrated.

16. Small, fluorescent adenosine-nucleotide peaks with sizes equivalent to those of PCR amplified fragments plus one nucleotide may be seen, especially if the concentrations of the PCR amplified fragments are high, most likely the result of the nontemplate addition of a single adenosine molecules to the 3' end of the PCR-amplified fragments *(16)*.

Acknowledgments

We thank Ms. Annemette Holbo Birk for technical assistance. The work was supported by grants to Juan Sanchez from Ellen and Aage Andersen's Foundation.

References

1. Gill, P. (2001) An assessment of the utility of single nucleotide polymorphisms (SNPs) for forensic purposes. *Int. J. Legal Med.* **114,** 204–210.
2. Andras, S. C, Power, J. B., Cocking, E. C., Davey, M. R. (2001) Strategies for signal amplification in nucleic acid detection. *Mol. Biotechnol.* **19,** 29–44.
3. Rozen, S., Skaletsky, H., Marszalek, J. D., Minx, P. J., Cordum, H. S., Waterston, R. H., et al. (2003) Abundant gene conversion between arms of palindromes in human and ape Y chromosomes. *Nature* **423,** 873–876.
4. Lindblad-Toh, K., Winchester, E., Daly, M. J., Wang, D. G., Hirschhorn, J. N., Laviolette, J. P., et al. (2000) Large-scale discovery and genotyping of single-nucleotide polymorphisms in the mouse. *Nat. Genet.* **24,** 381–386.
5. Broude, N. E., Zhang, L., Woodward, K., Englert, D., and Cantor, C. R. (2001) Multiplex allele-specific target amplification based on PCR suppression. *Proc. Natl. Acad. Sci. USA* **98,** 206–211.
6. Brownie, J., Shawcross, S., Theaker, J., Whitcombe, D., Ferrie, R., Newton, C., et al. (1997) The elimination of primer-dimer accumulation in PCR. *Nucleic Acids Res.* **25,** 3235–3241.
7. Mutter, G. L., and Boynton, K. A. (1995) PCR bias in amplification of androgen receptor alleles, a trinucleotide repeat marker used in clonality studies. *Nucleic Acids Res.* **23,**1411–1418.
8. Hu, G. (1993) DNA polymerase-catalyzed addition of nontemplated extra nucleotides to the 3' end of a DNA fragment. *DNA Cell Biol.* **12,** 763–770.
9. Magnuson, V. L., Ally, D. S., Nylund, S. J., Karanjawala, Z. E., Rayman, J. B., Knapp, J. I., et al. (1996) Substrate nucleotide-determined non-templated addition of adenine by Taq DNA polymerase: implications for PCR-based genotyping and cloning. *BioTechniques* **21,** 700–709.
10. Henegariu, O., Heerema, N. A., Dlouhy, S. R., Vance, G. H., and Vogt, P.H. (1997) Multiplex PCR: critical parameters and step-by-step protocol. *BioTechniques* **23,** 504–511.
11. Markoulatos, P., Siafakas, N., and Moncany, M. (2002) Multiplex polymerase chain reaction: a practical approach. *J. Clin. Lab. Anal.* **16,** 47–51.

12. Rees, W. A., Yager, T. D., Korte, J., and Von Hippel, P. H. (1993) Betaine can eliminate the base pair composition dependence of DNA melting. *Biochemistry* **32,** 137–144.
13. Hogan, M., LeGrange, J., and Austin, B. (1983) Dependence of DNA helix flexibility on base composition. *Nature* **304,** 752–754.
14. Pomp, D., and Medrano, J. F.(1991) Organic solvents as facilitators of polymerase chain reaction. *BioTechniques* **10,** 58–59.
15. Don, R. H., Cox, P. T., Wainwright, B. J., Baker, K., and Mattick, J. S. (1991) 'Touchdown' PCR to circumvent spurious priming during gene amplification. *Nucleic Acids Res.* **19,** 4008.
16. Brownstein, M. J., Carpten, J. D., and Smith, J. R. (1996) Modulation of nontemplated nucleotide addition by Taq DNA polymerase: primer modifications that facilitate genotyping. *BioTechniques* **20,** 1004–1010.

16

Y Chromosome SNP Analysis Using the Single-Base Extension

A Hierarchical Multiplex Design

María Brión

Summary

Single nucleotide polymorphisms (SNPs) are the most frequent polymorphisms described in the human genome, and their analysis is becoming an extensive routine in molecular biology, not only in the forensic field, but also in population and clinical genetics. In particular, SNPs located on the Y chromosome have a specific utility as forensic tools, and based on this fact, we have designed a strategy that allows us to identify the most frequent haplogroups in European populations. We selected 29 markers among the 245 binary polymorphisms described in the Y-Chromosome Consortium tree. The whole set was grouped into four multiplexes in a hierarchical way, allowing us to determine the final haplogroup using only one or two multiplexes. In this way, we only type in the best-case nine SNPs, and in the worst possible combination 17 SNPs, to define the haplogroup. The selected strategy to type the SNPs was a single-base extension method using the SNaPshot™ multiplex kit from Applied Biosystems, and detailed practical procedures are described here. With this hierarchical strategy adapted for European populations the massive typing of SNPs was avoided, and therefore the time and money involved in the study was also reduced.

Key Words: Y chromosome; SNP; multiplex PCR; single-base extension (SBE); SNaPshot.

1. Introduction

Single nucleotide polymorphisms (SNPs, including small insertions and deletions) are the markers of choice for many applications for localizing and identifying disease susceptibility genes, for understanding the molecular mechanism of mutation, for studying the origin of modern human populations, or for measuring the variability between them (*1,2*).

From: *Methods in Molecular Biology, vol. 297: Forensic DNA Typing Protocols*
Edited by: A. Carracedo © Humana Press Inc., Totowa, NJ

In particular, SNPs located on the Y chromosome have a specific utility as forensic tools for several reasons. First, in the case of the Y chromosome, as in autosomes, the SNPs are the most frequent kind of polymorphism. Second, because of their simplicity, SNPs can be analyzed from a very low quantity of DNA and are amenable to analysis with high-throughput technologies. Third, the low mutation rate of SNPs allows their use in paternity testing. Finally, there is the opportunity to genotype fragments smaller in size than those needed for existing deoxyribonucleic acid (DNA) polymorphisms. Nevertheless, because of the presence of only two alleles in each variable position in addition to the lack of recombination and the highly population specific distribution, shown in the Y chromosome, one often requires the analysis of large numbers of SNPs to obtain enough information.

Despite slow progress in the discovery of Y-chromosome variation until recently, now a large number of SNPs have been described, defining a highly resolved tree of NRY binary haplogroups *(3,4)*.

Checking the literature, we performed an extensive search, looking for the allele frequencies of each SNP in European populations. As a result of this search, a set of 29 SNPs were selected to determine the most frequent haplogroups present in European populations. **Figure 1** represents the maximum parsimony tree defined with these SNPs.

A large number of SNP genotyping methods are now available, and usually the choice of the appropriate method depends on the number of SNPs and the number of individuals that need to be typed. Because this study typed 29 SNPs, the selected genotyping strategy was a single-base (SBE) extension method using the SNaPshot multiplex kit (AB Applied Biosystems), which allows, with previous multiplex amplification and with an automatic sequencer, the quick development of a sufficiently large study, without investment in new technologies. The strategy adopted here for typing SNPs includes on one hand the development of four multiplex polymerase chain reactions (PCRs), and on the other hand the development of four multiplex SNaPshot reactions.

2. Materials

2.1. PCR

1. Oligonucleotides were purchased from Sigma-Genosys and MWG, desalted and lyophilized, and 100 μM stock aliquots were performed with deionized water and stored at $-20°C$.
2. AmpliTaq Gold™ with GeneAmp® 10X PCR buffer II (100 mM Tris-HCl, pH 8.3, 500 mM KCl) and 25 mM MgCl$_2$ Solution from AB Applied Biosystems, stored at $-20°C$.
3. GeneAmp® 10 mM dNTP Mix with dTTP from AB Applied Biosystems, stored at $-20°C$.

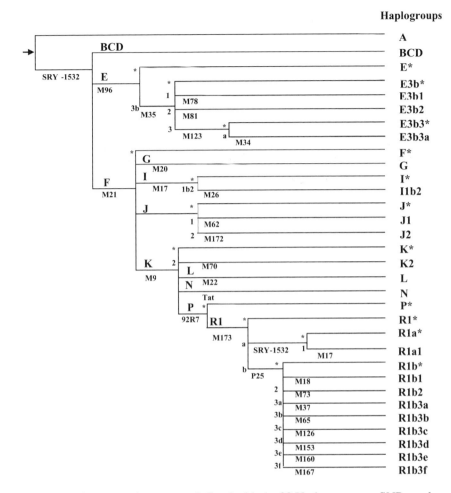

Fig. 1. Maximum parsimony tree defined with the 29 Y-chromosome SNPs analyzed.

2.2. PCR Product Cleanup

ExoSAP-IT® stored at –20°C and kept on ice while pipetting (Amersham Biosciences).

2.3. SBE Reaction

1. Oligonucleotides were purchased from Sigma-Genosys and MWG, purified by high-performance liquid chromatography and lyophilized, and 100 μM stock aliquots were performed with deionized water and stored at –20°C.
2. SNaPshot™ Multiplex kit (AB Applied Biosystems) stored at –15 to –25°C in a constant-temperature freezer

2.4. Postextension Treatment

Shrimp alkaline phosphatase (SAP) from Amersham Biosciences, stored at −20°C and kept on ice while pipetting

2.5. Analysis of the Amplified Products

The analysis was performed in an ABI PRISM® 3100 Genetic Analyser and the material required is listed below.

1. Performance Optimizer Polymer 4 or 6 (POP-4 or POP-6) stored at 4°C and kept at room temperature before being loaded in the genetic analyser (may cause eye, skin and respiratory tract irritation; *see* **Note 1**).
2. 36-cm array.
3. Matrix standard set DS-02 [dR110, dRGG, dTAMRA™, dROX™, LIZ™] stored at 4°C.
4. GeneScan-120 LIZ size standard stored at 4°C.
5. Hi-Di™ formamide stored at −20°C (it also may cause eye, skin, and respiratory tract irritation, in addition to cause damage to the central nervous system and the reproductive systems).
6. GeneScan® software, version 3.7.

All materials were purchased from Applied Biosystems.

3. Methods

The 29 SNPs were divided in four multiplex PCRs, in a hierarchical way according to their location on the Y-chromosome consortium tree. This means that for each sample, we only needed to amplify one or two multiplexes to determine the final haplogroup we can get with these SNPs.

Multiplex 1 included nine SNPs (*see* **Note 2**), which allowed for the detection of the major clades more frequent in Europe *(5,6)* and showed the second multiplex we needed to perform. Multiplex 2 included five SNPs and determined haplogroups G, I, and J. Multiplex 3 subdivides haplogroup E and included six SNPs. The last one, multiplex 4 subdivides haplogroup R1ab and included nine binary polymorphisms, five SNPs, three deletions, and one insertion.

3.1. PCR

The first step in the development of the multiplex PCR was the selection of the primers for each of the SNPs, trying to get amplicons with different size (**Table 1**). The primer 3 software (http://www-genome.wi.mit.edu/cgi-bin/primer/primer3_www.cgi) was used to check for the best place in the flanking region of each of the SNPs. The melting temperature of each primer was selected to be among 59 and 61°C to allow the multiplex amplification. In addition, possible secondary structures of the oligonucleotides were checked with the Oligonucleotide properties calculator software vs 3.02 (http://www.basic.nwu.edu/biotools/oligocalc.html).

PCR multiplexes were performed in a GeneAmp® PCR System 9700 thermal cycler (AB Applied Biosystems), in 25 µL of final volume. The reaction included 1X buffer, 300 µ*M* of dNTPs, 2 m*M* of $MgCl_2$, 2 U of Taq Gold polymerase, and 10 ng of genomic DNA, except multiplex 2, which was performed with 200 µ*M*, 1.5 m*M* of $MgCl_2$, and 0.5 U of Taq Gold. The cycling conditions were 95°C for 10 min, 32 cycles of 94°C for 30 s, 59°C for 30 s, and 70°C for 30 s, and a final extension at 65°C for 15 min. Primer sequences and detailed concentrations arc shown in **Table 1**. Some of the SNPs as M73 and M160 on one hand, and M17 and M18 on the other hand, are amplified in the same amplicon.

Because the size of the amplicons included in each multiplex is different, the PCR product can be detected in manual polyacrylamide gels to know whether all the SNPs have been successfully amplified or not. The smallest difference in size between two SNPs included in the same multiplex is 3 bp (**Table 1**); therefore, using 9% polyacrylamide gels (T = 9 and C = 5) silver stained, there are no problems distinguishing both fragments (**Fig. 2**).

3.2. PCR Product Cleanup

After PCR, unincorporated primers and dNTPs have to be removed because they can affect in the following primer extension reaction. To eliminate the excess of PCR primers and dNTPs, the product was cleaned up with ExoSAP-IT® (*see* **Note 3**). One microliter of the PCR product was mixed with 0.5 µL of ExoSAP-IT® kept on ice while pipetting and incubated at 37°C for 15 min and at 85°C for 15 min to inactivate the enzyme.

3.3. SBE Reaction

Mutation detection, through a SBE reaction, was performed by use of the SNaPshot Multiplex kit of Applied Biosystem. With this strategy, unlabeled primers placed with the 3' end immediately upstream to the SNPs are extended with a single ddNTP labeled with a fluorescence dye (**Table 2**). The development of multiplex SNaPshot reactions has been possible because the products were spatially separated tailing the 5' end of the minisequencing primers with varying lengths of poly (dC) nonhomologous tails (**Table 2**; *see* **Note 4**). In our case the smallest difference in size between two SNPs included in the same multiplex, with at least one of the polymorphic nucleotides in common, was four bases.

The same software as for PCR primers design were used to select the SBE oligonucleotides. Because the recommended annealing temperature for a

Table 1
SNP Primer Sequences, PCR Concentrations, and Amplicon Size

SNP	Primer (5'→3') Forward	Reverse	Size (bp)	Conc (µM)
Multiplex 1				
92R7	TGCATGAACACAAAAGACGTA	GCATTGTTAAATATGACCAGC	55	0.20
M70	TCATAGCCCACTATACTTTGGAC	CTGAGGGCTGGACTATAGGG	81	0.20
M22	GCTGATAGTCCTGGTTTCCCTA	TGAGCATGCCTACAGCAGAC	106	0.20
Tat	GACTCTGAGTGTAGACTTGTGA	GAAGGTGCCGTAAAAGTGTGAA	112	0.20
P25	GGACCATCACCTGGGTAAAGT	AGTGCTTGTCCAAGGCAGTA	121	0.20
SRY1532	TCCTTAGCAACCATTAATCTGG	AAATAGCAAAAACTGACACAAGGC	167	0.20
M173	GCACAGTACTCACTTTAGGTTTGC	GCAGTTTCCCAGATCCTGA	172	0.20
M213	GGCCATATAAAAACGCAGCA	TGAATGGCAAATTGATTCCA	208	0.30
M9	GCAGCATATAAAACTTTCAGG	AAAACCTAACTTTGCTCAAGC	340	0.35
Multiplex 2				
M201	TCAAATTGTGACACTGCAATAGTT	CATCCAACACTAAGTACCTATTACGAA	144	0.25
M26	AGCAGAAGAGACCAAGACAGC	GACGAAATCTGCAGCAAAAA	147	0.25
M170	TGCAGCTCTTATTAAGTTATGTTTTCA	CCAATTACTTTCAACATTTAAGACC	158	0.25
M172	TCCTCATTCACCTGCCTCTC	TCCATGTTGGTTTGGAACAG	187	0.25
M62	ACTAAAACACCATTAGAAACAAAGG	CTGAGCAACATAGTGACCCC	309	0.25

Multiplex 3				
M96	GTGATGTGTAACTTGGAAAACAGG	GGACCATATATTTTGCCATAGGTT	88	0.25
M34	CACAGTGTTTTCTCATGTTAATGC	GGGGACCCCAATAATCATAA	92	0.25
M81	TTATAGTTTCAATCCCTCAGTAATTTT	TGTTTCTTCTTGGTTTGTGTGAGTA	176	0.25
M35	GCATGGTCCCTTTCTATGGAT	GAGAATGAATAGGCATGGGTTC	198	0.25
M123	CACAGAGCAAGTGACTCTCAAAG	TCTTTCCCTCAACATAGTTATCTCA	248	0.25
M78	CTTCAGGCATTATTTTTTTGGT	ATAGTGTTCCTTCACCTTTCCTT	301	0.25
Multimplex 4				
M65	AAGGCTACCCATTCCCAAAT	AAGTCTGGCATCTGCAAAATC	71	0.15
M126	GTGCTTGAAACCGAGTTTGT	TCGGGAAACACAATTAAGCA	83	0.15
M73-M160	AAAACAATAGTTCCAAAAACTTCTGA	CCTTTGTGATTCCTCTGAACG	98	0.5
M37	ATGGAGCAAGGAACACAGAA	AAGAAAGGAGATTGTTTTCAATTTT	124	0.3
M167	GAGGCTGGGCCAAGTTAAGG	CTTCCTCGGAACCACTACCA	130	0.15
M17-M18	CTGGTCATAACACTGGAAATC	AGCTGACCACAAACTGATGTAGA	171	0.10
M153	TCTGACTTGGAAAGGGGAAA	TTTTCTCCTCATTATTGTCTTCA	239	0.5

Table 2
Fluorescence Dyes Assigned to Each ddNTP

ddNTP	Dye label	Color of analyzed data
A	dR6G	Green
T	dROX®	Red
G	dR110	Blue
C	dTAMRA®	Black

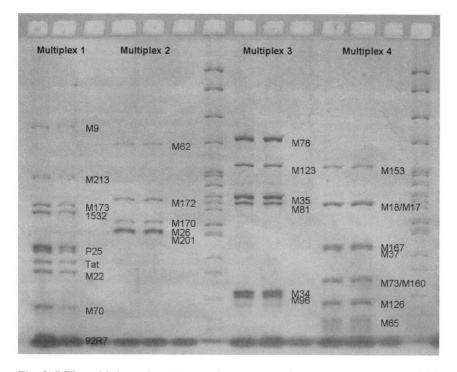

Fig. 2. PCR multiplexes in a silver-stained polyacrylamide gel. For each multiplex, two samples and a negative control were run. Lane 1 to 3 represent multiplex 1, lane 4 to 6 multiplex 2, lane 8 to 10 multiplex 3, and lane 11 to 13 multiplex 4. Lanes 7 and 14 show a pBR322 DNA-Msp I Digest molecular weight standard (New England BioLabs).

SNaPshot control oligonucleotide is 50°C, the melting temperature for the selected oligos was at least 50°C.

The nucleotide composition of the smaller oligonucleotides can modify significantly the electrophoresis mobility, so we tested all the used primers in singleplex, before being multiplexed, to ensure the spatial position of each of them.

The multiplex SBE reactions were performed in 5 µL of final volume, including 2 µL of multiplex SNaPshot kit and 1.5 µL of cleaned PCR product (*see* **Note 5**). Oligonucleotide sequences and concentrations are shown in **Table 3**. The cycling conditions were 96°C for 10 s, 50°C for 5 s, and 60°C for 30 s during 25 cycles.

Table 3 also shows the size of the oligonucleotides used with each SNP; however, during the analysis we have to take in account the single ddNTP extended besides the fluorescence dye, which will affect the mobility of the extended primers in the electrophoresis.

3.4. Postextension Treatment

Because unincorporated ddNTPs will coemigrate with the fragments of interest, to avoid interference in the SNaPshot products detection, the migration of ddNTPs has to be altered, removing the 5' phosphoryl groups (*see* **Note 6**). For this purpose, the final product was incubated with 1 U of SAP kept on ice while pipetting for 1 h at 37°C and 15 min at 85°C to inactivate the enzyme.

3.5. Analysis of the Amplified Products

SNapShot products were run on an ABI 3100 Genetic Analyser (Applied Biosystems). To prepare samples for the capillary electrophoresis, 1.5 µL of the minisequencing product was mixed with 10 µL of Hi-Di™ formamide and 0.2 µL of GeneScan-120 LIZ size standard. The mix was spin briefly and denatured by placing the plate at 95°C for 5 min. Until the samples are loaded in the analyzer, they have to be placed on ice or at 4°C.

Samples were analyzed using POP-4 as recommended by the manufacturer or POP-6 (*see* **Note 1**) with SNP36_POP4 default module independent of the polymer used. The parameters included in the run module are as follows: run temperature 60°C, prerun time and voltage 60 s and 15 kV, injection time and voltage 60 s and 2 kV, run time and voltage 1000 s and 15 kV. Data were analyzed with dye set E5 created with dR110, dRGG, dTAMRA™, dROX™, LIZ™ matrix standards

Analysis of files was performed according to the ABI PRISM GeneScan Analysis Software User's Manual, using the GeneScan 3.7 software (AB Applied Biosystems), and determining the size of the fragments was based on GeneScan-120 Liz size standard.

As in this case, when we are working with Y-chromosome SNPs, the interpretation of results becomes easy because we only have one allele for SNP and therefore we avoid any possible difficulty in the determination of heterozygous against homozygous (*see* **Note 7**)

Table 3
SNaPshot Primer Sequences and Concentrations

SNP		Minisequencing Primer (5'→3')	Size (bp)	Conc (µM)
Multiplex 1				
M22	For	CCGCCATTCCTGGTGGCTCT	20	0.10
P25	For	CCCCCCCTCTGCCTGAAACCTGCCTG	26	0.15
92R7	Rev	CCCGCATGAACACAAAAGACGTAGAAG	28	0.20
SRY1532	For	CCCCCTTGTATCTGACTTTTTCACACAGT	30	0.20
M70	Rev	CCCCCCCCTAGGGATTCTGTTGTGGTAGTCTTAG	34	0.15
M173	For	CCCCCCCCCCTTACAATTCAAGGGCATTTAGAAC	34	0.20
Tat	Rev	CCCCCCCCCCCCCCCCTGAAATATTAAATTAAAACAAC	42	0.20
M213	Rev	CCCCCCCCCCCCCCCCTCAGAACTTAAAACATCTGTTAC	45	0.25
M9	For	CCCCCCCCCCCCCCCCCCCCGAAACGGCCTAAGATGGTTGAAT	48	0.20
Multiplex 2				
M170	Rev	ACACAACCCACACTGAAAAAAA	22	0.45
M62	Rev	CCCCCC CAATGTTTGTTGGCCATGGA	27	0.50
M172	For	CCCCCCCCCCCAAACCATTTTGATGCTT	32	0.10
M26	Rev	CCCCCCCCCCCCCCCCATAGGCCATTCAGTGTTCTG	37	0.25
M201	For	CCCCCCCCCCCCCCCCGATCTAATAATCCAGTATCAACTGAGG	42	0.05
M34	Rev	TTGCAGACACCACCACATGTG	20	0.15

Multiplex 3				
M81	For	CCCCCCTAAATTTTGTCCTTTTTGAA	27	0.20
M78	For	CCCCCCCCCACACTTAACAAAGATACTTCTTTC	34	0.35
M35	Rev	CCCCCCCCCCCCCCCCCCCAGTCTCTGCCTGTGTC	36	0.03
M96	For	CCCCCCCCCCCGTAACTTGGAAAACAGGTCTCTCATAATA	40	0.05
M123	Rev	CCCCCCCCCCCCCCCCCCCTTCTAGGTATTCAGGCGATG	51	0.35
M167	For	CCCAAGCCCCACAGGGTGC	19	0.45
Multiplex 4				
M153	For	AAAGCTCAAAGGGTATGTGAACA	23	0.30
M17	For	CCAAAATTCACTTAAAAAAACCC	23	0.20
M18	For	CCCCAGTTTGTGGTTGCTGGTTGTTA	26	0.15
M126	For	CCCGCTTGAAACCGAGTTTGTACTTAATA	30	0.05
M37	For	CCGGAACACAGAAAATAAAATCTATGTGTG	30	0.35
M73	Rev	CCCCCCCCCCGATTCCTCTGAACGTCTAACCA	33	0.30
M65	Rev	CCCCCCCCCCCCCCCCCCCCCCACCCGCGGTAAG	36	0.05
M160	For	CCCCCCCCTTACAAGTTTAATACATACAACTTCAATTTTC	40	0.20

Each of the SNPs included in the multiplex is going to be represented after the analysis, as an electrophoretic peak with a different color depending on the base that has been extended. **Fig. 3** shows one example of each of the four multiplexes (*see* **Notes 8** and **9**).

4. Notes

1. According to the manufacturer, the SNaPshot multiplex kit should be used with POP-4™ polymer; however, we have realized that when the fragments are similar in size, the use of POP-6™ polymer results in a better resolution and discrimination in size.
2. Despite the four multiplexes that include 29 SNPs, **Fig. 1** shows 30 SNPs branches. The reason is because the SRY1532, included in multiplex 1, is one of the few SNPs showing recurrence, so it appears twice in the tree.
3. PCR product was also cleaned up according to the manufacturer's recommendations by mixing 15 µL of it with 5 U of SAP and 2 U of Exonuclease I (*Exo*I, Amersham Biosciences) and incubating at 37°C for 1 h and at 85°C for 15 min. In our experience, ExoSAP-IT® (Amersham Biosciences) gives clearer results, especially when small minisequencing primers are being used.
4. We have selected poly (dC) 5' tails because they are predicted to have minimal secondary structures. However, there are more available possibilities, such as the use of non-homologous tag sequences, as the published by Hirschorn et al. *(7)*.
5. To avoid the loss of material and possible contaminations, it is strongly recommended adding the SNaPshot kit and the oligonucleotides directly to the same tubes or plates where the clean-up has been conducted.
6. When the digestion with SAP does not remove all the ddNTP, in the electropherogram of the SNaPshot products some artefact peaks larger than 70 bp will appear (excess ddNTP also result in peaks of smaller sizes).
7. Because the intensity of the emitted fluorescence is different for each dye used to label ddNTPs, when the strategy includes autosomal markers, special consideration should be given to detect heterozygous.
8. In multiplex 1, the SNPs P25 and 92R7 are paralogous sequence variants originated for segmental duplications, where at least one of the variants is polymorphic *(8)*. This means that in the SBE reaction, the polymorphic position of each SNP can be extended with one ddNTP and the nonpolymorphic position with the same of another ddNTP. In the example represented in **Fig. 3A**, in the P25 the paralogous sequence variants are extended with two different ddNTP (C and A) and in the 92R7 with the same ddNTP (A).
9. In multiplex 2, the SBE reaction always shows the artifact blue peak indicated with an arrow in **Fig. 3B**. This artifact is generated in the M26 SNaPshot reaction because it also appears in the singleplex reaction of this SNP. Because M26 is a G to A transition, the artifact blue peak does not affect the interpreting of results. However, other SBE primers should be tried to avoid artifacts.

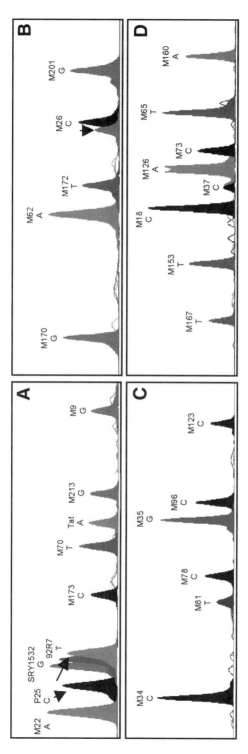

Fig. 3. Example of results for the four SNaPshot multiplexes from different samples. (A) multiplex 1 from sample assigned to haplogroup R1b, the P25 shows a duplicated pattern (see Note 8); (B) multiplex 2 from sample assigned to Hg 1*(xI1b2), M26 always shows an artefact blue peak (see Note 9); (C) multiplex 3 from sample assigned to Hg E3b2; (D) multiplex 4 from sample assigned to Hg R1b3f.

Acknowledgments

The technical assistance of Meli Rodríguez and Raquel Calvo is highly appreciated. This work was supported by the grants from the "Xunta de Galicia" (PGIDT01PXI20806PR) and from the "Ministerio de Ciencia y Tecnología" (DGCYT.P4.BIO2000-0145-P4-02).

References

1. Jorde, L. B., Watkins, W. S., and Bamshad, M. J. (2001) Population genomics: a bridge from evolutionary history to genetic medicine. *Hum. Mol. Genet.* **10,** 2199–2207.
2. Zhao, Z., Fu, Y. X., Hewett-Emmett, D., and Boerwinkle, E. (2003) Investigating single nucleotide polymorphism (SNP) density in the human genome and its implications for molecular evolution. *Gene* **312,** 207–213.
3. Y Chromosome Consortium. (2002) A nomenclature system for the tree of human Y-chromosomal binary haplogroups. *Genome Res.* **12,** 339–348.
4. Jobling, M. A., and Tyler-Smith, C. (2003) The human Y chromosome: an evolutionary marker comes of age. *Nat. Rev. Genet.* **4,** 598–612.
5. Rosser, Z., Zerjal, T., Hurles, M. H., Adojaan, M., Alavantic, D., Amorim, A., et al. (2000) Y chromosomal diversity within Europe is clinal and influenced primarily by geography, rather than language. *Am. J. Hum. Genet.* **67,** 1526–1543.
6. Semino, O., Passarino, G., Oefner, P. J., Lin, A. A., Arbuzova, S., Beckman, L. E., et al. (2000) The Genetic legacy of paleolithic homo sapiens sapiens in extant Europeans: a Y chromosome perspective. *Science* **290,** 1155–1159.
7. Hirschorn, J. N., Sklar, P., Lindblad-Toh, K., Lim, Y-M., Ruiz-Gutierrez, M., Bolk, S., et al. (2000) SBE-TAGS: an array-based method for efficient single nucleotide polymorphism genotyping. *Proc. Natl. Acad. Sci. USA* **97,** 12,164–12,169.
8. Sanchez, J. J. S., Brion, M., Parson, W., Blanco-Verea, A. J., Boersting, C., Lareu, M. V., et al. (2004) Duplications of the Y-chromosome specific loci P25 and 92R7 and forensic implications. *Forensic Sci. Int.* **140,** 147–250.

17

SNaPshot for Pharmacogenetics by Minisequencing

Klaus Bender

Summary

Genetic polymorphisms of genes coding for metabolic enzymes are helpful to predict how an individual may respond to medication or drugs. The described approach for the identification of genetic variations for the cytochrome P450 enzymes CYP2D6 and CYP2C19 has been designed for the rapid genotyping of relevant alleles (CYP2D6*1, -*3, -*4, -*6, -*7, and -*8 and CYP2C19*1, -*2, -*3, -*4, and -*5) by performing polymerase chain reaction amplifications of genomic regions containing the SNP followed by a single-tube multiplex single base extension (minisquencing) reaction. This multiplex assay can easily be expanded for additional genes and single nucleotide polymorphisms (SNPs). Minisequencing is a sensitive, reproducible, and time-saving method for SNP typing that can be performed using ordinary laboratory equipment.

Key Words: SNPs; pharmacogenetic; CYP2D6; CYP2C19; minisequencing.

1. Introduction

Single nucleotide polymorphisms (SNPs) are informative in the study of human genetic diversity and may be used in the diagnosis of disease-related alleles, pharmacogenetic typing, the identification of victims in mass disasters, and in population genetic studies. SNP typing can be performed by a variety of different methods *(1)*. The SNP analysis described in this chapter makes use of a DNA polymerase-mediated single-base extension (SBE). The reaction is robust, allowing specific genotyping of most SNPs at similar reaction conditions.

The typing of SNPs in the cytochrome P450 genes CYP2D6 and CYP2C19 is chosen as an example for a detailed explanation of this method. Because the proteins encoded by these genes are involved in the metabolism of many drugs, polymorphisms in the coding sequence can either modify the activity or lead to the inactivation of the enzymes. The reduction or loss of enzyme activity can

From: *Methods in Molecular Biology, vol. 297: Forensic DNA Typing Protocols*
Edited by: A. Carracedo © Humana Press Inc., Totowa, NJ

result in a nonresponse to medication or adverse drug reactions *(2,3)*. Therefore the prediction of the genotypes for drug-metabolizing enzymes may have an impact on the choice of the drug prescribed and could be helpful in the tailoring of medication that is specific to patients.

The method depends on the PCR amplification of the genomic region that contains the SNPs before the actual genotyping reaction is performed by multiplex minisequencing. The typing principle can be compared with a conventional sequencing reaction but makes use of a minisequencing primer annealing directly with its 3' end adjacent to the polymorphic site and using fluorescence-labeled ddNTPs rather than a mixture of dNTP and ddNTPs. The 3' end is extended with a single nucleotide that is complementary to the nucleotide at the site of the SNP. The assay itself involves three phases. First, the amplification of the target sequences by PCR; second, the removal of non-incorporated PCR primers and dNTPs; third, the minisequencing reaction (SBE) followed by separation and detection of the extended minisequencing primers by capillary gel electrophoresis (**Fig. 1**). By attaching oligo dT-tags with defined lengths to the 5' end of each minisequencing primer, the combined analysis of several SNPs can be performed in a single reaction tube *(4,5)*.

For the typing of the above-mentioned genes, a single PCR for CYP2D6 and a 4-plex PCR for CYP2C19 is performed. All PCR products are then pooled for exonuclease I and shrimp alkaline phosphatase (SAP) digestion. Minisequencing is performed by using the commercially available SNaPshot™ Kit (Applied Biosystems). The minisequencing products are analyzed by capillary gel electrophoresis. **Figure 2** summarizes the strategy for the combined typing of the most important SNPs for the two cytochrome P450 genes.

Minisequencing cannot be performed for the detection of whole gene deletions and duplications present in the CYP2D6 gene. These mutations can only be analyzed by using long-PCR technologies developed by Steen et al. *(6)* and Lundqvist et al. *(7)*, respectively.

2. Materials

1. PCR Thermocycler Gene® Amp PCR System 2400/9600 (Applied Biosystems).
2. Oligonucleotide primers (Invitrogen) (*see* **Note 1**).
3. 10 mM deoxy-ribonucleotide triphosphates (dNTPs) mixture (peqlab Biotechnology).
4. SAWADY "Mid Range PCR" Kit (peqlab Biotechnology).
5. Platinum Polymerase (Invitrogen).
6. 10X PCR Buffer, 50 mM MgCl$_2$ (Invitrogen).
7. Horizontal electrophoresis chamber for minimum gel length of 8 cm.
8. 10X TBE buffer: 109 g Tris-base, 55.6 g boric acid, 9.3 g ethylene diamine tetraacetic acid per liter.

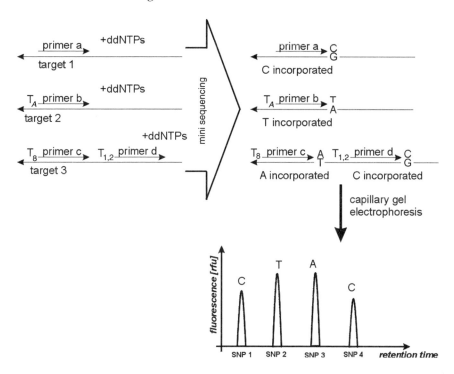

Fig. 1. Scheme of the minisequencing typing. The migration of the particular minisequencing primers corresponds to the difference in the length of the attached oligoT tails.

Gene	PCR	Fragments	Alleles analyzed	Purification		
CYP2D6	single	5000 bp	*1, *3, *4, *6, *7, *8	pooled for Exonuclease I and SAP digestion	minisequencing	CE
CYP2C19	4-plex	321 bp	*1, *2			
		271 bp	*1, *3			
		195 bp	*1, *4			
		229 bp	*1, *5			

Fig. 2. Strategy for the typing of relevant alleles for CYP2D6 and CYP2C19.

9. Universal agarose (e.g., peqGOLD, peqlab Biotechnology).
10. Ethidium bromide (10 mg/mL).
11. 6X DNA loading buffer: 0.25% cresolred, 30% glycerol in water.
12. DNA size markers (100-bp ladder DNA and λ DNA digested with *Hind*III).
13. Power supply capable of delivering a constant voltage between 60 and 200 V.
14. Long-wave ultraviolet transilluminator (312 nm).

15. Photographic equipment with filter for ultraviolet.
16. Exonuclease I (Amersham Pharmacia).
17. SAP (Roche Diagnostics).
18. ABI PRISM SNaPshot™ Kit (Applied Biosystems).
19. Genetic Analyzer ABI PRISM 310 (Applied Biosystems).
20. Formamide Sigma Ultra (F-5786).
21. ABI PRISM® dRhodamine Matrix Standards Kit (Applied Biosystems).
22. Matrix Standard Set DS-02 (Applied Biosystems).

3. Methods
3.1. PCR Amplification for the CYP2D6 Locus

1. The amplification protocol of the CYP2D6 gene is in general the protocol for the examination of gene duplications of CYP2D6 (7). The PCR is conducted in 50-μL reaction volumes containing 10–150 ng template DNA, 5 μL of 10X reaction buffer (500 mM Tris-HCl, pH 9.1, 140 mM $(NH_4)_2SO_4$, 17.5 mM $MgCl_2$), 350 μM dNTPs, 15 μM of each primer (**Table 1**), and 2.5 units of "Mid Range PCR" enzyme
2. Place the PCR tubes into a PerkinElmer Thermocycler Gene® Amp PCR System 2400/9600 with the following conditions: initial denaturation at 94°C for 2 min, 32 cycles of denaturation at 96°C for 30 s, primer annealing and extension at 68°C for 4 min, and a final extension step at 72°C for 10 min.

3.2. PCR Amplification for the CYP2C19 Locus

1. The 4-PlexPCR is conducted in a 50-μL reaction volume containing 10–150 ng template of DNA, 5 μL of 10X PCR buffer (200 mM Tris-HCl, pH 8.4; 500 mM KCl), 3 mM $MgCl_2$, 200 μM dNTPs, 10 μM of each primer (**Table 2**), and 2.5 units of Platinum Taq polymerase.
2. Place the PCR tubes into a PerkinElmer Thermocycler Gene® Amp PCR System 2400/9600 with the following conditions: initial denaturation at 94°C for 5 min, 37 cycles of denaturation at 96°C for 30 s, primer annealing at 57°C for 20 s, extension at 72°C for 45 s, and a final extension step at 72°C for 7 min.

3.3. Agarose Gel Electrophoresis

1. Agarose gel electrophoresis is conducted to check the presence and correct size of the amplified PCR products (*see* **Note 2**). Mix 5 μL of a 50-μL PCR with 1.3 μL of 6X DNA loading buffer for electrophoresis. Load the mixture into the slots of a 1–2% agarose gel prestained with ethidium bromide (0.3 μg/mL), prepared with 1X TBE, and run the gel with 60V for 30–60 min.
2. After running the gel examine the PCR fragments under ultraviolet light and photograph them for documentation (**Fig. 3**).

Table 1
Primers for CYP2D6 According to Lundqvist et al. *(7)*

Primer	Orientation	Ref. seq. acc. no.	Sequence (5' to 3')	Length (nt)
CYP2D6F	Forward	M33388	CCA GAA GGC TTT GCA GGC TTC A	22
CYP2D6R	Reverse		ACT GAG CCC TGG GAG GTA GGT A	22

Table 2
Primers for CYP2C19, CYP2C19*2, and *3 Primers According to Goldstein et al. *(8)*; CYP2C19*5 Primers According to Xiao et al. *(9)*; and CYP2C19*4 Primers According to Ferguson et al. *(10)*

Primer	Orientation	Ref. seq. acc. no.	Sequence (5' to 3')	Length (nt)
CYP2C19*2-A	Forward	M61854	CAG AGC TTG GCA TAT TGT ATC	21
CYP2C19*2-B	Reverse	"	GTA AAC ACA CAA CTA GTC AAT G	22
CYP2C19*3-A	Forward	"	AAA TTG TTT CCA ATC ATT TAG CT	23
CYP2C19*3-B	Reverse	"	ACT TCA GGG CTT GGT CAA TA	20
CYP2C19*4-A	Forward	"	TTA ACA AGA GGA GAA GGC TTC A	22
CYP2C19*4-B	Reverse	"	TTG GTT AAG GAT TTG CTG ACA	21
CYP2C19*5-A	Forward	"	TCC CTA TGT TTG TTA TTT CCA GG	23
CYP2C19*5-B	Reverse	"	GAG CAG CCA GAC CAT CTG TG	20

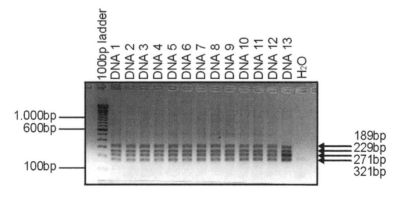

Fig. 3. Example for the 4-plex PCR of CYP2C19.

3.4. SNaPshot Minisequencing Protocol

3.4.1. Minisequencing Primer Design

1. Check both strands of each SNP target sequence to ensure that the plus- or the minus-strand minisequencing primer will not wrongly anneal somewhere else (*see* **Notes 3** and **4**).
2. The melting temperature (tm) of the minisequencing primer should be greater than the PCR annealing temperature, at least 50°C.
3. Check whether the minisequencing primers can form stable duplex molecules with each other at the given temperature in the experiment (*see* **Note 5**).
4. Check each primer for homodimers and hairpins by calculating the free energy alignment of a primer with itself.
5. Calculate a convenient length for the 5' oligo-dT tail for the proper separation of the minisequencing primers in the electrophoresis. A spacing of four to six nucleotides between two adjacent primers is sufficient (*see* **Note 6**).

3.4.2. Performing the Minisequencing

3.4.2.1. PURIFICATION OF PCR PRODUCTS

1. All reactions are performed in 0.2-mL tubes using a PerkinElmer Thermocycler Gene®Amp PCR System 2400/9600.
2. Remove the remaining primers and dNTPs by treating the PCR reactions with Exonuclease I- and SAP. PCR products from one or several single or multiplex PCR reactions can be combined. The total volume has to be adjusted to 15 µL with water.
3. Mix of PCR products

PCR products	x µL	max. 15 µL
H_2O	y µL	up to 15 µL
Total volume		15 µL

4. *Exo*I + SAP-mastermix

H_2O	3.24 µL
10X SAP buffer	0.36 µL
Exonuclease I (10 U/mL)	0.4 µL
SAP (1 U/mL)	2 µL
Total volume	6 µL

5. Digestion protocol

Mix of PCR products	15 µL
*Exo*I + SAP-mastermix	6 µL
Total volume	21 µL

6. Incubate the reaction for 60 min at 37°C, then inactivate the enzymes by heating to 75°C for 15 min. The reaction can be kept on ice. For longer storage, store at –20°C (*see* **Note 7**).

Table 3
Minisequencing Primers for CYP2D6 and CYP2C19 (Elongation Is Performed by Adding Oligo dT Tags to the 5' End of the Primers)

Primer	Primer Sequence (5' to 3')	Length (nt)
CYP2D6*3	GAC CCA GCT GGA TGA GCT GCT AAC TGA GCA C	31
CYP2D6*4	GCG ACC CCT TAC CCG CAT CTC CCA CCC CCA	30
CYP2D6*6	CAA CTT GGG CCT GGG CAA GAA GTC GCT GGA GCA G	34
CYP2D6*7	T8 TGG CCT GGG GCC TCC TGC TCA TGA TCC TAC	38
CYP2D6*8	T13 TGC CTT TGT GCC GCC TTC GCC AAC CAC TCC	44
CYP2C19*2	T21 GCA ATA ATT TTC CCA CTA TCA TTG ATT ATT TCC C	55
CYP2C19*3	T20 TGA AAA CAT CAG GAT TGT AAG CAC CCC CTG	50
CYP2C19*4	T28 GAG ACA GAG CAC AAG GAC CAC AAA AGG ATC CA	60
CYP2C19*5	T37 CGG GCC AGG CCC TCT CCC ACA CAA ATC C	65

3.4.2.2. MINISEQUENCING REACTION

1. Only a part of the digestion mix is used for minisequencing. For multiplex minisequencing all primers (**Table 3**) have to be adjusted to 1 μM in a premix solution (*see* **Note 8**).
2. Amplification protocol

Exo/SAP digested PCR products	4 μL
Minisequencing primer mix (1 μM)	0.5 μL
SNaPshot Premix	4.5 μL
Total volume	9 μL

3. Place the PCR tubes into a PerkinElmer Thermocycler Gene® Amp PCR System 2400/9600 with the following conditions: 25 cycles of denaturation at 96°C for 10 s, minisequencing primer annealing at 50°C for 15 s, extension at 60°C for 30 s (*see* **Note 9**).
4. To remove nonincorporated ddNTPs, add 1 μL of SAP to the each reaction, then incubate at 37°C for 60 min; the enzyme is then inactivated for 15 min at 75°C (*see* **Note 10**).

3.4.2.3. CAPILLARY GEL ELECTROPHORESIS

1. Mix 2 μL of the minisequencing reaction product with 20 μL of formamide in a 0.5-mL tube. Denature samples by placing them at 95°C for 5min. After cooling down to 4°C, load them into an ABI PRISM 310 Genetic Analyzer for allele discrimination.
2. In the present approach the modified module "GS POP6 Fast (1ml) E" and the Matrix "GS MatPOP6FastE" is used in conjunction with POP-6™ polymer. For electrophoresis with the POP-4™ polymer the module GS POP-4 (1 mL) E should

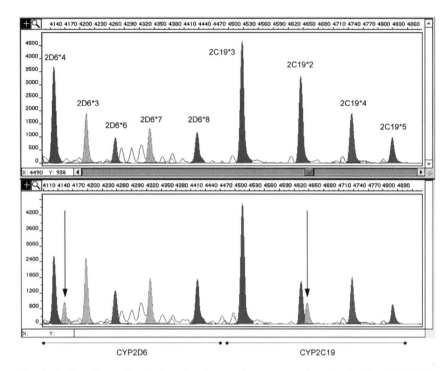

Fig. 4. A GeneScan displaying the electropherogram of peaks for the CYP2D6 and CYP2C19 gene. The upper panel shows an example for a wild-type constellation of all typed alleles. In the lower panel CYP2D6 is heterozygous for *1/*4 (arrow) and CYP2C19 is heterozygous for *1/*2 (arrow).

be used (*see* **Note 11**). In each case a suitable matrix for the fluorescent dyes used in the SNaPshot™ Kit has to be constructed with the ABI PRISM® dRhodamine Matrix Standards Kit (Applied Biosystems) according to the ABI PRISM 310 Genetic Analyzer User's Manual (P/N 403047).

3. Use the ABI GeneScan™ Analysis Software v.2.1 or later from Applied Biosystems to analyze results. A typical typing result is shown in **Fig. 4**.

4. Notes

1. Minisequencing primers have to be purified by HPLC to avoid "stutter" peaks representing incompletely synthesized primers.
2. It is not necessary to determine the exact concentration of the PCR products by spectrophotometry. Visible bands in an agarose gel are sufficient in most cases to perform a correct minisequencing reaction. In the majority of cases, low rather than high concentrations of PCR products produce clearer signals and less background. A dilution of the PCR reaction can be helpful.

3. To check whether a given minisequencing primer produces background signals and is well purified, test each primer separately before it is used in an multiplex assay. This should also be done after a new batch of primers has been ordered.

4. Run one negative control without template DNA when evaluating a new primer.

5. Calculation of all interactions between different minisequencing primers can be performed by using a corresponding computer program (e.g., FastPCR, free available in www.biocenter. helsinki.fi/bi/bare-1_html/download.htm). The programs computes the most stable interactions the strands can form, and returns free energy change ΔG for the reaction. If the free energy is negative, the DNA strands can interact in the experiment.

6. poly (dT), poly (dA), poly (dC) and poly GACT can be used as 5' nonhomologous tags.

7. Removal of residual primers and unincorporated dNTPs from the PCR also can be performed by using purification columns (e.g., MinElute PCR purification spin column, Quiagen). Attention has to be paid to the length of the PCR products, because the retention of very small amplicons (e.g., 55–90 bps) by columns can be critical.

8. To get more uniform signals for all typed SNPs in an multiplex or if a particular primer has a consistently low or high signal, increase or decrease the concentration of that primer in the primer premixture. The concentration can range between 0.05 μ*M* and 1 μ*M*. To adjust the amount of template DNA is usually not necessary.

9. Amplification can also be increased to 30 cycles compared with the original protocol from Applied Biosystems to make the system more sensitive. The increase the injection times for capillary gel electrophoresis or an increase of the amount of minisequencing product from 2 to 4 μL make the analysis more sensitive.

10. To minimize the costs for the analysis calf intestinal phosphatase can be used instead of SAP for the postextension treatment. Also, the amount of SNaPshot Premix in the minisequencing reaction can be reduced to 3.5 μL by filling up the reaction to the original volume of 4.5 μL with water.

11. To reduce the time for the electrophoresis run, the Fast GS Template E run module for GeneScan analysis can be used. This module requires the Fast Native Protocol polymer, but can also be performed with POP-6™ polymer.

12. For lower background signals, especially when multiple PCRs with many products are combined, the use of a higher concentration of exonuclease I results in lower peaks from an excess of PCR primers.

13. Unspecific signals larger than 70 bps are often caused by undigested ddNTPs. The use of a higher concentration of calf intestinal phosphatase /SAP or fresh enzyme is recommended.

14. Electropherograms from SNPs similar to a conventional Sanger sequencing reaction can be caused by the incomplete removal of dNTPs. Use fresh SAP.

15. To remove extra peaks or background peaks higher stringency thermal cycling conditions can be used: denaturation at 96°C for 10s, minisequencing primer annealing at 64°C for 5 s, and extension at 72°C for 30s.

16. If you have installed the data collection software for 5-dye detection, then the internal standard "GeneScan™-120 LIZ™ size" can be used to size the SNaPshot fragments in basepairs. The POP-4™ polymer is used in conjunction with the GS POP-4 (1 mL) E5 module. For matrix construction, use the Matrix Standard Set DS-02 (Applied Biosystems) according to the ABI PRISM 310 Genetic Analyzer User's Manual (P/N 4323050). For data analysis, the ABI GeneScan™ Analysis Software v.3.1 or higher is required.

References

1. Syvanen, A. C. (2001) Accessing genetic variation: genotyping single nucleotide polymorphisms. *Nat. Rev. Genet.* **2,** 930–942.
2. Ingelman-Sundberg, M. (2001) Pharmacogenetics: an opportunity for a safer and more efficient pharmacotherapy. *J. Intern. Med.* **250,** 186–200.
3. Pirmohamed, M., and Park, B.K. (2001) Genetic susceptibility to adverse drug reactions. Trends Pharmacol. Sci. **22,** 298–305.
4. Sanchez, J. J., Borsting, C., Hallenberg, C., Buchard, A., Hernandez, A., and Morling, N. (2003) Multiplex PCR and minisequencing of SNPs—a model with 35 Y chromosome SNPs. *Forensic Sci. Int.* **137,** 74–84.
5. Morley, J.M., Bark, J.E., Evans, C.E., Perry, J.G., Hewitt, C.A., and Tully, G. (1999) Validation of mitochondrial DNA minisequencing for forensic casework. *Int. J. Legal Med.* **112,** 241–248.
6. Steen, V. M., Andreassen, O. A., Daly, A. K., Tefre, T., Borresen, A.-L., Idle, J. R., and Gulbrandsen, A.-K. (1995) Detection of the poor metabolizer-associated CYP2D6(D) gene deletion allele by long-PCR technology. *Pharmacogentetics* **5,** 215–223.
7. Lundqvist, E., Johansson, I., and Ingelman-Sundberg, M. (1999) Genetic mechanisms for duplication and multiduplication of the human CYP2D6 gene and methods for detection of duplicated CYP2D6 genes. *Gene* **226,** 327–338.
8. Goldstein, J. A., and Blaisdell, J. (1996) Genetic tests which identify the principal defects in CYP2C19 responsible for the polymorphism in mephenytoin metabolism. *Methods Enzymol.* **272,** 210–218.
9. Xiao, Z. S., Goldstein, J. A., Xie, H. G., Blaisdell, J., Wang, W., Jiang, C. H., et al. (1997) Differences in the incidence of the CYP2C19 polymorphism affecting the S-mephenytoin phenotype in Chinese Han and Bai populations and identification of a new rare CYP2C19 mutant allele. *J. Pharmacol. Exp. Ther.* **281,** 604–609.
10. Ferguson, R. J., De Morais, S. M., Benhamou, S., Bouchardy, C., Blaisdell, J., Ibeanu, G., et al. . (1998) A new genetic defect in human CYP2C19 mutation of the initiation codon is responsible for poor metabolism of S-mephenytoin. *JPET* **284,** 356–361.

18

Methods for the Study of Ancient DNA

Christine Keyser-Tracqui and Bertrand Ludes

Summary

Whereas the analysis of ancient DNA (aDNA) has become an increasingly popular mode of investigation in both archaeological and evolutionary studies, this approach is complicated by the degraded nature of ancient nucleic acids, the presence of enzymatic inhibitors in aDNA extracts, as well as the risk of contamination during either excavation or manipulation of samples. Despite these difficulties, numerous methods have been developed to optimize the recovery, study, and authentication of aDNA. In this article, we describe the procedures used in our laboratory to extract and amplify informative DNA segments from prehistoric or protohistoric human samples, as well as the precautions and strategies implemented to avoid or at least detect contaminations.

Key Words: Ancient DNA; bone; inhibition; contamination; DNA markers.

1. Introduction

The interest in ancient deoxyribonucleic acid (aDNA) has grown considerably since it was first demonstrated that at least some molecules of aDNA have survived until today *(1,2)*. From these molecules, biologists and anthropologists have attempted to understand issues such as the social organization of past human populations, their cultural and funeral customs, their evolutionary histories, their migrations and interactions with other populations, and even their diseases *(3–6)*.

The analysis of aDNA sequences became possible with the invention of the polymerase chain reaction (PCR; ref. *7*). However, aDNA molecules tend to be damaged, which prohibits the application of usual procedures of nucleic acid analysis. Two types of damage are mainly likely to affect DNA over time: hydrolytic and oxidative damage. Hydrolytic damage results in deamination of bases and in depurination and depyrimidination, whereas oxidative damage

From: *Methods in Molecular Biology, vol. 297: Forensic DNA Typing Protocols*
Edited by: A. Carracedo © Humana Press Inc., Totowa, NJ

results in modified bases *(8)*. Both mechanisms reduce the number as well as the size of the fragments that can be amplified by PCR: the amount of DNA available for genetic typing is thus often in the picogram range, and the size of the amplified DNA fragment is rarely longer than 300–400 base pairs. The conditions under which the ancient specimens have been preserved may be of decisive importance. Low temperatures during the burial period as well as environmental stability, rather than simply presence or absence of water, increase the chance of DNA survival by slowing its breakdown by hydrolysis and oxidation.

Failure to amplify DNA may also result from the presence of inhibitors that interfere with the PCR. Archaeological samples may indeed contain low-molecular-weight compounds, supposedly derived from the burial environment, which coextract with the DNA molecules and potently inhibit the activity of the DNA polymerase. Among these inhibitors are Maillard products, byproducts of sugar reduction in which DNA may be entrapped *(9)*, and collagen type I *(10)*. Contamination of ancient specimens and molecular extracts by modern DNA represents another major limitation to ancient DNA analysis because, as a result of its higher concentration and quality, contemporary DNA amplification is favored over that of the endogenous DNA in the sample *(11)*. This is particularly the case when human remains are studied because human DNA is the most common source of contamination. Therefore, a number of criteria need to be fulfilled before an aDNA sequence determined from extracts of an ancient specimen can be taken to be genuine *(11,12)*.

Because many techniques developed for use with modern samples do not work equally well with ancient material, we describe here the experimental protocols and strategies developed in our laboratory to study the genetic relationships between human individual and/or populations from the past as well as the stringent criteria applied to ensure the reliability of the results obtained.

2. Materials

2.1. Biological Samples

The main source of DNA used in our laboratory for ancient investigations is bone. Bones are much more abundant than soft tissue remains and are generally better preserved. Moreover, it has been suggested that the adsorption of the DNA to an inorganic component of the bone called hydroxyapatite makes the DNA more stable *(8)*.

Teeth are also sometimes used owing to the relatively impervious outer enamel layer, which protects DNA from degradation and contamination. We usually apply either one of two methods to extract DNA from teeth. The first is simply powdering the tooth. The second requires sectioning the tooth before

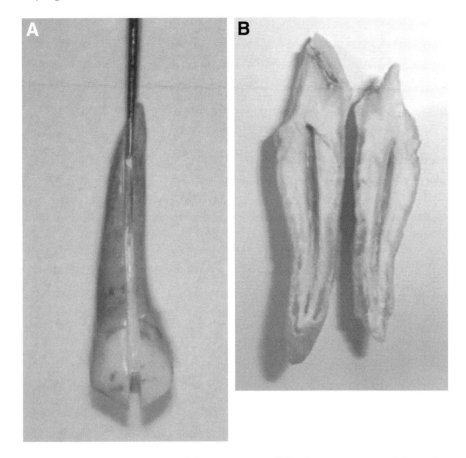

Fig. 1. The tooth is sectioned (**A**) then opened (**B**) prior to removal of the pulp.

removing the pulp (**Fig. 1**). The latter method is less destructive because the tooth can be glued back after pulp removal.

2.2. DNA Analyses

Compared with the standard apparatus of a molecular biology laboratory, we advocate additional equipment:

1. Germicidal ultraviolet (UV) sterilizing lamps + tubes (254 nm) positioned above every door of the laboratory.
2. High-speed grinding machine + accessories (collets, drill bit; Dremel®).
3. Cryogenic grinder (6800 Freezer/Mill, Spex CertiPrep).
4. Drill press (Practyl PC13-35).
5. Disposal perforator (Codman®).

2.3. Other Materials Required

1. Cleanmix kit (Talent).
2. Microconcentrators Microcon® YM-30 (Amicon).
3. DNA Away™ (Molecular BioProducts) or DNAZap™ (Ambion).
4. Aerosol-Resistant Tips (Molecular BioProducts).
5. Bovine serum albumin (BSA; Sigma).
6. AmpliTaqGold DNA polymerase (Applied Biosystems).

3. Methods

The sample preparation procedure described below only concern bone samples, these being preferably chosen as DNA sources in our studies. The DNA extraction procedure described optimizes the recovery of DNA and minimizes the impact of PCR inhibitors.

3.1. Bone Sample Preparation

3.1.1. Bone Sample Selection

The limiting factor for any aDNA study is the quality of the biological material tested (if the sample selected contains no amplifiable aDNA, then even the most efficient extraction procedure will not be successful). Careful sample choice is therefore prerequisite. There is no methodology for the rapid identification of bones from which DNA may be successfully extracted. Nevertheless, we have observed a correlation between macroscopic preservation of bone samples and DNA recovery. Our practice is thus to preferably choose heavy (dense) bone rather than more brittle bone, which has lost lipid and collagen and has therefore increased in porosity. Long bones (such as femur, tibia, and humerus) are preferred over rib or other thin bones. Moreover, compact (cortical) bone is preferred to spongy bone.

3.1.2. Bone Sample Cleaning

The preparation of most bone samples (which should take place in a room physically separated from downstream work areas) begins with cleaning. To get rid of modern DNA contamination, the surface of each bone sample is removed as follows:

1. Use a sterile scalpel blade to shave the surface of the bone sample and remove dirt, soil, and any other foreign material.
2. Prepare the high-speed grinding machine (Dremel®) and the drill bit (the whole unit previously UV irradiated) in the aspiration hood and abrade the surface of the bone sample 2 to 3 mL deep. The release of bone dust outside the hood is necessary to prevent DNA cross-contamination between ancient samples.
3. Wrap carefully the cleaned bone sample or fragment in a sterile paper.

3.1.3. Bone Sample Pulverization

Cleaned bone sample can be powdered in two ways:

1. To pulverize fragmentary pieces (such as skeletal elements from juvenile specimens or sections of bone diaphyses), we use a cryogenic grinder (Freezer mill) that preserves the chemical and structural features which would otherwise be degraded by the heat generated by milling. The bone sample, contained in a grinding vial, is immersed in liquid nitrogen, and then pulverized by the hammering of a magnetically driven impactor against the end plugs of the vial. Typical grinding time is 1 min with several rounds. Between each sample, the grinding vial is carefully cleaned by washing, application of DNA away™/or DNAZap™ and, finally, UV irradiation (*see* **Note 1**).
2. When long cortical bones are available, we preferably use a drill press. The long bone, wrapped in the sterile paper, is placed on the table of the column and kept in position with hold down clamps. The column supports a head containing a motor that turns a spindle at a controlled speed. The spindle holds a surgical drill bit that generates bone chips while avoiding overheating, a procedure that we believe is fundamental for correct DNA recovery (**Fig. 2**). The advantage of this method is that the bone morphology is not profoundly altered.

3.1.4. Bone Sample Decalcification

Once the bone powder is obtained, we generally operate as follows (all the steps are now carried out under a laminar flow hood):

1. Pour the powdered bone (2 g) into a sterile 50-mL tube.
2. Add 5 mL of an extraction buffer containing 5 mM ethylene diamine tetraacetic acid, 2% sodium dodecyl sulfate, 10 mM Tris-HCl (pH 8.0), 0.3 M sodium acetate, as well as 1 mg proteinase-K/mL (to solubilize DNA; *see* **Note 2**).
3. Vortex, seal the tube cap and incubate tube overnight at 50°C with continuous vertical rotation.

3.2. DNA Extraction and Purification

Whereas the organic extraction of proteins with phenol and/or chloroform/isoamyl alcohol is sometimes considered as unnecessary *(13,14)*, it constitutes an important step of our DNA recovery method.

3.2.1. Extraction of Nucleic Acids

1. The next morning, remove the sample from the incubator and add phenol/chloroform/isoamyl alcohol (25/24/1, v/v) to separate DNA from cellular debris.
2. Spin the sample tube at 1000g for 15 min.
3. Carefully remove the top aqueous layer with a P5000 pipet and transfer to a fresh 50-mL tube (the organic layer will be very dark and possibly contain an opaque precipitate constituted of fatty acids near the interface). Because the

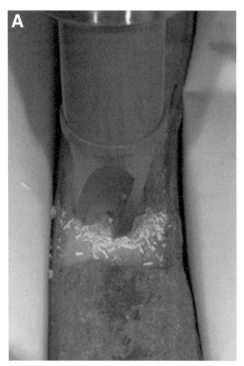

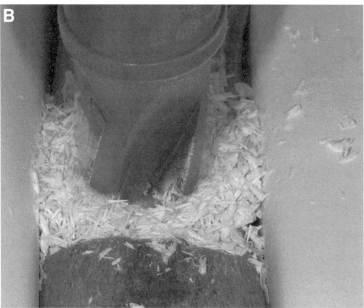

Fig. 2. The surgical drill bit (**A**) generates bone chips (**B**).

aqueous phase is a large volume, do not be concerned with recovering every microliter of this layer. A 1-mL pipet can be helpful to take the remainder of this phase, but avoid disrupting and drawing in the interface and the fatty layer below it.

3.2.2. Purification of Nucleic Acids

After extraction, the aqueous phase is purified with a commercially available CleanMix purification kit. This kit is based on a high capacity silica matrix that binds quickly to DNA and purifies it from some of its contaminants in the presence of the chaotropic agent guanidium thiocyanate. CleanMix spin columns are notably designated to trap PCR products that are larger than 100 pb and smaller than 10 kb. They are thus ideally suited for ancient DNA samples because these samples are generally degraded and the target regions for amplification generally quite small.

1. Add 2.5 mL of the Cleanmix-binding solution and 250 µL of the Cleanmix-high capacity purification resin to the extracted ancient DNA solution (*see* **Note 3**).
2. Put one Cleanmix filter into a 2-mL centrifuge tube. Transfer 500 µL of the mixture into the filter and spin for 30 s at 6000 rpm (until the column is empty). Discard the filtrate and repeat the process until all of the extracted solution has passed through the column.
3. Once the total volume of the sample has been placed into the column and spun through, wash the DNA by adding 500 µL of Cleanmix washing solution and centrifuging for 30 s. Repeat this step once.
4. Transfer the filter to a clean microcentrifuge tube. To elute DNA, add to the filter 400 µL of sterile water preheated at 65–70°C. Allow the DNA to resuspend for 2 min.
5. Spin the filter in the microcentrifuge tube for 2 min at 6000 rpm.

3.2.3. Concentration of Nucleic Acids

After the elution step, the diluted DNA is concentrated by passing through a Microcon YM30 filter containing an anisotropic membrane that retains macrosolutes (including DNA) while allowing low-molecular-weight solutes to pass through.

1. Transfer the eluted 400 µL into the sample reservoir without touching the membrane with the pipet tip.
2. Spin for 9 min at 7000*g* (the remaining volume on the membrane should approximate 30 µL).
3. Remove assembly from centrifuge; separate vial from sample reservoir.
4. Place sample reservoir upside down in a new vial, then spin 4 min at 1500*g* to transfer concentrate to vial.
5. Remove from centrifuge and separate sample reservoir.
6. Store the purified DNA sample at 4°C while in use and then place it at 20°C for long-term storage (successive freeze–thaw cycles can damage the DNA templates over time).

3.3. DNA Amplification

The DNA recovered using the procedure described above is then amplified using PCR. To enhance the efficiency of the PCR amplifications, we selected several strategies.

3.3.1. Addition of BSA in the PCR Mix

Amplification efficiency (yield of product) and specificity (absence of non-specific products) can be improved by the addition of an enhancer to the PCR. We usually use BSA, which has the ability to bind to enzyme inhibitors present in aDNA preparations. Our reaction mix is thus generally prepared as follows:

GeneAmp 10X PCR buffer	500 µL
25 mM MgCl$_2$ solution	300 µL
dATP (100 mM)	10 µL
dCTP (100 mM)	10 µL
dGTP (100 mM)	10 µL
dTTP (100 mM)	10 µL
BSA (20 mg/mL)	50 µL
Water	110 µL
Total	1000 µL

3.3.2. Hot Starting PCR

To increase the yield from PCR, it also is possible to use a hot-start procedure. Hot starting a PCR prevents the creation of primer oligomers and reduces the rate of mispriming during the initial heating up to the denaturation temperature. Although annealing is not a problem for routine PCR applications, room temperature extension is a major problem affecting the specificity of the amplification reaction when the PCR target is less than 100–500 copies.

Hot-start PCR is a simple modification of the original PCR process, whereby the enzyme is kept inactive until the PCR temperature is above normal primer annealing temperature. The yield of specific product increases because reactants are not wasted in the formation of unintended products. To hot start a PCR, we generally use a chemically modified form of Taq DNA polymerase called AmpliTaqGold, which is commercially available from Applied Biosystems. This enzyme is activated for PCR by heating at 95°C for 10 min.

3.3.3. Increasing the Number of Amplification Cycles

Another way to increase the sensitivity of the PCR is to raise the number of amplification cycles. This is routinely used by anthropologists and forensic scientists to analyze ancient DNA from bones *(15,16)*. We used, for example,

37 cycles instead of 28 to analyze short tandem repeats (STRs) from 2000- to 2400-yr-old skeletons *(6)*.

3.3.4. Stringent PCR

Amplification yield may also be increased by starting a PCR using stringent (high) annealing temperatures during the first three cycles, and then reducing the annealing temperature for the remaining cycles of the amplification. Although this results in low primer binding during the early cycles, mispriming is minimized, increasing the proportion of high-quality target sequences in each successive cycle. We used this approach to amplify DNA from ancient Central Asian horse specimens (article in preparation).

3.4. DNA Markers Selection and Analysis

DNA from archaeological specimens is usually of low average molecular size and low copy number because of various forms of damage (see **Subheading 1.**). For these reasons, primers that amplify short sequences are recommended. The short size of the STR markers (100–400 pb) makes them suitable for the investigation of degraded DNA. Moreover, these markers can be simultaneously amplified (notably with commercially available kits), reducing to an absolute minimum the amount of sample material necessary for kinship analysis. We generally use autosomal STR markers (*AmpFl*STR Profiler Plus kit, Applied Biosystems) to study close biological relationships (*see* **Notes 4** and **5**) and Y-chromosome STR markers (Y-Plex 6 kit, Reliagene or PowerPlex® Y system, Promega) to identify male lineages *(6)*. The maternal genetic inheritance is tested through sequencing of the hypervariable region (HVR-I) of the mitochondrial control region (D-loop). Mitochondrial DNA is especially useful because it is present at a high copy number in cells and is more likely to survive for prolonged periods compared with nuclear DNA. All these markers were also selected because of their ability to discriminate between aDNA and probable DNA contaminants (*see* **Subheading 3.5.6.**).

We also amplify the amelogenin locus (included in the human identification kits from Applied Biosystems or Promega). Amplification of this region leads to a single amplification product of 106 base pair (bp) for females and to two amplification products of 106 and 112 bp for males. This short marker is relatively easy to analyze, and it could represent a criteria of authenticity (morphological and genetic sex typing methods in accordance with each other).

Analysis of the amplification products will not be detailed here because it does not differ from classical genotyping or sequencing. Both can be performed in the laboratory alongside modern work because contamination is no longer a problem at this stage.

3.5. Contamination Precautions and Check for Contaminants

To minimize the chances of contamination and to identify contamination if it occurs, we use the following procedures:

1. All aDNA extractions and PCR set-ups should be conducted in a dedicated laboratory that undergoes regular decontamination. Modern DNA or PCR products are not introduced to this dedicated environment. We attempt to apply the "one-way traffic" rule: once you have entered a laboratory where modern DNA or PCR products are present, you cannot in principle return to the aDNA lab until the next day. This prevents contamination by aerosol particles. The laminar flow hoods as well as the top of the doors of each room are equipped with shortwave (254 nm) UV source. These UV sources are left switched on when nobody is working. All appliances, containers, pipets, racks, laboratory coats, and work areas (laminar airflow surfaces, PCR box) are cleaned and irradiated with UV light during this time. The extraction buffer (without proteinase K) and deionized distilled water also are irradiated by placing the tubes directly on the light source.

2. Personnel always wear laboratory coats and face masks and change gloves regularly. All general equipment (e.g., centrifuges) is dedicated to pre-PCR work (there is no shared equipment) and apparatus, pipets, or protective clothing from a post-PCR laboratory are never taken into the clean-room facility. All solutions, PCR reagents, and primers are kept in small carefully labeled aliquots dedicated solely for work with one ancient DNA collection. Pre- and post-PCR activities are spatially separated in the laboratory or performed in different laboratories.

3. Two parallel control reactions are used: an extraction control (blank) to check the purity of the extraction reagents with no bone added, and an amplification control to check the purity of the PCR reagents with no DNA added. The presence of amplified target in any of these negative control samples is evidence of contamination. Positive controls, comprising modern DNA, are not used to monitor the success of aDNA PCRs (but *see* **Note 5**).

4. Multiple DNA extractions (from a different skeletal element of the same individual when possible) and PCR amplifications are conducted at least several weeks or months apart. Only fully reproducible results are considered as authentic (*see* **Note 5**). aDNA sequences are characterized with respect to the lengths of the amplification products they lead to. In general, shorter fragments are easier to amplify, and the sequence obtained from these fragments contains fewer ambiguities.

5. All results are compared against a staff database: indeed, all archaeologists, anthropologists, and other workers who handle the skeletal material during excavation plus all personnel laboratory (including trainees and visitors) are typed for the various genetic loci examined by our group.

6. We use multiallelic markers (such as STRs), which allow the detection of contamination (*17*) as well as a multimarker approach: data obtained with biparentally, paternally, and maternally inherited markers should be consistent to be considered as genuine. Moreover, because we work in close collaboration with anthropologists, we often know the morphological sex of the sample studied,

which allows for comparison with the molecular sex obtained. Finally, genetic data from the ancient sample and likely descendant populations should be consistent and the mitochondrial sequences obtained should be those that can be reasonably expected considering the origin of people (e.g., Central Asia).

4. Notes

1. DNA away™ and DNAZap™ provide a convenient method to decontaminate a variety of surfaces in a matter of minutes. All nucleic acid is degraded to nucleotides, preventing any chance of false-positive amplification.
2. Ethylenediamine tetraacetic acid chelates calcium in the bone material and hence allows for its removal.
3. The binding solution that contains the chaotropic agent guanidium thiocyanate promotes the DNA association to the purification resin. For effective binding of DNA, the ratio of binding solution/sample should be 2:1 or higher, especially in the case of short fragments.
4. PCRs were performed according to the manufacturer's protocol (User's Manual, PE Applied Biosystems) except that 37 cycles were used instead of 28 in a reaction volume of 10 μL, reducing the volume of the DNA samples and improving the amplification yield.
5. Ideally, replicates should be analyzed by different laboratories. However, this procedure is usually time consuming, impractical, and difficult to arrange when many samples are studied. Therefore in our opinion, as long as replicate samples are extracted and analyzed according to stringent procedures, this type of reproducibility should not be insisted upon. This procedure is particularly relevant if the sample material is of limited quantity, unique, or extremely valuable.

References

1. Higuchi, R., Bowman, B., Freiberger, M., Ryder, O. A., and Wilson, A. C. (1984) DNA sequences from the quagga an extinct member of the horse family. *Nature* **312,** 282–284.
2. Pääbo, S. (1985) Molecular cloning of Ancient Egyptian mummy DNA. *Nature* **314,** 644–645.
3. Stone, A. C., and Stoneking, M. (1998) mtDNA analysis of a prehistoric Oneta population: implications for the peopling of the New World. *Am. J. Hum. Genet.* **62,** 1153–1170.
4. Raoult, D., Aboudharam, G, Crubézy, E., Larrouy, G., Ludes, B., and Drancourt, M. (2000) Molecular identification by "suicide PCR" of *Yersinia pestis* as the agent of Medieval Black Death. *Proc. Natl. Acad. Sci. USA* **97,** 12800–12803.
5. Clisson, I., Keyser, C., Francfort, H.-P., Crubézy, E., Samashev, K., and Ludes B. (2002) Genetic analysis of human remains from a frozen kurgan in Kazakhstan (Berel site, 200–300 B.C.). *Int. J. Legal Med.* **116,** 304–308.
6. Keyser-Tracqui, C., Crubézy, E., and Ludes B. (2003) Nuclear and mitochondrial DNA analysis a 2,000-year-old necropolis in the Egyin Gol valley of Mongolia. *Am. J. Hum. Genet.* **73,** 247–260.

7. Mullis, K. B., and Faloona, F. A. (1987) Specific synthesis of DNA in vitro via a polymerase-catalysed chain reaction. *Methods Enzymol.* **155,** 335–350.
8. Lindahl, T. (1993) Instability and decay of the primary structure of DNA. *Nature* **362,** 709–715.
9. Pääbo, S. (1989) Ancient DNA: extraction, characterization, molecular cloning, and enzymatic amplification. *Proc. Natl. Acad. Sci. USA* **86,** 1939–1943.
10. Scholtz, M., Giddings, I., and Pusch, C.M. (1998) A polymerase chain reaction inhibitor of ancient hard and soft tissue DNA extracts is determined as human collagen type I. *Anal. Biochem.* **92,** 463–471.
11. Handt, O., Höss, M., Krings M., and Pääbo S. (1994) Ancient DNA: methodological challenges. *Experientia* **50,** 521–619.
12. Cooper, A., and Poinar, H. N. (2000) Ancient DNA: do it right or not at all. *Science* **289,** 1139.
13. Yang, D. G., Eng, B., Waye, J. S., Dudar, J. C., and Saunders, S. R. (1998) Technical note: improved DNA extraction from ancient bones using silica-based spin columns. *Am. J. Phys. Anthropol.* **105,** 539–543.
14. Kolman, C. J. and Tuross, N. (2000) Ancient DNA analysis of human populations. *Am. J. Phys. Anthropol.* **111,** 5–23.
15. Gill, P., Ivanov, P. L., Kimpton, C., Piercy, R., Benson, N., and Tully, G. (1994) Identification of the remains of the Romanov family by DNA analysis. *Nat. Genet.* **6,** 130–135.
16. Schmerer, W. M., Hummel, S., and Herrmann, B. (1999) Optimized DNA extraction to improve reproducibility of short tandem repeat genotyping with highly degraded DNA as target. *Electrophoresis* **20,** 1712–1716.
17. Hummel, S., Bramanti, B., Schultes, T., Kahle, M., Haffner, S., and Herrmann, B. (2000) Megaplex DNA typing can provide a strong indication of the authenticity of ancient DNA amplifications by clearly recognizing any possible type of modern contamination. *Anthrop. Anz* **58,** 15–21.

19

Protocols for Ancient DNA Typing

Cristian Capelli and Frank Tschentscher

Summary

Molecular analysis of fossil and archaeological remains has been established as a powerful tool in providing new insight in phylogenetic investigations. The overlapping set of molecular modifications and degradation that forensic samples share with archaeological specimen suggests the application of similar technical approaches to the respective biological material. Polymerase chain reaction is the molecular technique of choice for the retrieval of specimen deoxyribonucleic acid (DNA) molecules. Because of intrinsic sensitivity, potential contaminations from exogenous DNA sources must be monitored through the entire process by the introduction of multiple blank controls. Cloning and sequencing of polymerase chain reaction products often is the only way to discriminate between contaminations and endogenous sequences as well as to identify variable positions from nucleotide modifications/DNA polymerase errors. Phylogenetic analysis and investigations of the pattern of substitutions are an additional and necessary step to validate the retrieved sequence. Comparison with available related samples (modern or extinct) is critical to correctly validate the results and to avoid artifactual data.

Key Words: Ancient DNA, cloning of PCR products, phylogenetic analysis, degradation, contamination, molecular archaeology.

1. Introduction

The investigation of evolutionary relationships among contemporary and extinct species for a long time has been conducted using classical morphological and functional comparisons. Both are still valuable and important methods, and it is somewhat regrettable that there are fewer scientists involved in these "classical" methods. However, the development of molecular techniques has provided new tools for species comparisons that is now bringing new and unexpected results (1). The pattern of difficulties faced by molecular analysis of fossil remains is similar to the one routinely encountered in genetic analysis of forensic specimens (2,3). The invention of polymerase chain reaction

From: *Methods in Molecular Biology, vol. 297: Forensic DNA Typing Protocols*
Edited by: A. Carracedo © Humana Press Inc., Totowa, NJ

(PCR) was the technical breakthrough in both application fields. This made feasible the retrieval of a minute amount of genetic material, but at the same time it raised issues regarding authenticity of results *(4,5)*. DNA modifications and contamination are the main issues in result validation *(6,7)*. Despite these limits, the scientific community has testified a large interest in archaeological molecular analysis, and this has contributed to the creation of a brand new discipline, "molecular archaeology" *(8–13)*.

PCR allows the retrieval of deoxyribonucleic (DNA) sequences of ancient and minute, often degraded remains (it was by the way the method that revolutionized the forensic analysis of biological stains; ref. *14*), but its critical sensitivity to low-amount DNA target also is a weak point, making the relevant analyses very prone to molecular contamination. Because of this, one should always seek to avoid contaminations and carefully spot its sources of it during the amplification procedure. Throughout the entire PCR procedure, negative controls must be introduced. The careful control of any possible labware used in the process also is mandatory to prevent cross contamination across various sections of the same laboratory. Disposable plastics, coats, and breathing masks are necessary. An ad hoc workspace with routine ultraviolet (UV) irradiation is necessary to avoid risks of contamination *(4,5)*, to a point that many laboratories involved in daily ancient DNA (aDNA) analysis are being quickly relocated into rooms with positive pressure.

The protocol we describe should be reproduced in compliance with as many of these precautions as possible. This protocol has been adopted, with minor variants, in a number of aDNA studies *(15–20)*. We start by a classical phenol–chloroform extraction followed by a silica purification step *(21,22)*. The organic extraction removes most of the protein molecules present in the sample. Often, especially in the case of bone extraction, several PCR inhibitors might be present as molecular constituents of the samples to test. The silica step is essential to bind the DNA and to get rid of inhibitors that tend to remain in the aqueous phase. The PCR folliws a hot-start approach to avoid mispriming and primer-dimers during the initial denaturing ramping phase.

2. Materials

1. 10% Sodium hypochlorite ("bleach").
2. Double-distilled (dd) water (in alternative autoclaved water exposed to UV light and filtered with centricon 30 can be used).
3. 0.5 M ethylene-diamine tetraacetic acid (EDTA), pH 8.0.
4. 5% Sarkosyl.
5. Proteinase K 10 µg/µL.
6. Phenol.
7. Chloroform:Isoamylalcohol 24:1.

  8. Amicon Centricon 30 centrifugal filter devices (Millipore, Billerica, MA).
  9. Silica (Sigma).
 10. HCl.
 11. 5 *M* guanidiniumisothiocyanate.
 12. 0.1 *M* Tris-HCl, pH 7.4.
 13. Ethanol 70%.
 14. Acetone.
 15. TE, pH 8.0.
 16. dNTPs.
 17. PCR buffer (supplied with the enzyme).
 18. *Taq* polymerase.
 19. Agarose reagents and equipment for electrophoresis.
 20. Primers of choice ,10 μ*M* each.
 21. *Sma*I (e.g. New England Biolabs).
 22. *Sma*I-specific buffer (New England Biolabs).
 23. T4 DNA polymerase (e.g. New England Biolabs).
 24. 10X T4 DNA polymerase buffer (New England Biolabs).
 25. 3 *M* Na-Acetate, pH 5.2.
 26. Glycogen 1 mg/mL.
 27. Ethanol 100%.
 28. *Sma*I-cut pUC18 vector, 25 ng/μL, (Pharmacia).
 29. T4 DNA ligase (New England Biolabs).
 30. ATP 500 μ*M*.
 31. Transformation and cell growth reagents.
 32. Sequencing reagents.

3. Methods

Several kits are currently available, based on, inspired by, or just competing with to the protocols we describe here. For example, a number of commercially available kits for DNA extraction from archaeological remains have been introduced, and different cloning systems, combined with various sequencing protocols, have been proposed. Our protocols are meant to just exemplify a basic approach, not necessarily the only one.

Most protocols have been conceived and or implemented by Matthias Hoss, Oliva Handt, and Matthias Krings at the Evolutionary Laboratory, Zoological Institute, University of Munich, Germany. They have been published in several articles *(15–20)*, as such or with alterations.

3.1. Extraction

Most samples in aDNA studies are bone remains. Therefore, our protocol specifically addresses this evidentiary sample. It is, of course, possible to any time modify or readapt the protocol to suit other materials. For example, the initial digestion step could be modulated to extract from samples with different characteristics, and the silica protocol could be easily introduced at some stage to remove inhibitors.

3.1.1. Sample Preparation

1. Compact, long bone is often better preserved. Cut out a bone section by a sterile saw blade, then rinse it with dd water, repeatedly.
2. Remove the surface of the bone by a scalpel or drill the bone and take the powder material from the inner part. It might be advisable to wash the surface of the piece with 10% sodium hypochlorite for 10 s, or less, and extensively rinse it with dd water. All of this is done to remove possible contaminants (from previous handling) from the sample surface.
3. Grind the bone fragment into fine powder. This is usually the most difficult part of this initial step. Commercially available freeze mills are the best option but are quite expensive. Any mechanical grinding is in principle an equally good option.
4. Weigh the ground bone and transfer 0.4 g to a 2-mL tube. Add 1 mL of 0.5 M EDTA, pH 8.0, 5% sarkosyl. Seal with plastic film and mount on a rotary wheel at room temperature (RT) for 48 h, or longer if need. You might want to refill with fresh EDTA after 2 d incubation. In that case, pellet by centrifugation, dispose of the saturated solution, and replace with fresh EDTA (1 mL).
5. After the EDTA treatment, add 10 µL of proteinase K (10 µg/µL) and incubate for another 48 h. More proteinase can be added if required and the incubation time prolonged accordingly.
6. Sample material is then pelleted by centrifugation for 1 min at maximum speed. We suggest keeping the pellet material for eventual subsequent re-extraction.

3.1.2. Organic Extraction

Extract the supernatant with a classical phenol:chlorophorm approach as follows:

1. Add 1 mL of phenol, equilibrated at pH 8.0, vortex, and then centrifuge 3 min at maximum speed. Transfer the aqueous phase to a clean tube—keep in mind that phase reversal caused by high salt concentration in the EDTA solution might occur so the phenol could built the upper layer.
2. Add 1 mL of phenol:chloroform/isoamylalcohol (24:1), vortex, and centrifuge. Move the upper aqueous phase to a clean tube. Note that the phenol and the chloroform:isoamylalcohol (24:1) are in a 1:1 ratio. Prepare and store at 4°C.
3. Add 1 mL of chloroform:isoamylalcohol (24:1), vortex, and centrifuge.
4. Move aqueous phase to a clean tube for the subsequent centricon 30 concentration step, following the supplier's recommendations for centrifugal speed. Wet the membrane for 15 min with 50 µL of dd water, add the aqueous phase from chloroform/isoamylalcohol step to the filter, and spin at recommended rpm.

(Note: the filter is sensitive to chlorophorm, so be careful not to carry it over from the previous steps. Avoid filter dehydration by overcentrifugation. After all the supernatant has been passed through the filter, wash twice with a corresponding volume of dd water.)

Finally, invert the filter to recover the DNA solution by a short centrifugation (2 min). Transfer the DNA solution to a 1.5-mL tube. The recovered volume should be approx 100 µL.

3.1.3. Silica Purification

Because inhibitors of PCR are often present, it is advised to purify the sample. We used a Silica purification process as described previously *(22)*.

3.1.3.1. PREPARATION OF REAGENTS FOR SILICA EXTRACTION

3.1.3.1.1. Silica

1. Dilute 4.8 g of SiO_2 (Sigma) in 40 mL of dd water (total volume) using a 50-mL tube, vortex, and sediment by leaving it on the lab bench for 24 h at RT.
2. Remove 35 mL of the supernatant and fill up to 40 mL with dd water. Resuspend silica pellet by vortexing and sediment for additional 5 h at room temperature.
3. Remove 36 mL of the supernatant and add 48 µL of HCl (32%, weight/volume, pH 2.0). Aliquot 0.5 mL in different tubes. The silica is stable for at least 6 mo when stored at RT in the dark.

3.1.3.1.2. Buffer L2

1. Dissolve 24 g of guanidinium thiocyanate in 20 mL of 0.1 *M* Tris-HCl, pH 7.4, in a 50-mL tube. To facilitate dissolution the tube with the solution can be heated a bit, but do not boil it!
2. Add 1 mL of silica. This will bind all the eventual contaminant DNA.
3. Spin down and transfer the supernatant in 50-mL tubes in aliquots of approx 20 mL each. Buffer L2 is stable at least 3 wk at RT in the dark.

3.1.3.2. SILICA PURIFICATION

1. Add 40 µL of the silica solution plus 1 mL of L2 buffer to the organically extracted solution. Vortex briefly and rotate for at least 15 min (as long as 1 h is feasible).
2. Centrifuge to pellet the silica.
3. Wash twice with 1 mL of ethanol 70% and once with acetone. In all steps, vortex, centrifuge to pellet again and remove the liquid. Avoid touching the pellet with the tip.
4. Dry for a short period at 56°C.
5. Elute the DNA twice, adding 65 µL of TE pH 8.0, per time by dissolving the pellet carefully with a pipette and incubating each time at 56°C for 15 min. Do not pipet up and down in the tip but dissolve by turning the tip gently in the silica. Pellet the silica by full speed centrifugation and collect the supernatant. The final

volume should range between 120 and 130 μL. Aliquot this in 3 different tubes, leaving the silica behind. Store extracts at –20°C. Usually 5 μL of the extract is used for subsequent PCR.

3.2. PCR Amplification

The use of a hot-start protocol is highly recommended *(23)*. Until a few years ago the only option was to mechanically separate the *Taq* polymerase enzyme from nucleotides, primers, and DNA by a wax layer that just melted as the initial denaturing step started *(24)*. Nowadays a number of genetically engineered enzymes or antibody-conjugated enzymes, active only at specific temperatures, are available. This makes PCR setup much easier and less prone to contaminations by reducing the necessary number of manipulations. We suggest using those enzymes as a valid alternative to previously described protocols.

The PCR can be set up in a final volume of 20 μL as follows:

10X PCR buffer	2 μL
Primer A, 10 pmolμL	0.5 μL
Primer B, 10 pmol/μL	0.5 μL
dNTPs, 25 m*M* each	0.1 μL
Taq polymerase, 5 UμL	0.2 μL
dd water	11.7 μL
DNA extract	5 μL

3.2.1. PCR Conditions

Forty cycles with 15 s 95°C/1 min primer-specific annealing temperature/ 1 min 72°C. Note that by using hot-start polymerases, an extended initial denaturing step has to be included.

If only faint bands are visible after agarose gel electrophoresis, one might consider reamplifying the PCR products. For this purpose, a modified freeze–squeeze protocol *(25)* can be applied to quickly recover the PCR products cut out of the agarose gel.

1. Cut out the desired product band with a razor blade and transfer it to a 1.5-mL microtube filled with 100 μL of dd water.
2. Melt it shortly on a heater (between 65 and 90°C) and snap freeze it in liquid nitrogen (alternatively, shock freeze using a dry ice/ethanol bath).
3. After thawing the solution, centrifuge it for 30 min with maximum rpm and use 0.5–5 μL for reamplification under the conditions described above but with only 25–30 cycles and increasing annealing temperature by 3°C.

3.3. Cloning of PCR products

We usually used the *Sma*I-cut pUC18 screening vector and performed blunt-end cloning of the PCR products. A preliminary requirement is not to have a

*Sma*I recognition site internal of your PCR product and to rule out a GGG, CGGG, or CCGGG at the 5' end of the amplification primers.

Despite our positive experiences with blunt-end cloning, it should be mentioned that another very efficient and easy method for PCR-product cloning is at hand nowadays. The so called "TA cloning method" takes advantage of the terminal transferase activity of *Taq* polymerase. The enzyme adds a single, 3'-A overhang to each end of the PCR product. This makes it possible to clone this PCR product directly into a linearized cloning vector with single, 3'-T overhangs. Note that DNA polymerases with proofreading activity, such as *Pfu* polymerase, cannot be used because they provide blunt-ended PCR products. TA cloning kits are available from different manufacturers.

To maximize your cloning rate, it is preferable to have a significant amount of PCR product. If not, a possibility is to try to reamplify the amplicon (refer to **Subheading 3.2.**).

The PCR should be optimized to avoid the amplification of unspecific bands. If this is the case, extract the band of interest from the agarose gel and reamplify it using the method described above.

3.3.1. T4 DNA Polymerase Reaction (Fill-In)

This reaction is necessary to fill-in eventual gaps left at the 3' end of the amplicon by *Taq* polymerase. Mix the following reagents in a 1.5-mL tube: 10 µL of PCR products (from the first amplification); 2 µL of 10X T4 DNA polymerase buffer (New England Biolabs); 1 µL of T4 DNA polymerase (3 units/µL) (New England Biolabs); and 7 µL of dd water. Leave the tube for 20 min at 12°C and then move it to 75°C for 10 min.

It is also possible to T4-treat the PCR band excised from an agarose gel (if the amount is enough):

Bring the purified band up in 10 µL of dd water (purification by, e.g., freeze–squeeze) and add 2 µL of 10X T4 DNA polymerase buffer (New England Biolabs); 1 µL of T4 DNA polymerase (3 units/µl) (New England Biolabs); 5 µL of dd water; and 2 µL of dNTPs (1 m*M* each). Leave the tube for 20 min at 12°C and then move it to 75°C for 10 min.

(Note: When using the PCR product directly from the PCR tube, nucleotides are in excess and are sufficient for the T4 treatment. Using the excised band, the addition of nucleotides is required.)

After the 75°C incubation, a precipitation step follows:

1. Bring the final volume to 100 µL, then add 10 µL of 3 *M* Na-acetate, pH 5.2; 2 µL glycogen (1 mg/mL); and 300 µL of ice-cold ethanol 100%.
2. Spin at 4°C at maximum speed for 40 min.
3. Wash pellet with 500 µL of 70% ethanol.

4. Discard the ethanol being careful to not dislodge the pellet and dry in a speed vac for 3 min.
5. Resuspend in 5 μL of dd water.

3.3.2. Ligation Reaction

The T4-treated, resuspended amplicons are then added to 1 μL of the pUC vector, 25 ng/μL, *Sma*I cut, not dephosphorilated; 1 μL of *Sma*I-specific buffer; 1 μL of *Sma*I, 10 units (New England Biolabs); 1 μL T4 DNA ligase (400 U/μL, New England Biolabs); and 1 μL of ATP (500 μ*M*). Leave at RT (16–25°C) overnight (approx 16 h). After incubation, precipitate and bring up in 20 μL dd water.

3.3.3. Transformation

After ligation and precipitation, competent cells require to be transformed with the ligated plasmid. We routinely used 40 μL of a suspension of readily competent *E. coli* SURE™ cells and transformed by electroporation:

1. To the 40 μL of *E. coli* suspension, add 10 μL of the ligation and transfer to a cooled cuvette for electroporation.
2. Electroporate at 1.6 to 1.8 kV, 200 Ohm, and 25 μFd.
3. Transfer the suspension to 1 mL of regular SOC medium for 20-25 minutes (at maximum to avoid sister clones). Gently shake at 37°C.
4. Plate 20–200 μL of the cell suspension on a selective medium afterward. In our experiments we used standard LB-agar plates with IPTG/X-gal (**26**). Incubate plates overnight at 37°C.

Note: Our regular transformation efficiency was around 4×10^8 transformants/μg circular plasmid; generally, we plated 50 μL of 1000 μL. The used plasmid contains the *E. coli* gene LacZ. The LacZ gene codes for the production of an enzyme called β-galactosidase. β-Galactosidase converts substrates such as X-Gal into a product of blue color. In order for the gene to be actively transcribed from the DNA and for the enzyme to be produced, the activator called IPTG is added.

Within the LacZ gene, there are multiple cloning sites (including the used *Sma*I site) where the plasmid may be cut and DNA may be added. Because of its location within the enzyme-coding sequence, the foreign DNA disrupts activity and function of the enzyme. The disrupted enzyme activity is observed as a white bacterial colony (if the enzyme is fully functioning meaning no insertion has taken place, each colony is of bright blue color). Very small inserts of foreign DNA may lead to light blue colonies.

3.3.4. Colony PCR Screening

The blue–white selection is a preliminary screening method to maximize the retrieval of cloned PCR products. The white colonies then have to be additionally screened by colony PCR to avoid sequencing of false-positive clones. Moreover, colony PCR generates a sufficient amount of the desired PCR product for sequencing. This protocol follows the one described *(27)*.

1. Per PCR add:

dd water	9.4 µL
BSA, 10 µg/µL	1.25 µL
10X *Taq* buffer	1.25 µL
Plasmid universal primers, 10 µ*M*	0.25 µL
	0.25 µL
dNTPs, 25 m*M* each	0.05 µL
Taq polymerase, 5 µ/µL	0.04 µL

2. Distribute the PCR master mix into reaction tubes.
3. Touch the selected colonies with a micropipet tip and pipet then, one by one, into the PCR tubes. To create a back-up plate, touch first an LB plate and then pipette in the PCR tube. PCR cycling should be performed as follows: an initial denaturation step of 90°C for 5 min then 30 cycles; 95°C for 30 s; (X°)C for 1 min (annealing temperature must be adjusted according to the used primers); 72°C for 1 min; and a final hold of 4°C until tubes are recovered from the PCR machine.
4. PCR products are loaded on a 2% agarose gel (3 µL of the 12.5 µL reaction volume). The colonies containing the insert should show a length equal to 144 base pair (bp) plus the insert length (if the pUC18 vector is used). Colonies of interest can be selected for the subsequent sequencing step.

3.4. Sequencing

Sequencing strategies are quickly evolving from four-lane-radioisotopes-X-ray films procedures to single-lane multifluorescent multichannel processing. Each laboratory has its own sequencing technology with optimized ad hoc protocols. We used 1.5 µL of the colony PCR to perform the sequencing reaction, without any prior purification step. In the case of a single lane multichannel detection system, a prior purification step removing unincorporated nucleotides and primers is necessary for subsequent sequencing steps. Critical information can be recovered by individual suppliers.

We also note that direct sequencing of the PCR product, avoiding a cloning step, is sometimes used in aDNA analysis. In principle, when dealing with animal remains, the probability of a contamination is very low so a direct sequencing approach can be a possibility. Additionally, polymerase-induced errors should be easily identified as overlapping peaks in the electropherograms. Sequencing of different amplification products should permit discrimination between those and endogenous variable positions.

3.5. Phylogenetic Analysis

When an ancient sequence is obtained, the phylogenetic plausibility of the finding should be checked. The crucial importance of this step is easily stressed by retelling the now classical example of the so-called dinosaur bone analysis *(8,9)*. The clamorous announcement was quickly called in doubt by the mere fact that the relevant sequence was clearly too closer to humans than to birds or reptiles as one would have expected. The whole case is a formidable caveat about the absolute need of result authentication. Consulting a database with contemporary species is part of the protocol when the consistency of the final consensus sequence to the original expectations is needed. At this stage, all apparent mutations should be retrieved in evolutionarily neighboring species. A large excess of unseen variants should be regarded as suspicious.

There is plenty of phylogenetic software to use for reconstructing relationships between "ancient" sequences and the rest of known sequences—some are available free of charge. Softaware programs differ one another with respect to the tree reconstructing method. PAUP (http://paup.csit.fsu.edu/index.html) (http://evolution.genetics.washington.edu/phylip/getme.html), Phylip, and tree-puzzle (http://www.tree-puzzle.del) are among the most used (see the attached web addresses for download information; ref. *28,29*).

4. Notes

aDNA is an extremely difficult field. Not only might it be painstaking to successfully establish a laboratory in the field, but ensuring authenticity of the results is every time challenging. Since the beginning, aDNA analysis has lived on a flimsy equilibrium between the "hall of fame" of sensational results (with the invariable footage of the daily press) and forceful retractions. In the past, sequences of extinct organisms (including lithified samples and amber entombed insects), millions of years old, have been described *(10,30)*, and they have triggered the hunt to older and even more spectacular preys. Some of these publications are clearly unlikely, but they were never retracted and the results are occasionally found in citation lists and textbooks *(9,11,31)*. Some of these results (the claims of DNA retrieval out of amber-entombed insects or bones of a dinosaur) have invariably ended up to inspire the media and the movie industry.

Another example for illusions inspired by aDNA reports are the claims of cloning a mammoth, which cannot work neither technically nor theoretically but of course raised dreams and hope by a broad spectrum of people *(32,33)*. Today we know that there is a theoretical upper limit for DNA preservation *(34)*, even if our methods are more sophisticated than earlier.

The recent dispute over DNA sequences obtained from 24,000-yr-old modern human (Cro-Magnon) has also suggested that the problem of authenticity is always open even if a research group acts in full conformity with the proposed criteria of authentication *(4,5,35–37)*.

How can one come to terms with the whole issue is hard to say. A newcomer in the field has better start working with animal samples before talking humans. The example of aDNA research on mammoth shows that there are many very well preserved specimen available, even proven to contain nuclear DNA *(38)*. These samples are less prone to contamination than human samples. The following rules should be adopted anyway.

1. In general it is decisive to control for possible contaminations throughout all steps of aDNA analysis, from extraction to PCR amplification. Several controls have to be added at each step. A blank control for the extraction has to be performed each time using the same extraction materials without adding samples. This control has to pass over all the extraction steps and must be included in subsequent amplification reactions. Additionally, two PCR controls, with no DNA added but containing the same reagents, have to be included to monitor eventual contaminants present in the reagents or occurring during amplification set-up. Similarly, if a reamplification is performed, a reamplification PCR control must be included.

2. Another laboratory's assistance should be always sought in the authentication process, if only to ensure that the whole sequence production process has been started afresh, with no contamination risks from the same source.

3. The samples we deal with are precious and unique and should therefore be treated with respect. There should always be a reason to believe that DNA might have survived in the material. Whether the often proposed determination of amino acid racemization by high-performance liquid chromatography is the method of choice is not clear *(39)*. The advantage of this method is that only minute amounts of the sample is needed; however, it is not proven that the racemization of certain amino acids directly permits predictions about DNA survival. Other hints to amplifiable DNA in a specimen could be the surrounding conditions at the place of excavation. A very good hint would also be successful DNA retrieval from other samples of the same layer at the excavation site. It might therefore be an option trying to extract and analyze DNA from less valuable bone fragments from the same site.

   Also because of its cellular abundance, mitochondrial (mt)DNA has been the target of choice in most ancient DNA analyses. Despite this, mtDNA bears the problem that there are translocated pieces in the nuclear genome of many species that might be mistaken for authentic organellar mtDNA sequences *(40)*. In order to avoid this, it was suggested to take explicit measures to authenticate mtDNA sequences in newly studied taxa or when any suspicious sequence is retrieved.

aDNA and molecular archaeology/evolution are fascinating fields that recruits enthusiastic young scientists, and we have no doubts about the fact that most problems affecting the field will be solved in the future. In the meantime, no chance to verify and critically question results should be missed.

Acknowledgments

The authors would like to thank Matthias Krings for helpful support in providing exhaustive clarification of the described protocols and Vincenzo Pascali for suggestions. F. Tschentscher is deeply grateful to Petra and Jakob Bärschneider for continuous support and understanding. C. Capelli would like to thank Sonia Bortoletto.

References

1. Hofreiter, M., Serre, D., Poinar, H. N., Kuch, M., and Pääbo, S. (2001) Ancient DNA. *Nat. Rev. Genet.* **2,** 353–359.
2. Jeffreys, A. J., Allen, M. J., Hagelberg, E., and Sonnberg, A. (1992) Identification of the skeletal remains of Josef Mengele by DNA analysis. *Forensic Sci. Int.* **56,** 65–76.
3. Gill, P., Ivanov, P. L., Kimpton, C., Piercy, R., Benson, N., Tully, G., et al. (1994) Identification of the remains of the Romanov family by DNA analysis. *Nat. Genet.* **6,** 130–135.
4. Capelli, C., Tschentscher, F, and Pascali, V. L. (2003) "Ancient" protocols for the crime scene? Similarities and differences between forensic genetics and ancient DNA analysis. *Forensic Sci. Int.* **131,** 59–64.
5. Cooper, A. and Poinar, H. N. (2000) Ancient DNA: do it right or not at all. *Science* **289,** 1139.
6. Gilbert, M. T., Willerslev, E., Hansen, A. J., Barnes, I., Rudbeck, L., Lynnerup, N., et al. (2003) Distribution patterns of postmortem damage in human mitochondrial DNA. *Am. J. Hum. Genet.* **72,** 32–47.
7. Gilbert, M. T., Hansen, A. J., Willerslev, E., Rudbeck, L., Barnes, I., Lynnerup, N., et al. (2003) Characterization of genetic miscoding lesions caused by postmortem damage. *Am. J. Hum. Genet.* **72,** 48–61.
8. Woodward, S. R., Weyand, N. J., and Bunnell, M. (1994) DNA sequence from Cretaceous period bone fragments. *Science* **266,** 1229–1232.
9. Zischler, H., Hoss, M., Handt, O., von Haeseler, A., van der Kuyl, A. C., Goudsmit, J., et al. (1995) Detecting dinosaur DNA. *Science* **268,** 1192–1193.
10. Cano, R. J., Poinar, H. N., Pieniazek, N. J., Acra, A., and Poinar, G. O. (1993) Amplification and sequencing of DNA from a 120-135-million-year-old weevil. *Nature* **363,** 536–538.
11. Gutierrez, G., Sanchez, D., and Marin, A. (1998) The most ancient DNA recovered from an amber-preserved specimen may not be as ancient as it seems. *Mol. Biol. Evol.* **15,** 926–929.

12. Mullis, K. B. and Faloona, F. A. (1997) Specific synthesis of DNA in vitro via a polymerase-catalyzed chain reaction. *Methods Enzymol.* **155**, 335–350.
13. Pääbo, S., Higuchi, R. G., and Wilson, A. (1989) Ancient DNA and the polymerase chain reaction: the emerging field of molecular archeology. *J. Biol. Chem.* **264**, 9709–9712.
14. Presley, L .A. and Budowle, B. (1993) The application of PCR-based technologies to forensic analysis, in *PCR Technology Current Innovations* (Griffin, H. G. and Griffin A. M., eds), CRC Press, Boca Raton, FL.
15. Hoss, M., Jaruga, P. , Zastawny, T. H., Dizdaroglu, M., and Pääbo, S. (1996) DNA damage and DNA sequence retrieval from ancient tissues. *Nucleic Acids Res.* **24**, 1304–1307.
16. Handt, O., Krings, M., Ward, R. H., and Pääbo, S. (1996) The retrieval of ancient human DNA sequences. *Am. J. Hum. Genet.* **59**, 368–376.
17. Krings, M., Stone, A., Schmitz, R. W., Krainitzki, H., Stoneking, M., and Pääbo, S. (1997) Neandertal DNA sequences and the origin of modern humans. *Cell* **90**, 19–30.
18. Krings, M., Geisert, H., Schmitz, R. W., Krainitzki, H., and Pääbo, S. (1999) DNA sequence of the mitochondrial hypervariable region II from the neandertal type specimen. *Proc. Natl. Acad. Sci. USA* **96**, 5581–5585.
19. Greenwood, A. D., Capelli, C., Possnert, G., and Pääbo, S. (1999) Nuclear DNA sequences from late Pleistocene megafauna. *Mol. Biol. Evol.* **16**, 1466–1473.
20. Krings, M., Capelli, C., Tschentscher, F., Geisert, H., Meyer, S., von Haeseler, A., et al. (2000) A view of Neandertal genetic diversity. *Nat. Genet.* **26**, 144–146.
21. Boom, R., Sol, C. J. A., Salimans, M. M. M., Jansen, C. L., Wertheim-van Dillen, P. M. E., and van der Noordaa, J. (1990) Rapid and simple method for purification of nucleic acids. *J. Clin. Microbiol.* **28**, 495–503.
22. Hoss, M. and Pääbo, S. (1993) DNA extraction from Pleistocene bones by a silica-based purification method. *Nucleic Acid Res.* **21**, 3913–3914
23. Nuovo, G. J., Gallery, F., MacConnell, P., Becker, J., and Bloch, W. (1991) An improved technique for the in situ detection of DNA after polymerase chain reaction amplification. *Am. J. Pathol.* **139**, 1239–1244.
24. Chou, Q., Russell, M., Birch, D. E., Raymond, J., and Bloch, W. (1992) Prevention of pre-PCR mis-priming and primer dimerization improves low-copy-number amplifications. *Nucleic Acids Res.* **20**, 1717–1723.
25. Tautz, D. and Renz, M. (1983) An optimized freeze-squeeze method for the recovery of DNA fragments from agarose gels. *Anal. Biochem.* **132**, 14–19.
26. Ausubel, F. A., Brent, R., Kingston, R. E., Moore, D. D., Seidman, J. G., Smith, J. A., et al., eds. (1995) *Current Protocols in Molecular Biology*. John Wiley & Sons, New York, NY.
27. Kilger, C., Krings, M., Poinar, H., and Pääbo, S. (1997) "Colony sequencing": direct sequencing of plasmid DNA from bacterial colonies. *BioTechniques* **22**, 412–414.

28. Strimmer, K. and von Haeseler, A. (1997) Likelihood-mapping: a simple method to visualize phylogenetic content of a sequence alignment. *Proc. Natl. Acad. Sci. USA* **94,** 6815–6819.
29. Schmidt, H. A., Strimmer, K., Vingron, M., and von Haeseler, A.(2002) TREE-PUZZLE: maximum likelihood phylogenetic analysis using quartets and parallel computing. *Bioinformatics* **18,** 502–504.
30. Golenberg, E. M., Giannasi, D. E., Clegg, M. T., Smiley, C. J., Durbin, M., Henderson, D., et al. (1990) Chloroplast DNA sequence from a miocene Magnolia species. *Nature* **344,** 656–658.
31. Austin, J. J., Smith, A. B., and Thomas, R. H. (1997) Paleontology in a molecular world: the search for authentic ancient DNA. *Trends Ecol. Evol.* **12,** 303–306.
32. Stone, R. (1999) Siberian mammoth find raises hopes. *Questions Sci.* **286,** 876–877.
33. Tschentscher, F. (1999) Too mammoth an undertaking. *Science* **286,** 2084.
34. Lindahl,T.(1993) Recovery of antediluvian DNA. *Nature* **365,** 700.
35. Caramelli, D., Lalueza-Fox, C., Vernesi, C., Lari, M., Casoli, A., Mallegni, F., et al. (2003) Evidence for a genetic discontinuity between Neandertals and 24000-year-old anatomically modern Europeans. *Proc. Natl. Acad. Sci. USA* **100,** 6593–6597.
36. Abbott, A. (2003) Anthropologists cast doubt on human DNA evidence. *Nature* **423,** 468.
37. Barbujani, G. and Bertorelle, G. (2003) Were Cro-Magnons too like us for DNA to tell? *Nature* **424,** 127.
38. Greenwood, A. D., Lee, F., Capelli, C., DeSalle, R., Tikhonov, A., Marx, P.A., et al. (2001) Evolution of endogenous retrovirus-like elements of the woolly mammoth (*Mammuthus primigenius*) and its relatives. *Mol. Biol. Evol.* **18,** 840–847.
39. Poinar, H. N., Hoss, M., Bada, J. L., and Pääbo, S. (1996) Amino acid racemization and the preservation of ancient DNA. *Science* **272,** 864–866.
40. Thalmann, O., Hebler, J., Poinar, H. N., Pääbo, S., and Vigilant, L. (2004) Unreliable mtDNA data due to nuclear insertions: a cautionary tale from analysis of humans and other great apes. *Mol. Ecol.* **13,** 321–335.

Index

279